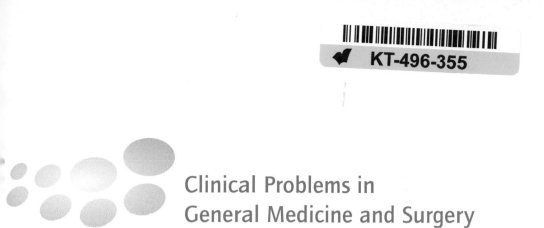

Clinical Problems in
General Medicine and Surgery

Commissioning Editor: Laurence Hunter
Project Development Manager: Hannah Kenner
Project Manager: Frances Affleck
Designer: Sarah Russell

Clinical Problems in General Medicine and Surgery

SECOND EDITION

Peter Devitt
Associate Professor
Department of Surgery
Royal Adelaide Hospital
Adelaide, Australia

Juliet Barker
Assistant Professor
Department of Medicine
University of Minnesota
Minneapolis, USA

Jonathan Mitchell
Clinical Fellow in Hepatology
Institute of Liver Studies
Kings College Hospital
London, UK

Christian Hamilton-Craig
Medical Registrar
St Vincent's Hospital;
Associate Lecturer
University of New South Wales
Sydney, Australia

Foreword by **Roy Pounder**
Professor of Medicine
Royal Free & University College Medical School
London, UK

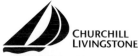

CHURCHILL
LIVINGSTONE

EDINBURGH LONDON NEW YORK OXFORD PHILADELPHIA ST LOUIS SYDNEY TORONTO 2003

CHURCHILL LIVINGSTONE

© Harcourt Brace Jovanovich Group (Australia) Pty Ltd 1992
© 2003, Elsevier Science Limited. All rights reserved.

First edition 1992
Second edition 2003

ISBN 0 440 07323 6

British Library Cataloguing in Publication Data
A catalogue record for this book is available from the British Library

Library of Congress Cataloging in Publication Data
A catalog record for this book is available from the Library of Congress

Note
Medical knowledge is constantly changing. Standard safety precautions
must be followed, but as new research and clinical experience broaden our
knowledge, changes in treatment and drug therapy may become necessary
or appropriate. Readers are advised to check the most current product
information provided by the manufacturer of each drug to be administered
to verify the recommended dose, the method and duration of
administration, and contraindications. It is the responsibility of the
practitioner, relying on experience and knowledge of the patient, to
determine dosages and the best treatment for each individual patient.
Neither the Publisher nor the editor assumes any liability for any injury
and/or damage to persons or property arising from this publication.

The Publisher

The
Publisher's
policy is to use
**paper manufactured
from sustainable forests**
II

Printed in China

Contents

THE PROBLEMS:

Foreword

Clinical Problems in General Medicine and Surgery provides a succession of amazing clinical challenges for the reader. It's like a series of medical and surgical emergency shifts, where every patient has something substantial that's wrong with them. It is like real life – that is, the clinical problems are undiagnosed and they present with a series of symptoms, physical signs and abnormal investigations. And things often get worse before the patient improves. Scary stuff for the doctor in charge so best learned in advance, ideally in an armchair!

The book is written for the senior medical student or junior doctor – but it is exciting reading even for a more senior physician. The clinical problems evolve and the reader is challenged to understand the illnesses and to interpret the results of investigations and the patients' response to treatment. The authors have created the clinical cases and ask the questions, but they also provide very full explanations for the correct answers. The style is good: it explains the answers in full sentences, not just lists to be remembered. If you understand the problem, it is easier to remember the facts.

This is the second edition of *Clinical Problems in General Medicine and Surgery* and it has taken account of the really dramatic changes of the last decade – particularly in imaging, resuscitation, surgical technique and therapeutics. The book is also up-to-date in its use of publishing technology, with frequent links to useful additional information available through the Internet.

Congratulations to Peter Devitt, Juliet Barker, Jonathan Mitchell and Christian Hamilton-Craig for producing a wonderful tool to improve healthcare. *Clinical Problems in General Medicine and Surgery* is a real contribution to helping doctors to understand how to manage acutely ill patients, and that has to help everyone.

Roy Pounder MA MD DSc FRCP
Professor of Medicine
Royal Free & University College Medical School
London, UK

Preface

First published in 1992, *Clinical Problems in General Medicine and Surgery* was principally written for senior medical students and interns, about to or already experiencing the real world of medical practice. It was a departure from 'traditional' medical texts in that the book dealt with the real problems of clinical medicine through scenarios encountered in the emergency department, on the wards and in outpatient clinics. How to manage the comatose patient? How to manage the young man with chest pain? What to do with the rowdy, confused patient on the ward, or the jaundiced patient in the clinic?

Perhaps it was this hands-on approach that maintained its popularity through the 1990s, if not the often-heard comment 'it was the single book that got me through Finals'. But, more importantly, this book should be recognized as an invaluable guide to the clinical care of patients.

For this new edition the basic ethos has not changed. The book still relies on real-life medical scenarios to illustrate important everyday principles in clinical medicine. The successful format of case presentation, interspersed by questions and answers, and a final synopsis of key material has been maintained in the second edition. With the assistance of two new editors, J.M. and C.H-C., and a multitude of colleagues across three continents, every problem has been revised and updated. New images reflect the extensive changes in the field of minimally invasive diagnostics. Searching questions have been added to guide the reader towards further self-directed learning and the worldwide web now features highly as an important source of further information.

Despite the technological progress of the last decade, the principles of history and examination remain the cornerstone of sound medical practice. So often our advanced technology can only be appropriately applied if the clinician has taken the correct history. Furthermore, despite medical advances, many diseases remain disabling or lethal. In this setting, a clinician's empathy with the patient's situation and the ability to counsel the patient honestly and effectively is of paramount importance. These aspects of clinical care have been emphasized throughout this edition.

The book does not purport to be an exhaustive text on clinical medicine. Nor is it a replacement for real experience and the hands-on teaching of expert clinicians. It is designed as a valuable source of information and practical aid to the management of clinical problems. But more than this, we hope the problems instil in the reader a sense of excitement and curiosity to drive them to further learning and, if it is half as much fun and thought provoking for the reader as it has been for us in the writing, then we will have succeeded in our aims.

P.D.   J.B.   J.M.   C.H-C.

Acknowledgements

We are grateful to our many colleagues who have helped put this book together. Our particular thanks go to those who gave up precious time to review the problems from the first edition and to comment on, update and occasionally rewrite the material. Particular thanks go to Roger Pepperell, Stephen Lam and Gabriel Lee who produced new problems. Those individuals who helped are listed below.

Roger Ackroyd, Sheffield **(Problem 18)**

Anthony Antoniou, London **(Problems 8, 46)**

Kim Bannister, Adelaide **(Problems 47, 48)**

Adrian Bauze, Adelaide **(Problem 32)**

Nick Buckley, Canberra **(Problem 53)**

Michael Chia, Adelaide **(Problems 37, 43)**

Brendon Coventry, Adelaide **(Problem 11)**

Tom Creed, Bristol **(Problems 20, 23, 42)**

Nick Davies, Bournemouth **(Problem 16)**

Will Davies, London **(Problem 31)**

Andrew DeBeaux, Edinburgh **(Problem 13)**

Paul Drysdale, Adelaide **(Problem 50)**

Robert Fitridge, Adelaide **(Problems 27, 28, 29, 30)**

Gordian Fulde, Sydney **(Problems 53, 61)**

Mitra Guha, Adelaide **(Problem 58)**

Tabitha Healey, Adelaide **(Problem 57)**

Nigel Jones, Adelaide **(Problem 55)**

Richard Krisztopyk, Bath **(Problem 1)**

Paul Leeder, Oxford **(Problem 3)**

Robert Ludemann, Portland, Oregon **(Problems 2, 21)**

Suren Krishnan, Adelaide **(Problem 6)**

Jim Kollias, Adelaide **(Problem 5)**

Robert Kennedy, Belfast **(Problem 10)**

Stephen Lam, Adelaide **(Problem 64)**

Gabriel Lee, Perth **(Problem 63)**

Ian Leitch, Adelaide **(Problem 12)**

John Miller, Adelaide **(Problem 25)**

Andrew Mitchell, Oxford **(Problems 33, 34, 35)**

Charles Mulligan, Adelaide **(Problem 56)**

Simon Noble, Cardiff **(Problems 9, 10, 26, 36)**

Colm O'Boyle, Hull **(Problem 4)**

Roger Pepperell, Melbourne **(Problems 65, 66)**

Suzannna Proudman, Adelaide **(Problem 60)**

Mark Reding, Minnesota **(Problem 36)**

Tony Roberts, Adelaide **(Problem 59)**

Karen Rowland, Adelaide **(Problem 61)**

David Shaw, Adelaide **(Problem 40)**

Justine Smith, Portland, Oregon **(Problem 52)**

Rick Stapledon, Adelaide **(Problem 39)**

Jim Sweeney, Adelaide **(Problem 24)**

Anne Tonkin, Adelaide **(Problem 49)**

Michelle Thomas, Adelaide **(Problem 15)**

Philip Thompson, Adelaide **(Problems 51, 54)**

William Tam, Adelaide **(Problem 14)**

Victoria Wheatley, Cardiff **(Problem 7)**

Michael Wines, Sydney **(Problem 19)**

Glenn Young, Adelaide **(Problem 37)**

The visual material in the book has come from many sources and in particular we would like to thank Dr Elizabeth Coates (Fig. 62.1), Dr Ian Kirkwood (Figs 49.3, 57.4) Dr Robert Fitridge (Figs 27.3–29.3) Dr Jamie Taylor (Figs 25.1–25.3, 25.5, 25.6) Dr Angela Barbour (Fig. 5.2), Dr Jim Kollias (Fig. 5.4), Dr Roger Ackroyd (Figs 18.1, 18.2), Dr Mark Schoeman (Figs 22.1, 22.2), Dr Chris Jones (Figs 36.1, 36.2), Professor Nigel Jones (Fig. 55.4), Dr Charles Mulligan (Figs 56.1–56.5), Professor Roger Pepperell (Figs 66.1, 66.2) and Dr John Reece (Figs 19.3, 19.4).

The retinal photograph (Fig. 52.1) came from the Casey Eye Institute, Portland, Oregon and the coronary angiograms were provided by Claudio La Posta, Chief Radiographer in the Cardiovascular Investigation Unit at the Royal Adelaide Hospital. The paracetamol nomogram is reproduced by permission of the Clinical Services Unit of the Royal Adelaide Hospital.

Normal range of values

Normal values will vary between laboratories. The following ranges are used for the cases described in this book.

HAEMATOLOGY

Haemoglobin	Male:	135–180 g/l
	Female:	115–165 g/l
PCV	Male:	42–52%
	Female:	37–47%
MCV	80–96 fl	
MCH	27–31 pg	
MCHC	300–360 g/l	
Platelets	150–400 x10^9/l	
Leucocytes	4.0–11.0 x10^9/l	
Granulocytes	2.0–7.5 x10^9/l	
Lymphocytes	1.0–4.0 x10^9/l	
Monocytes	0.2–1.2 x10^9/l	
ESR	Adult male:	0–10 mm/hr
	Adult female:	0–20 mm/hr
	Elderly:	0–35 mm/hr

CLINICAL CHEMISTRY

Sodium	135–145 mmol/l	
Potassium	3.8–5.2 mmol/l	
Chloride	99–110 mmol/l	
Bicarbonate	22–30 mmol/l	
Anion gap	10–18 mmol/l	
Osmolarity	272–283 mmol/l	
Glucose	3.0–5.4 mmol/l (fasting)	
Urea	3.0–8.0 mmol/l	
Creatinine	0.05–0.12 mmol/l	
Uric acid	Male:	0.25–0.45 mmol/l
	Female:	0.15–0.40 mmol/l
Total calcium	2.20–2.55 mmol/l	
Ionized calcium	1.17–1.27 mmol/l	
Phosphate	0.70–1.3 mmol/l	
Albumin	36–46 g/l	
Globulins	25–36 g/l	
Cholesterol	<5.5 mmol/l	

Conjugated bilirubin	1–4 µmol/l	
Total bilirubin	6–24 µmol/l	
GGT	1–55 U/l	
Alkaline phosphatase	30–120 U/l	
LDH	105–230 U/l	
AST	1–45 U/l	
ALT	1–45 U/l	
Lipase	0–300 U/l	
Amylase	30–110 U/l	
C-reactive protein	0–5 mg/l	

SERUM IRON STUDIES

Ferritin	Male:	20–250 µg/l
	Female:	10–150 µg/l
Iron	Male:	8–35 µmol/l
	Female:	10–35 µmol/l
Transferrin	25–50 µmol/l	
Transferrin saturation	Male:	10–55%
	Female:	10–35%

COAGULATION STUDIES

INR	1.0–1.2
APTT	25–33 seconds
Bleeding time	2–8 minutes

THYROID FUNCTION TESTS

TSH	
euthyroid	0.4–5.5 mU/l
hypothyroid	>4.5 mU/l
hyperthyroid	<0.3 mU/l
Free T4	
euthyroid	16–26 pmol/l
upper borderline	27–30 pmol/l
on adequate T4	15–35 pmol/l
Free T3	
euthyroid	2.1–5.3 pmol/l
upper borderline	8.1–10.0 pmol/l
hyperthyroid	>10.0 pmol/l

ARTERIAL BLOOD GAS ANALYSIS (on inspired room air)

pO_2	65–83 mm Hg
pCO_2	35–45 mm Hg
pH	7.35–7.45
Calculated bicarbonate	22–32 mmol/l

LIPID STUDIES

Total triglyceride	0.3–2.0 mmol/l
Total cholesterol	desirable <5.5 mmol/l
HDL cholesterol	0.9–2.0 mmol/l
IDL cholesterol	desirable <3.7 mmol/l
Total cholesterol/ HDL cholesterol	desirable <3.5

SERUM CARDIAC ENZYMES

Creatine kinase	20–180 U/l
CK–MB isoenzyme 1	0–4%
Troponin (cTnT)	<0.03 ng/ml

OTHERS

Serum B12	180–1000 ng/l
Serum folate (fasting specimen)	2.8–15.0 µg/l

The Internet

Listed below are a few websites that we have found particularly useful.

www.e-medicine.com
A huge online textbook of medicine with a vast array of superb peer reviewed articles, clinical cases and links.

www.surgical-tutor.org.uk
An excellent resource for surgical training includes tutorials, revision notes, images and case studies.

www.nlm.nih.gov
The American National Library of Medicine. A huge government information resource including access to PubMed.

www.medicalstudent.com
This brilliant online medical library has links to literally hundreds of sites including online textbooks and atlases all subdivided into subject matter.

www.ncbi.nlm.nih.gov/entrez/query.fcgi?db=PubMed
This is the website for those wanting to do a literature search. This is the database of the National Library of Medicine and commonly referred to as 'PubMed'.

In the 10 years since the first edition of this book was published the Internet has revolutionized the way that we learn, communicate and share information in medicine. In this second edition of the book we have embraced this information revolution. The editors and contributors are spread throughout three continents and without the high-speed communication of the Internet and email, this edition would have had a long and tedious gestation. All the problems have been produced in a paperless environment and content, images and comment have gone from editor to editor to publisher over the Internet. From many angles the electronic medium has been invaluable.

We have tried to reflect some of these changes in the book. Although reference is still made to important papers (many of which can be accessed online), every problem refers to at least one website which we have found valuable and useful.

Those we have quoted range from large sites from major medical organizations such as **www.asge.org** through patient-oriented sites like **www.asthmalearninglab.com** to huge web educational resources like **www.e-medicine.com.** Some are commercial sites with pharmaceutical sponsors, others are posted by private individuals and healthcare professionals.

These lists are in no way exhaustive, but merely reflect what the editors have found interesting and feel offer useful information. Websites vary in quality and some are here today, gone tomorrow. The main aim is to stimulate you, the reader, to explore a subject matter using this vast resource at your fingertips.

Start with a good search engine such as **www.yahoo.com** or **www.google.com** and use broad search terms to begin. Search especially for national associations in each subject, for instance the American Heart Association or British Society of Gastroenterology. Most of these websites have lots of information for non-members although many require free registration. Also, look on the websites of the major journals. An increasing number offer free full text articles online including **www.bmj.com** (all articles free) and **www.nejm.com** (articles free after 6 months). The website **www.freemedicaljournals.com/** gives an up-to-date list of free journals.

A word of warning is given to the reader. The very nature of the Internet means that there is a huge amount of inaccurate, misleading and, at times, frankly dangerous information posted. Beware of unsubstantiated claims on private and commercial sites. Reliable and creditable information is most likely to found at the large non-profit making sites and those run by well-known medical organizations. If in doubt, look for the credentials of the author or institution, their qualifications and the date on which the material was produced.

Difficulties with postoperative fluid balance in a 65-year-old man

A 65-year-old man is admitted with abdominal pain. He has been ill for 12 hours prior to admission with severe and constant lower abdominal pain, which started on the left side. He has vomited twice.

Twenty-four hours previously he had had a colonoscopy and polypectomy. Two polyps were removed, one from the sigmoid and the other from the transverse colon. The procedure was uneventful and the patient went home the same day. Prior to this episode his general health was good and his past medical history unremarkable.

On examination he looks ill with a temperature of 38.5°C, a dry coated tongue and a loss of skin turgor. He feels thirsty and has a tachycardia of 110 bpm and a blood pressure of 110/70 mm Hg (lying). On sitting, his pulse goes up to 130 bpm and his systolic blood pressure drops to 90 mm Hg. Examination of his cardiovascular and respiratory systems reveals no significant abnormalities. Abdominal examination shows a mildly distended abdomen with no scars and no respiratory movements. The abdomen is rigid to palpation, dull and tender to percussion and no bowel sounds are heard on auscultation.

Q1 What is your interpretation of the history and physical findings?

The provisional diagnosis is this patient probably has a perforated colon as a complication of the procedure performed the previous day.

Q2 How are you going to manage this problem?

Blood is collected for haematological and biochemical screen and an intravenous cannula inserted for fluid replacement. Abdominal and chest radiographs are ordered. A urinary catheter is inserted and 300 ml concentrated urine drains. His blood results are as follows:

Investigation 1.1 Blood results			
Haemoglobin	164 g/l	White cell count	13.6 x 10⁹/l
Platelets	350 x 10⁹/l		
Sodium	149 mmol/l	Calcium	2.16 mmol/l
Potassium	3.4 mmol/l	Phosphate	1.15 mmol/l
Chloride	112 mmol/l	Total protein	65 g/l
Bicarbonate	29 mmol/l	Albumin	38 g/l
Urea	10.0 mmol/l	Globulins	27 g/l
Creatinine	0.12 mmol/l	Bilirubin	19 μmol/l
Uric acid	0.21 mmol/l	ALT	25 U/l
Glucose	4.4 mmol/l	AST	39 U/l
Cholesterol	3.6 mmol/l	GGT	17 U/l
LDH	110 U/l	ALP	74 U/l
Amylase	65 U/l		

The chest radiograph is shown in Figure 1.1.

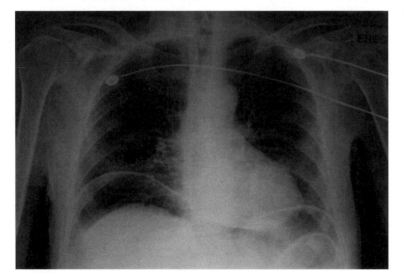

Fig 1.1

Q3 Comment on the chest radiograph and blood results.

The patient undergoes an exploratory laparotomy. The patient will need central intravenous
access broad-spectrum antibiotics and fluid
replacement.

Q4 What fluid replacement would you give before the operation?

A purulent peritonitis is found at laparotomy and 300 ml purulent fluid is aspirated from the lower part of the abdominal cavity. The source of the peritonitis is found to be a perforation of the transverse colon.

He undergoes a resection of the transverse colon, a primary anastomosis and formation of a 'split' ileostomy. This is a defunctioning ileostomy, i.e. it remains in continuity with the distal bowel. Because of peritoneal contamination a tube drain is inserted into the abdominal cavity, down to the site of the operation. A nasogastric tube is inserted because in cases of extensive peritonitis gastrointestinal stasis is expected for 3 or 4 days after the operation.

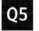 **What would you expect his fluid requirements to be in the first 24 hours after surgery?**

The morning after his operation the patient looks reasonably well and is afebrile. He continues on prophylactic intravenous antibiotics and is on patient-controlled narcotic analgesia. His blood pressure is 130/90 mm Hg and his pulse rate is 90 bpm. His fluid balance chart for the 18 hours since admission is as follows:

Investigation 1.2 Fluid balance chart on admission		
Fluid input	**Fluid output**	
IV fluids 4200 ml	Urine total	400 ml
	Urine last 4 hours	22/16/12/0 ml
	Nasogastric tube	700 ml
	Wound drain	200 ml
	Ileostomy	300 ml

With a bolus of 500 ml isotonic saline you get the urine output up to 50 ml over the next hour. You then order a maintenance regimen of 1 litre of isotonic saline to be followed by 1 litre dextrose 5% at 100 ml/hour and a replacement regimen of isotonic saline at 50 ml/hour using an infusion pump. You then hand over to your fellow intern and take your afternoon off.

When you see your patient the next morning you notice he was given an additional 1 litre dextrose 5% when his urine output fell over a 4-hour period to less than 20 ml/hr. He feels thirsty and there is loss of skin turgor. When you check the patient his blood pressure is 110/65 mm Hg on lying and 90/60 mm Hg on sitting. His pulse rate is 100 bpm and he has a dry tongue. His fluid balance chart for the previous 24 hours shows:

Investigation 1.3 Fluid balance 24 hours later		
Fluid input	**Fluid output**	
IV fluids 4500 ml	Urine total	800 ml
	Urine last 4 hours	15/13/9/8 ml
	Nasogastric tube	2500 ml
	Wound drain	300 ml
	Ileostomy	3000 ml

The early morning electrolytes are as follows:

Investigation 1.4 Electrolytes			
Sodium	138 mmol/l	Potassium	2.6 mmol/l
Chloride	102 mmol/l	Bicarbonate	29 mmol/l
Urea	7.0 mmol/l	Creatinine	0.08 mmol/l

Q6 Comment on this man's fluid balance and electrolytes. What fluids are you going to give the patient over the next 24 hours?

The patient's ileus persisted for another 7 days and he was given total parenteral nutrition. Twelve days after the operation he was tolerating a light diet, was managing his ileostomy satisfactorily and was discharged home to await closure of his ileostomy.

ANSWERS

A1 The patient has generalized peritonitis, probably secondary to a perforated colon.

Peritonitis is inflammation of the peritoneal cavity. Initially this will have been a localized process, hence the site of the abdominal pain reported earlier in the illness. Fibrinous adhesions form rapidly and together with the omentum and small bowel loops may contain the inflammatory process.

If inflammation continues, local defences fail and generalized peritonitis supervenes. At this stage patients are severely ill, with fever, dehydration and absent bowel sounds. The slightest movement, even percussion, is painful.

Perforation secondary to diagnostic colonoscopy is uncommon and occurs in 0.1–0.5% of cases. Typically the bowel is perforated by excess pressure in a fixed bowel loop, such as the sigmoid, resulting in a longitudinal antimesenteric split, or from the tip of the endoscope pushing directly through the bowel wall.

The risk of perforation after colonoscopic polypectomy is 0.5–1.0%. It is more common in the right colon, where the bowel wall is thin. Diathermy injury can lead to immediate perforation or it can be delayed by up to 48 hours as the thermal injury leads to slow bowel wall necrosis.

A2 This man is clinically dehydrated and has signs of peritonitis. You need to:

- Insert an intravenous cannula and start immediate resuscitation with 1 litre isotonic saline over 1 hour. The rate of fluid replacement can be adjusted once you have his laboratory results back.
- Administer oxygen by face mask (2–3 l/min).
- Give appropriate analgesia (he will require an opiate).
- Collect blood samples for haematological and biochemical (electrolyte) analysis.
- Arrange for a chest and abdominal radiograph.
- Administer a broad-spectrum antibiotic.
- Contact a surgeon to give an opinion on the management of his peritonitis.

A3 The chest radiograph shows that there is gas under the left and right hemidiaphragms. This finding supports the diagnosis of a perforated viscus. Subdiaphragmatic (or subphrenic) gas is seen in 90% of such cases and is best seen on an erect chest radiograph. On the right side, the subdiaphragmatic area is occupied by the liver, so subphrenic gas is readily identified. On the left side care should be taken not to confuse gas in the fundus of the stomach or splenic flexure with free subphrenic gas.

The blood results reveal that:

- The elevated white cell count supports a diagnosis of inflammation and infection. The absolute number is increased and a differ-

A N S W E R S – cont'd

ential white count will show an excess of neutrophils.

- The high haemoglobin is probably a reflection of dehydration. This would be supported by an elevated haematocrit or packed cell volume.
- The biochemical values are abnormal: the high urea, chloride and sodium are all features of dehydration.

A4 This patient has had a substantial loss of fluid from the circulating volume into the bowel and peritoneum. Initial fluid prescription is intended to correct this existing deficit:

- The 'lost' fluid is isotonic and best replaced by isotonic saline ('normal' or 0.9% saline).
- Initially 2 litres of isotonic saline can be given over 1 hour.

The total volume lost is difficult to determine exactly, but is likely to be 3–4 litres. A patient who is subjectively thirsty, with reduced skin turgor and dry mucous membranes, may have lost up to 10% bodyweight of fluid, which needs to be replaced. A patient who has a tachycardia and orthostatic hypotension, such as the patient described here, may have an acute deficit of up to 20% of the circulating volume.

An ECF deficit of up to 3 litres can be adequately sustained by shift of fluid from the ECF to the intravascular space. Beyond this, upto 4 litres, there are signs of mild tachycardia and postural hypotension. Once fluid deficit reaches 5–6 litres the pulse becomes rapid, thready and hypotension and circulatory collapse ensue.

Resuscitation should be guided by improvement in clinical signs. This means stabilizing blood pressure, reducing tachycardia and producing a urine output of 30–50 ml per hour. Careful monitoring of the patient is vital during this time, particularly in the elderly, or in patients who may have associated cardiac disease. The use of a central venous line will allow accurate measurement of central venous pressure in such patients, who may need nursing in an intensive care unit.

A5 Fluid requirement over this time can be separated into maintenance and replacement fluids.

Maintenance fluid can be predicted with reasonable accuracy. Under normal circumstances a 65 kg man needs 2.5–3.0 litres of water, 100–150 mmol sodium and 60–90 mmol potassium to replace normal losses of water and electrolytes through urine, faeces, expired air and perspiration. Pyrexia will increase insensible losses from the skin and lungs, up to 20% more for each degree.

In normal circumstances the daily water and electrolyte requirements are met by appropriate volumes of isotonic (0.9%) saline and 5% dextrose. Isotonic saline contains 154 mmol of sodium ions in 1 litre. Thus 0.5–1.0 litre will provide enough sodium for 24 hours, and 2–2.5 litres 5% dextrose make up the additional water. The addition of 20 mmol of potassium to each litre of fluid will provide enough potassium.

In this case, the stress of surgery leads to stimulation of the hypothalamo–pituitary–adrenal axis with production of antidiuretic hormone (ADH) and aldosterone. This leads to renal conservation of sodium and water and by way of exchange there is loss of potassium. This produces a urine sodium concentration of <10 mmol/l and osmolality >450 mosm/kg. Under these conditions the patient will need only 2 litres of 5% dextrose without sodium. Usually more potassium is released by tissue damage at the time of surgery than is lost in the urine and so potassium supplement is best guided by serum electrolyte level. Remember that pyrexia and tachypnoea can increase loss from perspiration and expired air.

Replacement fluid is intended to replace any losses recorded in the first 24 hours on a volume for volume basis with a fluid of similar composition. Such replacements are ideally calculated and replaced on an hourly basis, but 4-hourly is generally accepted to be more practical. Nasogastric losses are lower in sodium but not potassium and can be replaced with 0.45–0.9% saline with 20 mmol/l of potassium. Ileostomy losses have a slightly higher sodium level and similar potassium level and can be replaced with normal (0.9%) saline with 20 mmol/l of added potassium.

When large volumes of fluid are required, remember regular measurement of electrolytes is needed to monitor and tailor electrolyte replace-

ANSWERS – cont'd

ment and, more importantly, regular clinical examination to assess fluid status.

Infusion pumps should be used when fluid measurement needs to be precise. Pumps accurately deliver the correct volume of fluid over time, rather than the traditional bag of fluid hung from a drip stand. This is particularly important in elderly patients whose fluid status is precarious and who have a risk of cardiac failure with over-zealous fluid therapy.

A6 Your fluid prescription should begin with an evaluation of fluid losses and gains over the previous 24 hours and a careful clinical examination. These reveal that the patient has lost more fluid than he has received; he is in negative fluid balance and hypokalaemic. He has clinical features of recurrent hypovolaemia, with oliguria, tachycardia, postural hypotension and loss of skin turgor.

His fluid requirements include maintenance and replacement fluids, including fluid to restore his existing hypovolaemia and correction of the hypokalaemia. A fluid bolus of up to 2 litres of normal saline per hour should be given to restore urine output to at least 50 ml/hr. During this time the patient must be frequently assessed to ensure urine output returns and avoid over-expansion of the intravascular compartment and heart failure. Potassium is predominantly an intracellular ion, and provided there is no

acid–base disturbance, the serum potassium concentration reflects the total body pool. This patient's serum potassium is 1 mmol/l below normal and the total body deficit of potassium is likely to be 10%. Using central access, 20 mmol/hour can be replaced without risk of cardiac arrhythmia. For this potassium level at least 80 mmol of replacement will be required along with ongoing maintenance to compensate for ongoing loss. After the initial replacement, further replacement should be guided by a repeated serum potassium estimation.

Maintenance fluids are prescribed as already described: 2 litres 5% dextrose (with 20 mmol potassium per litre). Replacement should be the same in volume and electrolyte content as the losses they replace; particular attention should be paid to increased nasogastric and ileostomy losses, which have been 5.5 litres in the previous 24 hours, but clearly inadequately replaced. In general terms the gastrointestinal losses need to be replaced, litre-for-litre with isotonic saline. Sodium (50–100 mmol/l) and chloride (100–140 mmol/l) losses from the stomach and small intestine (ileostomy) can be matched reasonably accurately with isotonic saline. Potassium (5–15 mmol/l) must be added to the replacement fluids. In reality, losses of this magnitude in such a complex clinical setting will be replaced on an hour-by-hour basis and serum electrolyte concentrations monitored frequently.

REVISION POINTS

Fluid balance
Approximately 60% of bodyweight is made up of water.

In a 65 kg man, this is 40 litres:
- Two-thirds (24 l) is intracellular fluid (ICF).
- One-third (16 l) is extracellular fluid (ECF).
  - intravascular (3 l)
  - interstitial (12 l)
  - transcellular (digestive tract, CSF, joints, aqueous humor, etc.) (1 l).

Volume changes may be due to:
- External losses (haemorrhage, vomiting or diarrhoea).
- Internal redistribution of extracellular fluid: for example, sequestration within the gut lumen (so-called 'third-space' loss). This leads to loss of effective ECF into a relatively non-functioning compartment. Only on resolution of the disease is this fluid eventually mobilized back into the effective ECF. Faced

continues overleaf

REVISION POINTS – cont'd

with such losses the body's priority is to maintain the intravascular compartment for adequate circulation.

Fluid management requires understanding and calculation of three principal factors:
- correction of existing abnormalities
- maintenance of daily requirements
- replacement of ongoing losses.

Some examples of abnormalities include:
- intra-abdominal sepsis (isotonic fluid shifts from ECF to 'third space')
- diarrhoea and vomiting (electrolyte and water loss)

- dehydration (loss of ICF will lead to compensatory cardiovascular changes).

Patients' fluid requirements can rarely be predicted accurately and can change dramatically from hour to hour. Successful fluid management relies on careful anticipation of expected fluid losses and appropriate replacement. Repeated clinical assessment with measurement of pulse, blood pressure and urine output, to determine whether patients are hypovolaemic or overloaded, must be combined with regular measurement of electrolyte concentrations.

ISSUES TO CONSIDER

- How accurately can you clinically assess the extent of dehydration?
- What fluid solutions are available for use in the management of patients with fluid and electrolyte disturbances?
- Consider the differences in these solutions and work out the best combination of fluid and electrolytes for dehydration, paralytic ileus and vomiting caused by gastric outlet obstruction.
- What complications commonly occur as a result of inappropriate fluid prescriptions on surgical wards?

FURTHER INFORMATION

www.studentbmj.com/back_issues/0497/data/0497ed1.htm A didactic page on fluid balance.

A middle-aged man with postoperative fever

Your patient, a 58-year-old man, is about to undergo surgery for a carcinoma of the rectum. He does not have any significant past medical history. He is not on any medications and has never smoked cigarettes.

Operations are classified according to the potential for bacterial contamination of the wound and hence their risk of infection.

 Q1 What are the categories and how would this operation be classified?

This patient is in a high-risk category for the development of septic complications after surgery.

Q2 What steps should be taken preoperatively to reduce the risk of wound infection?

Appropriate measures are taken to reduce the chance of wound infection. The surgeon resects the rectal tumour with difficulty and performs a stapled end-to-end anastomosis 8 cm above the dentate line.

Five days post procedure, the patient begins to complain of pain in the wound. He has a low-grade fever, but his pulse and pressure are normal. He is mobile and is tolerating a light diet. On physical examination his chest is clear, and the abdominal wound is tense, fluctuant, erythematous and tender at the superior aspect. The remainder of his examination is normal.

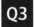 **Q3** What is your diagnosis and what should you do?

The wound is incised and a small amount of pus drained. The patient improves, but on the morning of discharge, the patient reports 'just not feeling well'. The nursing observation chart for the last few days is shown (Figure 2.1).

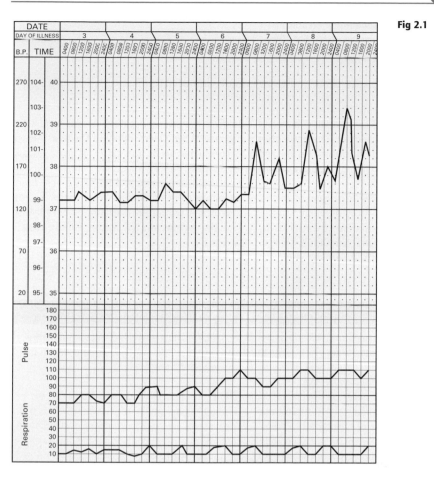

Fig 2.1

Q4 What is shown on the chart and what are you going to do?

From the history and casenotes it is ascertained that the patient underwent a large bowel resection 10 days earlier and the operation notes record that the procedure was 'difficult'. Apart from the changes noted on the nursing observation chart, nothing else abnormal is found on examination. In particular, his abdomen is soft and the wound infection has resolved.

A rectal examination is performed. You note some fullness posteriorly and the anastomosis cannot be felt. You arrange a number of investigations, including a CT scan (Figure 2.2).

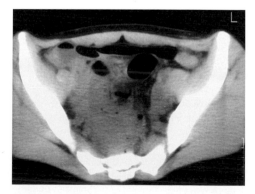

Fig 2.2

Your other investigations are unremarkable apart from an elevated white cell count of $18 \times 10^9/l$.

Q5 What does the scan show and what is your plan of action?

The patient is returned to the operating room and the abscess drained per rectum. The antibiotics are continued until his temperature settles and the patient is discharged home 3 weeks after his operation.

An anastomotic leak was diagnosed in this patient as the source of intra-abdominal sepsis. Anastomotic leaks may declare themselves by discharge of faecal material through a drain or by systemic signs of sepsis. A contrast study can confirm the site and extent of the leak. Compromise of the blood supply to the anastomosis is considered to be the cause of most anastomotic leaks. Not all anastomotic leaks will lead to abscess formation, and many are only found on routine contrast studies. When a pelvic abscess develops it will often discharge spontaneously into the rectum and no further intervention is necessary.

ANSWERS

A1 As part of your preoperative work-up of any patient about to undergo surgery, you want to identify any risk factors that may have an untoward influence on postoperative recovery. One important aspect is the assessment of the risk of infection (particularly chest, wound and operative site). The type of operation has a considerable bearing on the risk of infection. There are four categories into which operations are classified according to their risk for the development of wound infection. These are:

● clean
● clean-contaminated
● contaminated
● dirty.

Clean cases (e.g. hernia repair) where the gastrointestinal, respiratory or gynaecologic tract are not entered have low infection rates (<0.5%) with any contaminant likely being of skin origin. Clean-contaminated cases such as cholecystectomy for cholelithiasis have mild infection rates of 1–5% and are associated with entry into the foregut or biliary tree, areas considered to be sterile. Contaminated cases involve procedures on the colon (including the appendix), where the high bacterial content produces a 10–30% infection rate. Dirty cases are any cases where purulence is drained. Your patient is about to undergo an operation on a part of his gut with a normally high bacterial flora content – that is, it will be a 'contaminated' procedure.

A2 The important and most likely sources of infecting organisms are the colon and the skin. The bowel is prepared by emptying it of its faecal content, most commonly by using an isotonic, electrolyte-rich lavage. The patient drinks 3–4 l of the solution the day before surgery, producing a large catharsis. Hypovolaemia may be induced by this procedure and patients are instructed to also consume absorbable electrolyte solutions. Alternatively, if the patient is not particularly fit the preparation is done as an inpatient with simultaneous intravenous fluid replacement.

On the morning of surgery the patient will be given a shower using a bactericidal soap and the surgical site clipped immediately prior to operation.

Approximately 1 hour to surgical incision, the patient will be given a dose of intravenous broad-spectrum antibiotics (e.g. a second-generation cephalosporin), the goal being adequate tissue penetration of antibiotic at the time of the incision.

For clean and clean-contaminated cases, the role of prophylactic antibiotics is not so clear cut. Several other factors enter into the overall risk of postoperative infection and influence decisions

A N S W E R S – cont'd

on the usage of prophylactic antibiotics. For example, an inguinal hernia repair would not usually require antibiotics, but if mesh was incorporated into the procedure, the patient would probably be given a single dose of an antibiotic as a prophylactic measure. Emergency procedures have a higher risk than those performed electively. Patients in a poor state of health, with malignancy, immunosuppression (diabetes) or malnutrition are at increased risk. Antibiotics are more likely to be used in these groups of patients.

A3 The patient has a surgical wound infection. Incision and drainage of the wound are necessary. Incision should be extensive enough to allow easy drainage of the wound and easy wound care. If small and localized, such an infection may be treated at the bedside. Saline-soaked gauze can be used to dress the wound. Debridement may be necessary in more severe cases. If the patient has a cellulitic component to the wound infection or has a systemic response to the infection, antibiotics will be necessary. Patients who have prosthetic devices (e.g. joint replacements), are at risk of prosthesis infection (a catastrophic complication) and will need antibiotics.

A4 Over the last 72 hours the patient has had multiple fever spikes with associated tachycardia. The patient most likely has an underlying infection and a complete work-up is necessary. This should include:
- a full history and physical examination
- complete blood picture
- blood cultures taken when febrile
- urine culture
- chest radiograph.

As the patient has undergone a low anterior resection of the rectum, an intra-abdominal fluid collection may have accumulated in the pelvis or subdiaphragmatic spaces with leakage from the anastomosis being the most likely source. Therefore, CT scan of the abdomen and pelvis is also needed.

A5 The CT view of the pelvis in this patient shows an abscess behind the rectum. There are pockets of gas within the abscess cavity. This suggests that an anastomotic leak has occurred and the patient has had a septic response to this leak. The patient should be started on a broad-spectrum antibiotic and the abscess drained.

R E V I S I O N   P O I N T S

Postoperative fever, focusing on infection

Aetiology
Six different sites are considered:
- The pulmonary tract. Generally seen in the immediate postoperative period secondary to atelectasis or subsequently pneumonia.
- Urinary tract (common in patients with indwelling catheters).
- Cellulitis in venous access sites.
- Surgical wound infections generally present 3–7 days postoperatively.
- Intra-abdominal sepsis from abscess is considered after the 5th–7th postoperative day.
- Occasionally the blood may become seeded with bacteria (bacteraemia or septicaemia depending on the clinical presentation). This

is usually from contamination of central catheters particularly in critically ill patients in intensive care units.

Prevention
The most important aspect of therapy.
Preoperative identification of risk factors:
- category of surgical procedure
- co-morbidities (e.g. diabetes, prosthetic heart valve).

Measures taken to reduce risk of infection:
- prophylactic use of antibiotics
- bowel preparation
- improvement in general state of patient:
  - chest physiotherapy and use of bronchodilators in patients with chronic obstructive pulmonary disease

continues overleaf

REVISION POINTS – cont'd

– correction of any anaemia or malnutrition
- use of topical antiseptic measures at site of operation
- good surgical technique and use of prophylactic perioperative antibiotics
- early ambulation and aggressive pulmonary toilet
- appropriate analgesia to aid good respiratory effort and mobilization
- early removal of indwelling catheters as soon as the patient can void.

Diagnosis

The work-up of a postoperative fever is directed at the five most common sources. After a complete physical examination with careful inspection of the surgical wound, blood test and cultures may be added. Chest X-ray and urinalysis are generally considered and if intra-abdominal abscess is suspected, CT scan or ultrasound can be diagnostic and can be used in treatment.

Management

When a focus of infection is determined, antibiotic usage should be tailored to likely organism(s) and risk of systemic sepsis.
- a localized collection is best drained
- antibiotics should be given when:
  – there is evidence of spreading infection
  – the patient is septic
  – host defences are reduced (e.g. immunosuppression)
  – any infection would have grave consequences (e.g. presence of a prosthetic heart valve or joint replacement).

ISSUES TO CONSIDER

- What are the important differences between the terms 'bacteraemia', 'septicaemia' and 'septic shock'?

- How would you counsel this patient before his operation? What else does he need to know about, apart from the risk of wound infection?

- There are other potential risks and complications, related specifically to this operation and to major surgery in general. How would you go about reducing the risk of some of these other potential problems?

FURTHER INFORMATION

www.emedicine.com/MED/topic2702.htm
A textbook description of the diagnosis and management of intra-abdominal abscesses.

Postoperative hypotension

You are called to see a 65-year-old man on the surgical ward. He is 5 days post emergency left hemicolectomy for an obstructing carcinoma. The senior nurse is concerned that the patient has become increasingly confused over the day and his blood pressure has now dropped to 80/50 mm Hg.

Q1 What important causes of postoperative hypotension must you consider?

As you leave the warm and friendly confines of the residents' bar and go towards the ward, you appreciate that if that patient is confused you may not get much of a history from him.

Q2 In trying to establish the cause of the hypotension, what other sources of information should you seek before you examine the patient?

The patient has no prior medical history of note. He had been making an uneventful recovery from his surgery although his gut has not yet started functioning. You note from his charts that a tachycardia has been developing over the last 24 hours and his urine output has dropped from over 30 ml per hour to 10 ml per hour over the last 3 hours. His temperature is 39.4ºC. You read the operation record and note that the procedure was uncomplicated and a primary anastomosis was performed. A broad-spectrum antibiotic was given prophylactically and continued for 48 hours.

You attend to the patient. He is mildly confused and is unable to answer your questions appropriately. His skin is pale and clammy and his pulse is faint but regular at 120 bpm.

Q3 What will you look for in your examination?

He already has peripheral venous access and a triple-lumen central line which was inserted during the operation. Both insertion sites look clean and dry. His JVP is not visible and his tongue is dry. He has a tachypnoea of 28 breaths per minute. His heart sounds are normal. His lung examination reveals dull percussion note and absent breath sounds in the lower third of the left lung.

The right lung has some crepitations at the base. The remainder of the lung fields are clear.

His abdomen is mildly distended, but soft with minimal tenderness to deep palpation. There are no localizing signs. The abdominal wound looks clean and dry. Bowel sounds are absent. His urine appears concentrated but clear. His calves are not tender or swollen.

Q4 What do you think is wrong? How will you manage this patient initially? What investigations would you like to perform?

The following blood results become available.

Investigation 3.1 Blood results			
Haemoglobin	152 g/l	White cell count	$17.0 \times 10^9/l$
Platelets	$350 \times 10^9/l$	Neutrophils 88%	$15.0 \times 10^9/l$
PCV	0.39	Lymphocytes 7%	$1.2 \times 10^9/l$
MCV	86.9 fl	Monocytes 3%	$0.5 \times 10^9/l$
MCH	29.5 pg	Eosinophils 1%	$0.2 \times 10^9/l$
MCHC	340 g/l	Basophils 1%	$0.2 \times 10^9/l$
Sodium	140 mmol/l	Calcium	2.16 mmol/l
Potassium	5.4 mmol/l	Phosphate	1.15 mmol/l
Chloride	106 mmol/l	Total protein	59 g/l
Bicarbonate	18 mmol/l	Albumin	32 g/l
Urea	15.3 mmol/l	Globulins	27 g/l
Creatinine	0.21 mmol/l	Bilirubin	16 µmol/l
Uric acid	0.24 mmol/l	ALT	40 U/l
Glucose	4.4 mmol/l	AST	42 U/l
Cholesterol	3.5 mmol/l	GGT	17 U/l
LDH	151 U/l	ALP	70 U/l
Arterial blood gas analysis on room air			
pO_2	67 mm Hg	pCO_2	37 mm Hg
pH	7.30	Base excess	−9.5

Q5 What do these results tell you?

A 12-lead ECG and cardiac troponin are both within normal limits. A chest X-ray is performed (Figure 3.1).

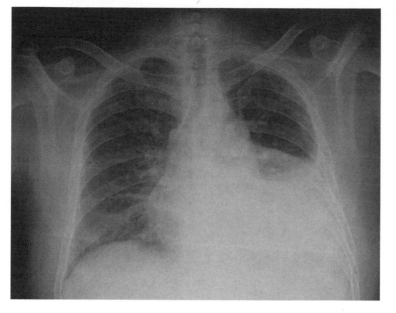

Fig 3.1

 Q6 What abnormalities are shown on the X-ray? What do you think has caused this appearance? What are you going to do now?

The patient responds well to your resuscitation measures and his hypotension corrects with intravenous fluid. He is started on broad-spectrum intravenous antibiotics, avoiding aminoglycosides due to concern about nephrotoxicity. The effusion is observed. His condition remains stable and one week later when his sepsis is under control and his renal function has returned to normal, a contrast-enhanced CT scan of the chest and abdomen is performed. One sequence is shown (Figure 3.2).

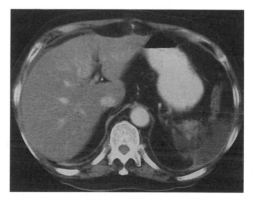

Fig 3.2

Q7 What abnormalities are shown on the CT scan?

The collection is drained percutaneously under radiological control. The material is sanguinous and a sample sent for culture grows coliforms, sensitive to the antibiotics you have prescribed. A drain is left in the cavity (and removed after a week). His condition rapidly improves over the next 48 hours. A contrast study is performed which does not show any evidence of anastomotic leakage. The postoperative recovery progresses without further mishap.

ANSWERS

A1 The confusion and hypotension suggests this patient is suffering from shock. Shock is defined as inadequate tissue perfusion. There are several potential causes in this case:

1 Hypovolaemia
This is an important cause of hypotension in the postoperative patient. In this case it could be due to:
- haemorrhage
- gastrointestinal 'third-space' losses (e.g. ileus) with inadequate fluid replacement and subsequent dehydration.

2 Sepsis
There are many potential sites for infection in the postoperative setting. Look for the presence of a fever which, in the case of an infected collection, may be 'swinging' in nature.

This patient had emergency surgery for a colonic obstruction. The risk of persistent intra-abdominal infection is high. If an anastomosis was performed in the emergency situation, there is a significant risk of an anastomotic leak.

Other potential sources of infection are the chest (retained sputum and inadequate cough reflex), the urinary tract (catheterization) and from intravenous access sites.

3 Low cardiac output
Cardiogenic shock following an acute myocardial infarct is a common cause for sudden hypotension and requires exclusion. Look for serial ECG changes and a rise in cardiac enzymes, including troponins.

Pulmonary embolus also occurs in the postoperative period and if suspected will need to be excluded with spiral CT.

Other cardiac causes include arrhythmias.

4 Anaphylaxis
Attention must be paid to any medication or blood transfusion that has been commenced over the postoperative period. Penicillin hypersensitivity is common, but be aware that 10% of patients have a cross-sensitivity with cephalosporins.

Anaphylaxis will require emergency treatment with fluid resuscitation, adrenaline (epinephrine) and hydrocortisone.

A2 Additional information may be available from several sources.

1 As the patient is confused and may not be able to give much history, the nursing staff may be able to provide information on:
- any symptoms (e.g. chest pain, dyspnoea, chilling or rigors)
- any evidence of blood loss such as bloody return from an nasogastric tube, bloody vomitus, melaena or bright red blood per rectum.

2 The patient record should be studied:
- The vital signs: recent changes in blood pressure and temperature (the presence of a fever will suggest underlying infection and septic shock).
- The fluid balance chart. A negative fluid balance and falling weight over the preceding days is in favour of dehydration.
- Any medications or blood products the patient has recently received. A recent transfusion or change in antibiotics may point toward anaphylaxis as a cause of shock.

3 Ask for the medical records and review the patient's past medical history. Regardless of the cause of the current deterioration, this will be important knowledge in the current management of the patient.

A3 You must do a speedy, efficient but thorough assessment of the patient looking for clues as to the underlying cause of the shock. There are multiple possibilities. A postoperative patient after emergency colonic surgery may have an anastomotic leak or an intra-abdominal collection. However, shock could also be due to line infection, a urinary tract infection, pulmonary embolus, upper gastrointestinal bleed or myocardial infarction.

In a methodical manner you will:
- look for evidence of circulatory collapse
- try and identify the underlying cause of the collapse.

Start by taking the pulse and recheck the blood pressure yourself (and measure any orthostatic drop). As you feel the pulse you should check the

ANSWERS – cont'd

perfusion of the peripheries by observing the temperature of the hands and feet.

1 Sepsis
Look for evidence of systemic vasodilatation such as warm, flushed peripheries and a hyperdynamic circulation. In other forms of shock, such as volume depletion or haemorrhage, there is peripheral vasoconstriction and the extremities are cool and 'shutdown'. Look also for sources of infection such as:
- Abdomen: intra-abdominal collection secondary to anastomotic leak. Look for peritonism.
- Wound: look for cellulitis, swelling, discharge.
- Venous access sites: discharge, erythema. How long have the cannulae been in?
- Chest: pneumonia, effusion.
- Heart: endocarditis.
- Urinary tract: indwelling catheters.

2 Hypovolaemia
- Look for evidence of dehydration such as dry mucous membranes, lack of skin turgor.
- Look at the nature and amount of urine in the urinary drainage bag.
- Haemorrhage may not be immediately obvious. Examine drains, gastric aspirates and perform a rectal examination if colonic bleeding is suspected.

3 Cardiogenic
A raised JVP may indicate cardiac failure or pulmonary embolism. Look also for other signs of heart failure such as the presence of pulmonary oedema.
- Examine the legs for evidence of deep venous thrombosis.

4 Anaphylaxis
- Look for a skin rash, angioedema and the presence of wheeze.

A4 The presence of fever, tachycardia, hypotension, dehydration and confusion indicate this patient is most likely to have severe sepsis.

The development of pyrexia, tachycardia, tachypnoea and abnormal white cell count is defined as Systemic Inflammatory Response Syndrome or SIRS. When SIRS occurs in the presence of infection, this is termed sepsis.

In the more advanced cases, there may be evidence of organ dysfunction. Where two or more organ systems are affected this is termed Multiple Organ Dysfunction Syndrome or MODS. Where MODS occurs in the presence of an identified source of infection, this is termed severe sepsis or sepsis syndrome. Infection and hypotension that fails to respond to initial resuscitation is termed septic shock.

The patient requires prompt resuscitation:
- Commence high-flow oxygen. Attach pulse oximeter.
- Ensure there is adequate intravenous access.
- Commence rapid intravenous fluid replacement. Either crystalloid (e.g. isotonic saline) or colloid would be appropriate. Initially, the patient is likely to require a large amount of fluid quickly, e.g. 1000 ml isotonic saline over 15–30 minutes. Subsequent fluid replacement should be guided by the patient's blood pressure, tachycardia, urine output and central venous pressure. Patients who do not respond quickly to resuscitation or in whom assessing the adequacy of resuscitation is difficult should be transferred to an intensive care unit for closer monitoring.
- Collect venous blood samples for a complete blood picture and biochemistry, clotting screen, cross-match and blood culture. If central lines are in situ, blood cultures should be taken through the lines (all ports) and also peripherally. If the lines look infected or are old they should be replaced.
- Perform arterial blood gas analysis looking for evidence of acidosis, hypoxia and high lactate (a measure of poor tissue perfusion).
- If not already in place, insert a urinary catheter to monitor fluid status and renal perfusion. Send a urine specimen for culture. Consider a central line if not already inserted and resuscitation difficult.
- Attach to cardiac monitor. Perform an ECG and arrange a chest X-ray.

ANSWERS – cont'd

- Give a broad-spectrum antibiotic intravenously. The choice of antibiotic should be guided by local protocol and the suspected source of the patient's infection.
- Further specimens should also be sent for infection screen. These may include sputum, and any pus or drain fluid.

A5 The results suggest the following:
- Dehydration (high haemoglobin, increased urea and creatinine).
- Infection (leucocytosis due to neutrophilia).
- Renal dysfunction (raised urea and creatinine).
- Metabolic acidosis.
- Hypoxia.

The renal dysfunction is probably prerenal in origin, due to hypovolaemia and poor perfusion. The low pH, high base deficit and low bicarbonate level point to a metabolic acidosis, consistent with severe sepsis. Hypoxia could be due to a postoperative basal atelectasis, chest infection, diaphragmatic splinting secondary to abdominal surgery or respiratory depression secondary to decreased consciousness or excessive opiate use.

A6 There is opacification of the left lower zone. The presence of a meniscus and the preservation of the diaphragm and cardiac border suggest that this is a moderate-sized pleural effusion. This could be due to a postoperative pneumonia or an underlying intra-abdominal infection.

Although intra-abdominal infection with a sympathetic pleural effusion and now systemic sepsis is most likely, you still do not know exactly what is happening. The patient could have a nosocomial infection of the bloodstream from infection of his central catheter. As he is seriously ill, he requires broad-spectrum intravenous antibiotics along with his resuscitation. Whichever antibiotic regimen is used, it must be reviewed on a regular basis and altered according to response and to the results of microbiological (particularly blood) cultures. If there is any suggestion of renal impairment, you should try and avoid using aminoglycosides. However, aminoglycosides can be used in settings where the risk of uncontrolled sepsis outweighs the risk of renal impairment or failure. In such circumstances, the dose should be adjusted to the calculated glomerular filtration rate (using the Cockroft–Gault nomogram) and the serum concentrations of the drug monitored closely.

Once the patient has been resuscitated, further imaging studies need to be performed. The preferred investigation is an abdominal CT scan with percutaneous drainage and insertion of a catheter into any identified localized collection. If the patient's condition worsens or there is evidence of peritonitis, surgical intervention may be required. If an anastomosis has leaked, either the anastomosis may need to be dismantled and exteriorized or a proximal (diverting) ostomy fashioned.

A failure to respond to initial resuscitation suggests the need for management in an intensive care unit, with facilities for invasive monitoring, vasopressor support and mechanical ventilation.

A7 The scan shows a view through the upper abdomen. Contrast has been given to outline the stomach. Posteriolateral to the stomach is a loculated collection of fluid. There are several bubbles of gas in the collection. This is likely to be an infected collection – that is, an abscess. It is the likely explanation for the (sympathetic) pleural effusion.

REVISION POINTS

Shock

Definition
Inadequate tissue perfusion.

Aetiology
- Hypovolaemic.
- Cardiogenic.

continues overleaf

R E V I S I O N   P O I N T S – cont'd

- Septic.
- Anaphylactic.
- Neurogenic.

Signs
- Cold, clammy, confused.
- Tachycardia, tachypnoea.
- Reduced urine output (oliguria).
- A normal systolic blood pressure does *not* exclude shock. A young patient can lose up to 30% of their blood volume (~1.5 l) before a drop in blood pressure occurs.

Treatment
- Administer IV fluid. Replace what is lost. Aim for 10–20 ml/kg initial bolus.
- High-flow oxygen.
- Look for cause of shock that requires specific treatment (e.g. haemorrhage, anaphylaxis).

- Monitor blood pressure, oxygen saturations, urine output and central venous pressure to assess response to resuscitation.
- Consider transfer to intensive care facility.

Sepsis
- Identify and treat site of infection.
- Systemic infections and high-risk patients require appropriate intravenous antibiotics
- Infected lines need to be removed
- Infected collections need to be drained.

High-risk sepsis
- Elderly.
- Malnourished.
- Diabetic.
- Immunocompromised: particularly any neutropenic patient, patients with haematological malignancies or BMT, solid organ transplant recipients, those on corticosteroids.

ISSUES TO CONSIDER

- How would your management of this case differ if the CT scan had not yielded an intra-abdominal collection?
- What other forms of haemodynamic monitoring are available on the intensive care department? What are the limitations of CVP monitoring?
- What are the differences between crystalloids and colloids as resuscitation fluids?

FURTHER INFORMATION

www.rcsed.ac.uk/Journal/vol45_3/4530010.htm
An excellent review article on SIRS from the Royal College of Surgeons of Edinburgh.

www.biomedcentral.com/1364-8535/4/S16
One of many articles fuelling the debate between the colloid camp and the crystalloid camp!

Postoperative confusion

A 57-year-old man on the surgical ward has become acutely confused and agitated at 3 a.m. It is 5 days since he had a total gastrectomy for adenocarcinoma of his stomach. The nursing staff are concerned that he is frightening the other patients. You are woken by a telephone call from a member of staff who asks you to give a verbal order for haloperidol.

Q1 What are you going to tell the nurse?

When you arrive at the ward it is obvious from the noise and bustle which is your patient. He is sitting up in bed with one leg dangling out of the side and he is trying to pull his drip out. A harassed nurse is attempting to restrain him, while another is waving an ampoule of haloperidol and the drug chart in your face.

The patient is agitated and inappropriately attentive to his surroundings. He focuses on everything that is happening but cannot seem to make sense of the situation. When you talk to him he swears at you and mumbles incoherently. He is easily distracted and is unable to carry out a conversation. He is clearly disorientated and you wonder if he is hallucinating. The nurse informs you that the previous evening he had spent much of the night awake but had not been rowdy. During the day he had been drowsy and slept. However, since about 10 p.m. he has become confused and agitated.

Q2 What are the possible causes of this man's postoperative confusion? What factors may have put him at risk?

On examination he has a low-grade fever of 37.7°C and a pulse rate of 110 bpm. His blood pressure is 150/100 mm Hg. His respiratory rate is 30 breaths per minute. Cardiovascular and respiratory examinations are otherwise normal. His abdominal wound appears clean and is not infected. His abdomen is soft and non-tender and there are occasional bowel sounds. He has no focal neurological signs. His calves appear normal with no evidence of deep venous thrombosis.

He had a normal contrast study (to check anastomotic integrity) earlier in the day and has been taking in 30 ml per hour of water and ice-chips. On analysis of his fluid balance chart his fluid status appears satisfactory. He has no abnormal fluid losses.

He has been receiving a low-dose morphine infusion for analgesia. His bowels were open yesterday and were quite loose and malodorous. He is on no other medications. He has had a low-grade temperature and tachycardia for 24 hours. A urine analysis done in the last 12 hours is normal. From the case notes you learn that he has no significant past medical history. He is a non-smoker and his alcohol intake is unknown.

A CT scan prior to surgery demonstrated a localized tumour on the greater curve of the stomach with no evidence of local or distant spread. There were also changes on the CT scan consistent with liver cirrhosis. The operation note recorded an uneventful procedure and the stomach and all obvious tumour were successfully removed prior to the creation of a roux-en-Y anastomosis. The liver was small and nodular.

 Q3 How would you describe this man's clinical state?

 Q4 What investigations may be helpful at this stage?

You note that preoperative blood tests revealed an MCV of 104.9 fl and a GGT of 119 IU/l. The rest of his preoperative work up was unremarkable.

His postoperative course has been otherwise uncomplicated. Plans were being made for discharge within the next 3 or 4 days. The results of your investigations are shown below.

Investigation 4.1 Summary of results	
Complete blood picture:	normal
Electrolytes, urea, creatinine, liver function tests:	normal
Arterial blood gases:	normal
Chest X-ray:	bibasal atelectasis

Q5 What do you think is happening to this patient? Would any other history be helpful?

You decide to try and obtain some further information about the patient and call his partner. She says that to her knowledge he does not abuse drugs or take benzodiazepines, but he does drink 'quite a bit'. When asked what that means she says that he would drink a bottle of wine every evening on weekdays and more on weekends. She also thought he might drink during his lunch breaks. She says that she had told him to reduce his drinking, but he has never listened to her.

Q6 How does this extra information affect your assessment? What is your management plan for this patient?

With appropriate management, the patient's symptoms of alcohol withdrawal settle over the next 48 hours.

 Q7 What other damage may he have suffered as a result of his alcohol abuse?

Q8 What should be done for this man before discharge?

The patient admitted to alcohol abuse but said that he would deal with the problem privately and was discharged from the ward 10 days after his operation.

ANSWERS

A1 The patient has postoperative confusion. You tell the nurse on the end of the telephone that you will come to the ward and the patient must be assessed before any sedative or hypnotic is given. You will need to:

- Talk to the nurses to establish the duration and severity of confusion.
- Read the casenotes to determine premorbid pathology, preoperative blood analyses and results of other preoperative investigations.
- Read the operative record looking for any intra-operative difficulties or unusual findings,

and determine the postoperative course thus far.
- Talk to relatives if available.
- Examine observations chart, and any recent blood results.
- Talk to and examine the patient.

A2 Postoperative confusion can be caused by a variety of conditions. It is more common in the elderly, in the medically unfit and debilitated, and after emergency surgery. Examples of precipitating causes include:

Box 4.1 Precipitating causes of postoperative confusion

Sepsis	Intra-abdominal abscess
	Wound infection
	Pneumonia
	Urinary tract infection
Hypoxia	Chest infection
	Pulmonary embolus
	Pre-existing pulmonary disease
Metabolic abnormalities	Hyponatraemia
	Hypo- or hyperglycaemia
	Acidosis
	Alkalosis
Cardiac	Myocardial ischaemia
	Arrhythmias
	Congestive cardiac failure
Hypotension	Haemorrhage
	Dehydration
Cerebrovascular event	Stroke
Exacerbation of medical conditions	Hypothyroidism
	Pre-existing cognitive disorders
	Pre-existing dementia
Drug withdrawal	Alcohol
	Benzodiazepines
	Narcotics
Narcotic analgesic effect	Opiate sedation causing hypoventilation
Pain	

ANSWERS – cont'd

Specific surgical causes of confusion occur most commonly on days 5–10 after upper gastrointestinal procedures. It is important to be aware of potentially catastrophic complications when assessing this patient. They include:

- anastomotic dehiscence
- delayed haemorrhage from a ligated vessel or staple line
- intestinal volvulus
- duodenal stump blow-out.

As hospitalization takes the patient out of his or her usual environment withdrawal from drugs of addiction is not uncommon. The most frequent examples are alcohol and benzodiazepine withdrawal but narcotic withdrawal is also sometimes seen.

Elderly patients are particularly at risk of postoperative confusion often precipitated by relatively 'mild' abnormalities. These factors are often cumulative. In addition, if there is pre-existing mild dementia the stress of surgery and the placement of the patient in a foreign environment will often precipitate an acute state of confusion.

A3 This man has clouding of consciousness with hyperactivity, agitation, disorientation, incoherence, irritability and reversal of the sleep–wake cycle (awake at night and asleep during the day). He may be hallucinating but it is difficult to be sure. It would seem he has delusional ideas and is moderately aggressive. This is a classical case of delirium.

In the current American Psychiatric Association classification DSM–IV, the cardinal features of delirium are:

- An underlying medical condition.
- Disturbed consciousness. The patient's attention span is reduced.
- Development of cognitive impairment: perception, memory, language and orientation may be disturbed.
- Short duration of onset.

Delirium is an organic brain syndrome and should be considered a medical emergency. It is seen commonly in both medical and surgical patients, and more so in the elderly. Delirium occurs in up to 65% of surgical patients.

Causes of apparent confusion such as deafness, dysphasia, blindness and depression must be excluded (check that patients have their spectacles and ensure that any hearing aids are working).

Patients are often sleepy and quiet during the day only to decompensate at night and are frequently the cause of much commotion in the ward in the middle of the night. On occasion they may need to be sedated or even shackled for their own safety and that of everyone concerned, the nursing staff included. Before this is done, it must be recognized that these patients are acutely unwell and need full assessment to establish the underlying cause of the confusion.

Not all patients with confusion or delirium are noisy and aggressive or become the focus of attention. Some are quiet. This state may only be picked up by casual conversation with the patient during routine care. Although this mode of presentation is not as dramatic as the rowdy patient, the problem may still be equally as serious.

A4 Following a full examination, you should consider the following investigations:

- Complete blood picture for anaemia and leucocytosis.
- Electrolytes and renal function for electrolyte imbalance and renal failure.
- Glucose.
- Culture blood, urine, drain fluids, etc.
- ECG for evidence of myocardial ischaemia.
- Chest X-ray for evidence of infection.
- Arterial blood gases for hypoxia and acid–base disturbance.

A5 The patient has no known pre-existing medical problems. He has had no major postoperative complications. Other than the low-grade fever, tachycardia, tachypnoea and the basal atelectasis there are no abnormalities on examination. His blood tests are unremarkable. This excludes major cardiovascular disturbance, fluid or electrolyte abnormality and hypoxia. An anastomotic leak is unlikely following a normal contrast study. An abdominal CT scan could be considered if it was thought that the patient had an intra-abdominal collection.

A N S W E R S – cont'd

A withdrawal state would be in keeping with these findings and the low grade fever and tachycardia would be consistent. An alcohol or benzodiazepine withdrawal syndrome would be most likely. Alcohol abuse would be supported by the preoperative macrocytosis and mildly raised GGT. Further history concerning the patient's alcohol intake should be obtained. The patient should also be re-examined for tremor and clinical evidence of liver disease.

Further information should be sought including contacting relatives (even in the middle of the night) for additional history of alcohol abuse or benzodiazepine use as well as gaining an impression of his preoperative cognitive function.

If it is unclear what is happening to the patient you should consider further investigations and contact senior medical staff for advice (never be afraid to ask for help).

A6 This extra history is in keeping with the diagnosis of alcohol withdrawal. His history of alcohol consumption is high and his actual alcohol intake is likely to be higher than stated.

The patient requires the general supportive measures that are given to any delirious patient:
- Nurse separately in a well-lit room.

- Try to maintain the same nursing staff as far as possible.
- Frequently reorientate the patient. Visitors should introduce themselves.
- Protect the patient from his confusion.
- Maintain fluid and nutritional status.
- Provide sedation as necessary.

In this situation, a benzodiazepine would be the most appropriate treatment. Benzodiazepines have a wide therapeutic window, and have similar CNS effects to alcohol (predominantly GABA-ergic). Short-acting benzodiazepines (e.g. lorazepam, oxazepam) are safer in patients with severe liver disease, but in this patient symptomatic control will best be achieved with a longer acting drug such as diazepam.

Reference should be made to your hospital's alcohol withdrawal protocol. A dose of oral diazepam (e.g. 10–20 mg) should be administered. The patient should then be reassessed in 30 minutes and the dose can then be repeated if the symptoms of alcohol withdrawal are still profound. Assessment of the severity of alcohol withdrawal symptoms should be made using the Clinical Institute Withdrawal Assessment (CIWA-AR) reproduced in Table 4.1.

Table 4.1 Clinical Institute Withdrawal Assessment

Score	Symptom groups and grades		
	Nausea and vomiting	Tactile disturbances	Tremor
0	Nil	None	No tremor
1	Mild nausea	Mild (numbness, burning, paraesthesia, itching)	None visible but may be felt 'tip to tip'
2		Mild itching	
3		As above but moderate	
4	Intermittent with dry heaves	Moderate tactile hallucinations	Moderate
5		Severe tactile hallucinations	
6		Severe tactile hallucinations	
7	Constant nausea with frequent vomiting	Severe and continuous tactile hallucinations	Severe, even without arms extended

A N S W E R S – cont'd

Table 4.1 Clinical Institute Withdrawal Assessment – cont'd

	Anxiety	Visual disturbances	Agitation
0	Nil	Nil	Nil
1	Mild	Very mild light sensitivity	More than normal
2		Mild sensitivity	
3		Moderate sensitivity	
4	Moderate, guarded	Moderate visual hallucinations	Moderate: fidgety, restless
5		Severe visual hallucinations	
6		Extremely severe hallucinations	
7	Severe panic	Continuous hallucinations	Severe: paces back and forth Unable to keep still
	Headache/fullness in head (not lightheadedness)	Auditory disturbances	Paroxysmal sweats
0	Nil	Nil	Nil
1	Very mild	Very mild harshness of sound, the ability to frighten	Barely
2		As above, mild	As above
3	Moderate	Moderate	
4		Moderate auditory hallucinations	Beads of sweat on forehead
5	Severe	Severe auditory hallucinations	
6		Extremely severe hallucinations	
7	Extremely severe	Continuous hallucinations	Drenching
	Orientation		
0	Orientated, able to do serial additions		
1	Unable to do serial additions, sure of date		
2	Disorientated for date by no more than 2 days		
3	Disorientated for date by more than 2 days		
4	Disorientated for place and/or person		

The CIWA-AR Scoring System for Alcohol Withdrawal: Patients are assessed by observation and direct questioning. A total score is obtained. Reassessment is performed regularly to assess the response to treatment. Adapted from *Br J Addict* 1989;84:1353–7.

A N S W E R S – cont'd

Doses of sedative can be repeated until the score is less than 10. The key to effective and safe treatment of alcohol withdrawal is continuous and regular reassessment.

Occasionally the administration of oral benzodiazepines will be ineffective or impossible. Intramuscular administration of a quick-acting sedative such as lorazepam may be appropriate. The administration of intravenous sedatives in this situation is extremely dangerous and should only be performed in a high dependency setting. Intravenous infusions should never be administered outside of an intensive care environment.

Major tranquillizers such as haloperidol may be of use in patients with florid hallucinations but can lower the seizure threshold so should be avoided in patients with a history of withdrawal fits.

High-dose thiamine should always be given to patients with suspected alcohol abuse and confusion (to treat or prevent Wernicke's encephalopathy).

The patient should be closely monitored for deterioration. Keep an open mind for additional diagnoses. For example, although the patient is on broad-spectrum antibiotics, he may have sepsis in addition to his probable alcohol withdrawal.

A7 In addition to the alcohol dependence syndrome with its attendant psychological, social and physical problems (including withdrawal syndromes), alcohol abuse causes damage to or affects many of the body's systems. Commonly recognized features are shown in Box 4.2.

Box 4.2 Features of alcohol abuse

Cardiovascular

- Alcohol-induced cardiomyopathy
- Beriberi (rare)
- Cardiac arrhythmias (e.g. atrial fibrillation)

Gastrointestinal

- 'Chemical' gastritis
- Carcinoma of the oesophagus
- Liver disease – fatty liver, acute alcoholic hepatitis, cirrhosis, hepatoma
- Acute and chronic pancreatitis

Neuromuscular

- Seizures
- Wernicke–Korsakoff syndrome
- Cerebellar degeneration
- Peripheral neuropathy
- Myopathy

Respiratory

- Aspiration pneumonia
- Tuberculosis

Hematological

- Macrocytosis or macrocytic anaemia (marrow toxicity or folate deficiency or liver disease)
- Thrombocytopaenia or leucopaenia (marrow toxicity, folate deficiency or hypersplenism)

A N S W E R S – cont'd

Box 4.2 Features of alcohol abuse – cont'd

Metabolism
- Hyperlipidaemia
- Hyperuricaemia (which may precipitate gout)
- Obesity

Bone
- Osteoporosis and osteomalacia

A8 The patient should be counselled about his alcohol abuse and referred to an appropriate service for further management. Various services are available, but some patients will elect to be managed by their local doctor, or decline any help. Whatever service is offered and sought, it must be available on a continuing basis to review and support the patient, as the problem of alcohol dependence is not one that can be dealt with quickly.

The patient's exact alcohol intake and drinking pattern needs to be established. The psychological and social problems of alcohol abuse (e.g. relationship, sexual, family, employment, accidents) need to be investigated. Psychological and physical features of alcohol dependence need to be detected. Safe levels of alcohol consumption need to be decided.

R E V I S I O N   P O I N T S

Postoperative confusion

Incidence
Up to 65% of surgical patients,
Risk factors
- advanced age
- alcoholism
- chronic medical conditions
- major surgery
- malignancy
- cognitive disorder
- postoperative complications.
Cardinal features of delirium
- medical condition
- altered consciousness
- cognitive impairment
- short duration of onset.
Clinical management
- Exclude causes of apparent confusion (deafness, dysphasia, depression, blindness).
- Exclude major underlying postoperative complications.
- Treat cause(s).

- Prescribe sedative only when appropriate history, examination and investigations have been performed.
Alcohol abuse
A common problem in the community.

The intake required to cause physiological dependence will vary with:
- age
- sex
- build
- metabolism.

Excessive social drinking is on a continuum with alcohol dependence. In the latter situation the person becomes both psychologically and physically addicted to alcohol and will therefore experience withdrawal symptoms on cessation of alcohol. This case demonstrated alcohol withdrawal of moderate severity. More severe withdrawal syndromes include withdrawal seizures and the life-threatening delirium tremens.

One of the main problems with alcohol abuse in regard to treatment is often its identification. Identifying features of withdrawal when a patient

continues overleaf

REVISION POINTS – cont'd

is hospitalized is one method of detection. Other ways in which alcohol abuse presents to medical staff includes trauma, unexplained falls and unexplained dyspepsia or gastrointestinal bleeds.

Alcohol-related organ damage, e.g. acute hepatitis or pancreatitis, may lead to emergency hospitalization.

ISSUES TO CONSIDER

- What pharmacological treatments are available for alcoholism?
- What is the Wernicke–Korsakoff syndrome, how is it identified and how do you treat it?
- What other nutritional deficiencies can present as a result of chronic alcoholism?

FURTHER INFORMATION

Sullivan J T, Skykora K, Schneiderman J. **Assessment of alcohol withdrawal: the revised Clinical Institute Withdrawal Assessment for Alcohol Scale (CIWA-Ar)**. *British Journal of Addiction* 1989;84:1353–7.

www.asam.org/publ/withdrawal.htm Pharmacological guidelines for the management of alcohol withdrawal from the American Society of Addiction Medicine.

Swelling in the neck in a 58-year-old man

A 58-year-old man presents with a 2-month history of a swelling in the neck. This has been getting slowly bigger and is not painful. He has no other symptoms and the history is otherwise unremarkable. The swelling is shown in Figure 5.1.

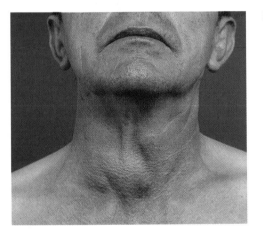

Fig 5.1

Q1 Describe the abnormality in the photograph.

Q2 What further information would you like from the history?

His general health is good and he has no difficulty in breathing or swallowing, nor has he noticed any change in his voice. There is nothing to suggest thyroid dysfunction. As you take the history, you notice that the swelling moves up and down as the patient talks.

On closer examination of the neck, you find that the swelling moves up when you ask him to swallow some water and it does not move when he protrudes his tongue. The swelling is non-tender, firm, smooth surfaced and appears to arise from the lower pole of the right lobe of the thyroid. The swelling is not attached to any adjacent structures and there are no enlarged lymph nodes. The trachea is not deviated. The left lobe of the gland appears normal and percussion does not reveal any obvious retrosternal extension. There is no bruit. His blood pressure is

130/90 mm Hg and the heart rate is 90 and regular. He has neither tremor nor increased sweatiness. There are no signs of thyroid eye disease. The examination of the chest and abdomen is unremarkable.

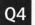   **What are the possible causes of this man's problem?**

The patient appears to be euthyroid and you are reasonably confident that this is a solitary nodule in the right lobe of the thyroid.

Q4   **What investigations would you organize?**

The thyroid function tests are normal and no thyroid antibodies are found. An aspiration of the swelling is performed and the cytological examination is shown in Figure 5.2.

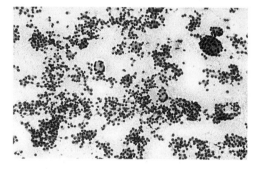

Fig 5.2

Q5   **What does the cytology of the aspirate reveal?**

An ultrasound scan is performed (Figure 5.3).

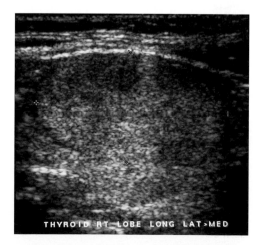

Fig 5.3

Q6 What does the scan show?

Your investigations have provided sufficient information to allow you to counsel the patient.

The scan confirms that the trachea is displaced to the left, but there is no compression.

Q7 What are you going to tell him?

The patient agrees to surgery, and a right hemithyroidectomy is planned. The patient asks

about the nature and possible complications of the surgery.

Q8 What do you tell him about the surgery?

A right hemithyroidectomy is performed, with identification and preservation of the recurrent laryngeal nerve and parathyroid glands. The opened operative specimen is shown in Figure 5.4.

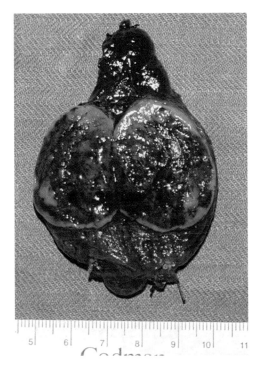

Fig 5.4

Q9 What does the specimen show?

Histologically, the lesion was 4.6 cm in diameter and comprised of follicular cells. There were areas where tongues of follicular cells could be seen extending through the capsule. There was no evidence of invasion into blood vessels. It was concluded that the lesion was an invasive follicular carcinoma.

Q10 What advice will you now give the patient?

Arrangements were made for complete thyroidectomy and subsequent thyroid tissue ablation with ^{131}I. The patient was then placed on replacement thyroxine. A bone scan and CT scan of the chest were arranged and did not find any evidence of metastatic disease. The patient was followed up periodically and remained disease free.

ANSWERS

A1 There is a smooth, surfaced swelling at the base of the neck on the right side. The swelling is in the anterior triangle and about 4 cm in diameter. The trachea appears to be displaced to the left. The overlying skin is normal. This may well be a swelling arising in the right lobe of the thyroid gland.

A2 You want to know if the patient has:
- any symptoms suggestive of excessive thyroid hormone production (metabolic, cardiovascular, neuropsychiatric or ocular manifestations). This may occur in cases of toxic adenoma. Alternatively, the thyroid mass may be incidental, but the presence of thyrotoxicity may modify treatment plans
- any symptoms suggestive of local pressure effects on adjacent structures in the neck (dysphonia, dysphagia, dyspnoea, stridor)
- a family history of thyroid cancer (i.e., medullary or papillary carcinoma)
- had previous exposure to ionizing radiation
- lived in an area of endemic goitre or has a family history of goitre.

A3 The differential diagnosis of this thyroid mass in order of most to least common is:
- prominent nodule in a multinodular (colloid) goitre
- true solitary nodule:
  - cyst
  - adenoma
  - carcinoma
  - focal area of Hashimoto's thyroiditis.

Even when it is thought that the nodule is a true solitary nodule, further investigation will show that 50% of cases will be multinodular goitres with a prominent nodule, which has been mistaken for a solitary nodule. Most solitary thyroid nodules will be hyperplastic nodules, some will be cysts, and the minority (<5%) will be malignant.

A4 The following investigations are required:
- thyroid function tests (T3, T4 and TSH) and thyroid antibodies
- ultrasound:
  - shape, size and consistency of the swelling
  - definition of the rest of the gland (impalpable lumps)
  - enlarged cervical lymph nodes
  - tracheal displacement or compression
- fine needle aspiration for a cytological diagnosis.

It is unlikely that this patient is grossly hyper- or hypothyroid, but his thyroid status must be checked, because endocrine dysfunction will modify management.

Cytology by fine needle aspiration (FNA) is the most specific, sensitive and cost-effective of all thyroid investigations. If the lump is a simple thyroid cyst, this can be aspirated to dryness, thus eliminating the lump and provide immediate reassurance to the patient. For solid lesions, the cytology result may demonstrate malignant cells (that is, papillary, medullary or anaplastic carcinoma) which will decide on definitive management. In cases of cellular follicular lesions, cytological assessment is less accurate and it may be difficult to distinguish between a well-differentiated tumour and a benign lesion. If a large amount of colloid is present with a small number of bland follicular cells, the diagnosis is more in keeping with a benign colloid cyst or hyperplastic nodule.

ANSWERS – cont'd

A5 The cytological examination shows sheets of follicular cells with very little colloid. There are many clusters of bland epithelial cells which form well defined circular follicular structures in the centre and to the right of the picture. There is no clear evidence of malignancy.

When follicular structures are identified on a fine needle aspirate of a thyroid nodule, the differential diagnosis includes a hyperplastic colloid nodule (dominant nodule in a multinodular goitre), adenoma and follicular carcinoma. Reliable distinction is not possible on cytological appearances from a FNA, and further investigations are required. Follicular carcinomas do not necessarily show nuclear atypia and encapsulated varieties can only be distinguished from adenomas by finding capsular or vascular invasion on a tissue section.

A6 The ultrasound scan reveals a well circumscribed solitary solid lump in the lower pole of the right lobe of the thyroid. The rest of the gland is normal and there is no deviation or compression of the trachea. It is almost certainly a tumour, but probably benign.

A7 You should tell the patient that he has a growth in his thyroid gland. The gland appears to be functioning normally, but the lump is solid and solitary and might be a cancer although you favour a benign or innocent growth. The only way you will be able to tell exactly what the lump is, will be to perform an operation and remove the lump. This will involve removal of the right half of his thyroid gland. Once the pathologist has given you a more definitive diagnosis, you will be able to discuss further treatment with the patient should it be required. At this stage, it is probably unnecessary to have a detailed discussion on thyroid malignancy, since the lump is likely benign.

The main difficulty with cytology is in distinguishing benign from malignant follicular lesions. Under these circumstances, hemithyroidectomy is usually necessary.

A8 The details you provide on the procedure should include:
- Hemithyroidectomy is a safe operation.

- There will a small incision in the lower part of the neck.
- The right half of the thyroid gland will be removed.
- The left half of the gland will not be touched.
- The left side will provide sufficient functioning thyroid tissue such that the patient should not require ongoing thyroid replacement.
- The resultant scar should be neat and inconspicuous.
- There are risks associated with the procedure. Those:
  - associated with anaesthesia
  - related to any operation (infection, bleeding)
  - specific to thyroid surgery.

The specific risks associated with surgery to the thyroid gland include:
- Bleeding into the neck (fewer than 1 in 100 cases).
- Voice changes (fewer than 1 in 10 cases). These may be due to:
  - laryngeal trauma during intubation
  - recurrent laryngeal nerve injury
  - trauma to the external branch of the superior laryngeal nerve.
- Hypocalcaemia (parathyroid gland injury – rare).

Voice changes related to nerve injury are usually the result of neuropraxia and most spontaneously resolve within 3 months.

A9 The right lobe of the thyroid has been opened longitudinally. There is an encapsulated tumour 3 cm in diameter which occupies most of the lobe. The tumour is pinkish-red and vascular with areas of haemorrhage. Gross examination does not show any evidence of capsular invasion. If this is malignant, it is more likely to be a follicular than a papillary tumour.

A10 You will need to explain the following to the patient:
- A cancer has been excised.
- You believe it has been completely removed although further surgery is required.

ANSWERS – cont'd

- These tumours have a good prognosis (85% 10-year survival).
- The risk of a further focus in the remainder of the thyroid is less than 10%.

You would recommend to the patient that:
- Removal of the remainder of the thyroid gland be undertaken (a completion thyroidectomy) to facilitate any further treatment and observation.

- Any further treatment would involve radio-iodine ablation (involves swallowing one tablet).
- He will be on lifelong thyroxine (most differentiated thyroid cancers are TSH-dependent and the thyroxine will suppress the secretion of TSH and so reduce the incidence of recurrence).
- He should have a CT scan of the neck and chest and a bone scan to check for metastatic disease.

REVISION POINTS

Management of a lump in the thyroid

Aims

To establish if the lump is solitary or not
- If solitary, to ascertain if it is a carcinoma.

Process

- Define the anatomy and morphology of the gland (clinical examination and ultrasound).
- Measure thyroid function (T4, T3 and TSH).
- Establish a tissue diagnosis: fine needle aspiration cytology and/or biopsy (FNA has 95% accuracy).
- Exclude certain pathology when indicated (e.g. thyroid antibodies for Hashimoto's thyroiditis).

Follicular carcinoma of the thyroid

Incidence

- <1:100 000 population.
- <10% of all primary thyroid neoplasms (i.e. rare but important).
- Peak age incidence 40–50 years.

Risk factors include

- Endemic goitre.
- Radiation exposure.
- Autoimmune thyroiditis.

Presentation

- Lump in the thyroid.
- Effect of a metastatic deposit, e.g. a pathological fracture.

Diagnosis

- Abundant follicular cells and little colloid on FNA (usually difficult to distinguish between a benign and malignant aspirate).
- Hemithyroidectomy to confirm diagnosis.

Treatment

- Total thyroidectomy.
- Ablation of any remaining thyroid tissue with radioactive iodine (^{131}I) for poor prognosis tumours.
- Thyroxine (replacement and TSH suppression).

ISSUES TO CONSIDER

- How would your management differ if the FNA reported a papillary carcinoma?
- What other thyroid malignancies exist and how are they treated?
- Why is there such a high incidence of thyroid cancer near to the Chernobyl nuclear plant?

FURTHER INFORMATION

www.british-thyroid-association.org Website of the British Thyroid Association, with a number of useful links.

www.aace.com The website of the American Association of Clinical Endocrinologists, with clinical guidelines for the management of thyroid carcinoma.

www.thyroidmanager.org An excellent, extensive site covering all aspects of thyroid disease and designed for medical professionals.

A 26-year-old man with a swelling below the ear

A 26-year-old man comes to see you with a 2-month history of a painless swelling below his left ear. The lump has been getting slowly larger but he has not noticed any other swellings. There is no change in the size of the lump with eating nor does it become painful.

There has been no discharge from the lump and the patient's health is otherwise good. In particular he has no night sweats nor loss of weight. His past medical history is unremarkable. Figure 6.1 shows the swelling.

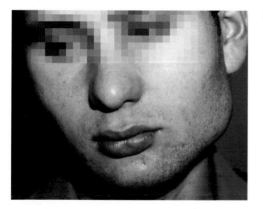

Fig 6.1

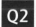 **Q1** Describe the photograph.

You now undertake a more formal examination.

Q2 What are you going to look for on examination?

On examination there is a 3 cm diameter smooth-surfaced swelling situated over the angle of the left jaw. It is not attached to the overlying skin and no punctum is visible. The lump appears to be fixed to the underlying tissue and is firm in consistency. There are no other palpable neck swellings and the left external auditory meatus appears normal. Intra-oral examination shows that the patient has good, well cared-for dentition. The buccal and gingival mucosa appears healthy. The orifices to both parotid ducts are normal.

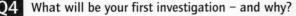

Q3 What is the likely pathological diagnosis and why? What other conditions could produce a similar swelling?

From your examination you are reasonably confident that this is a salivary gland tumour and as such, is likely to be benign.

Q4 What will be your first investigation – and why?

A CT scan is performed. One of the slices is shown in Figure 6.2.

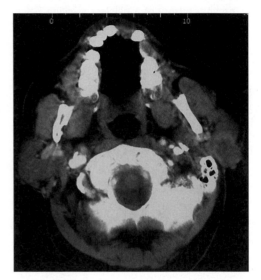

Fig 6.2

Q5 What does the CT scan show?

Cytological examination of a fine needle aspiration confirms that the lump is a pleomorphic adenoma.

Q6 What are you going to advise the patient?

The patient undergoes a superficial parotidectomy at which time all five branches of the facial nerve are clearly identified and preserved. The patient makes an uneventful postoperative recovery and the tumour is confirmed histologically as a pleomorphic adenoma which was completely removed.

ANSWERS

A1 The photograph shows a swelling approximately 3 cm in diameter over the angle of the left jaw. The swelling is smooth-surfaced and the overlying skin appears normal.

A2 You will want to ascertain the following characteristics of the lump:
- site, shape, size, surface and attachments
- relationship to nearby anatomical structures (mandible and pre-auricular groove)
- its anatomical layer (skin, subcutaneous tissue and muscle)
- consistency
- whether it impinges on adjacent structures (facial nerve).

In addition, you should perform a general screening physical including looking inside the mouth, in the left ear and examine for lymphadenopathy.

A3 This is probably a pleomorphic adenoma of the parotid gland. The tumour appears to arise from the region of the superficial lobe of the gland.

Any lump in this region that is not obviously part of the skin (e.g. epidermoid cyst) should be assumed to be arising from the parotid gland until proven otherwise. The pleomorphic adenoma is the most common tumour of the parotid gland and is most often found in the superficial lobe of the gland. Other conditions to consider include:
- Benign lesions of the parotid:
  - cystadenolymphoma (Warthin's tumour)
  - monomorphic adenoma
  - oncocytoma
  - sialadenitis (with or without an associated calculus)
  - lymphoepithelial lesions (associated with Sjögren's syndrome and with some incidence of conversion to mucosa-associated lymphoma).
- Carcinoma of the parotid.
- Non-parotid lesions:
  - lipomas
  - epidermoid cyst
  - lymph nodes (chronic infection, e.g. tuberculosis, lymphoma; secondary malignancy, e.g. from an oropharyngeal primary; or part of

a generalized inflammatory lymphadenopathy, e.g. AIDS-related lymphadenopathy).

The majority of salivary tumours are benign and most are found in the parotid gland. When tumours occur in the submandibular, sublingual or minor salivary glands, they are more likely to be malignant. Benign tumours tend to present as a painless lump, whereas patients with a malignant neoplasm may have a lump that is painful, rapidly growing in size and showing evidence of invading adjacent structures such as the facial nerve.

A4 In lesions in the region of the parotid gland the first investigation is a CT scan. The CT scan will provide a clear definition of the site of the lesion, its vascularity and occasionally, the diagnosis (e.g. a lipoma has a characteristic lack of radiodensity). The scan will provide important anatomical information including any possible extension of a lesion into the deep lobe of the parotid. If the lesion is malignant, the CT scan may provide information on spread into adjacent lymph nodes in the neck. Fine needle aspiration biopsy is performed next, but cytological diagnosis is very difficult in salivary gland tumours and generally the final histological diagnosis is best established by appropriate (superficial or total) parotidectomy.

A5 The CT scan shows both parotid glands. The superficial lobes can be seen clearly. Within the substance of the superficial lobe of the left parotid gland there is a well-circumscribed tumour. There is no extension of tumour into the deep lobe of the gland.

A6 You will explain the diagnosis to the patient. He has a slow-growing tumour in the parotid gland, and while it will not metastasize, it will get larger and may eventually undergo malignant transformation. The tumour has a tendency to infiltrate outside its capsule and local excision of the lump would be associated with a high risk of local recurrence. For that reason you would advocate a superficial parotidectomy and you would discuss the risk of damage to the facial nerve. The branches of the facial nerve run

ANSWERS – cont'd

between the superficial and deep lobes of the gland. Some degree of bruising of the nerve is common during operation, and you would warn the patient that he is likely to get some temporary facial weakness after the operation. You should warn the patient that he may develop gustatory sweating (Frey's syndrome), i.e. the patient may notice that when he eats, that side of his face on which the surgery was performed begins to sweat. This occurs in about 25% of cases but is troublesome in less than 5%. The condition is thought to arise when parasympathetic fibres responsible for innervating the parotid gland are damaged, and subsequently regenerate and take control of local sweat glands.

REVISION POINTS

Pleomorphic adenoma of the parotid gland

Prevalence
- 80% of salivary gland tumours occur in the parotid.
- 80% of the tumours are benign.
- The majority of tumours are pleomorphic adenomas.
- Most are in the superficial lobe of the parotid gland.

Presentation
Slow growing and painless swelling in the parotid region.

Examination
- Ensure the lump arises from the parotid gland.
- Check facial nerve function.
- Examine the mouth and exclude any intra-oral pathology.
- Examine the oropharynx, particularly the region of the tonsil, as deep lobe parotid tumours will displace the superior pole of the tonsil medially.
- Examine the external auditory canal, particularly in the young, for congenital abnormality with fistulous openings in the external ear canal.

Management
- CT imaging will define the tumour.
- FNA for cytology may confirm the diagnosis.
- Usually benign and cured by adequate resection. Enucleation of the tumour is associated with local recurrence. These tumours tend to have a macroscopic bosselated surface and microscopic evidence of finger-like protrusions with a pseudocapsule. Complete excision requires removing a cuff of normal parotid tissue around the tumour.
- Malignant tumours may need adjuvant radiotherapy and although its use for benign tumours is controversial it may well be indicated as adjuvant therapy after surgery for recurrent pleomorphic adenomas.

Complications
- Facial nerve palsy. This nerve runs between superficial and deep lobes of the gland. Any weakness is usually temporary and due to neuropraxia and usually resolves within a few weeks.
- Frey's syndrome.
- Sialocele (subcutaneous accumulation of saliva).

ISSUES TO CONSIDER

- How would you investigate a patient with suspected salivary gland calculi?
- What advice would you give a patient who attends your clinic with a probable dental abscess?

FURTHER INFORMATION

www.baoms.org.uk The website of the British Society of Oral and Maxillofacial Surgeons with information on a wide variety of disorders and links to related sites.

www.parotidtumour.org.uk/salivaryglands/indepth.htm An independent website with lots of information and links for professionals and patients alike.

Swelling in the neck

A 73-year-old woman attends your surgery for the first time in several months. She had noticed a swelling on the left side of her neck about 3 weeks ago but during this period it has enlarged somewhat. The lump has not caused her any pain and she feels that her health has been fairly stable recently. She denies any significant weight loss. She is a long-term smoker of 30 cigarettes a day and drinks about 60 grams of alcohol daily. Her 'smoker's cough' is unchanged and she expec- torates some clear sputum every morning. She experiences 'bronchitis' most winters but this generally settles with a course of antibiotics. In the past she has had a cholecystectomy and hysterectomy and a myocardial infarction 3 years ago. On examination you notice that she is unkempt and her oral hygiene is poor. She has tar-staining of her fingers consistent with her smoking history. You examine her neck and see what is shown in Figure 7.1.

Fig 7.1

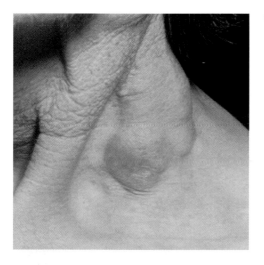

Q1 Describe the photograph.

Palpation reveals a hard, non-tender fixed mass with an irregular surface and a second similar mass without the associated skin changes more posteriorly.

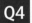**Q2**   What further action is necessary to determine the cause of this swelling?

A detailed history from this woman does not reveal any further symptoms. In particular she has no dyspepsia, loss of appetite, nausea, vomiting or change in bowel habit. She is breathless on moderate exertion but this has been stable for the last 6 months.

A full examination reveals several other enlarged cervical lymph nodes on the left, particularly in the submandibular region. She has a normal cardiovascular system with widespread polyphonic expiratory wheezes bilaterally. Abdominal and breast examination are unremarkable. Inspection of her tongue reveals the following (Figure 7.2):

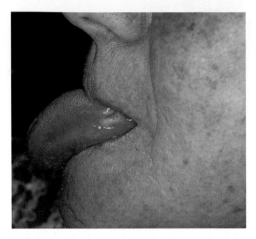

Fig 7.2

Q3   Describe the photograph.

Further inspection of the oral cavity revealed dental caries and an area of leucoplakia.

Q4   What would you like to do now? What will you tell the patient?

ANSWERS

A1 In the left posterior triangle of the neck, at the level of the middle of the sternocleidomastoid muscle there is an irregular mass. There is an area of induration on its lower aspect.

Characterization of neck swellings

- Position: where is it in relation to other structures?
- Size and shape. You should measure it.
- Consistency and character: is it hard or soft, fixed or mobile?
- Colour and temperature: hot or cold, erythematous?
- Is it painful? Ask before touching and be gentle.
- Does it move with swallowing (thyroglossal

cyst) or come and go (pharyngeal pouch)?
- Does it transilluminate?
- Is it pulsatile (e.g. carotid aneurysm)?

A2 Any hard, fixed, irregular cervical mass is likely to be due to malignant infiltration of lymph nodes. You should take a detailed history and a further examination to ascertain the likely origin of any cancer.

- A history of constitutional symptoms such as sweats, fever or pruritus in association with generalized lympadenopathy, particularly in a younger person, would suggest a diagnosis of lymphoma.

ANSWERS – cont'd

- Anyone over the age of 50 is more likely to have a primary carcinoma. Solid tumours metastasizing to cervical lymph nodes may originate anywhere within the head and neck, upper gastrointestinal tract, lung and breasts. You should enquire about weight loss, worsening respiratory symptoms or new gastrointestinal symptoms. Examination of the mouth, nose, oropharynx, thorax, breasts and abdomen are needed.

A3 An area of ulceration is visible on the lateral aspect of the tongue. The edge of the ulcer is thickened and raised.

A4 This woman is likely to have carcinoma of the tongue with metastatic spread to cervical lymph nodes.

Immediate investigations should include a full blood count, routine biochemistry, coagulation screens, chest X-ray and fine needle aspiration of the neck mass or a biopsy of the tongue lesion to confirm the diagnosis histologically.

She should be referred to a specialist team, as this has been shown to give the best results from treatment with respect to function and survival. The stage and grade of the cancer must be ascertained in order that treatment can be planned. The stage refers to the extent of spread of the tumour and detailed imaging of the head and neck may be needed (MRI or CT). The grade of the tumour is determined by detailed histological examination and may help to predict its future behaviour and response to treatment. With this information the team can plan a treatment programme for her. The available treatment modalities include surgery, radiotherapy and chemotherapy. In this case the presence of metastatic disease precludes any chance of cure, so the aims of treatment are to prolong and maintain quality of life.

You should explain this to your patient in simple terms: for example, she has a cancer of her tongue which has spread into the glands in her neck, and that you will be performing a number of tests to be sure your diagnosis is correct. You will then be able to talk further about treatment. You should allow her time to ask questions. Bear in mind that she is unlikely to remember much of what you have said on this occasion. Include family members or friends if possible, as they may be able to go through things with her at a later date. It may be helpful to write down the plans for immediate management so that she can refer to this when she gets home. She will need to return for the results of your investigations and you should emphasize that you will discuss the treatment and answer her questions at this point.

REVISION POINTS

Swellings in the neck

Common:
- thyroid
- lymph nodes
- salivary glands
- skin and subcutaneous lesions (e.g. epidermoid cyst, lipoma, abscess).

Less common:
- thyroglossal cyst
- branchial cyst.

Rare:
- chemodectoma
- aneurysms.

Diagnosis

History:
- duration
- recent change in size
- pain
- discharge
- associated symptoms (e.g. hyperthyroidism)
- a rapidly growing painless swelling in an older person suggests malignancy.

Physical characteristics:
- site, shape, size, surface, consistency and attachments
- anatomical surroundings
- anatomical layer (e.g. skin or subfascial).

continues overleaf

REVISION POINTS – cont'd

Investigations:

- fine needle aspiration (FNA) for cytological examination
- imaging (ultrasound or CT)
- open biopsy (skin lesions)
- swellings in the skin and subcutaneous tissues should not require FNA or imaging to establish a diagnosis
- imaging is reserved for thyroid and salivary swellings (and other rarer causes, e.g. congenital cysts).

Carcinoma of the tongue

Incidence
Head and neck cancers account for 5% of adult malignancies.

Risk factors
- smoking
- alcohol
- poor dental hygiene
- spices
- chewing betel nut or tobacco
- syphilis
- male sex (m:f 2:1)
- age >50
- leucoplakia as malignant lesion.

Histology
The vast majority are squamous carcinoma.

Presentation
- persistent oral ulcer or mass
- symptoms due to primary (pain, dysphagia, dysarthria)
- local spread to cervical nodes
- distant metastases via haematogenous spread rare
- high risk of other tumours of aerodigestive tract.

Prognosis
- dependent on stage and grade at presentation
- small localized tumours are amenable to curative treatment (5-year survival as high as 80%)
- 30% have lymph node metastases at presentation
- further 25% will develop lymph node metastases within 2 years
- death generally due to recurrent local or lymphatic disease.

Treatment
- surgery and/or radiotherapy remain the mainstays of treatment
- adjunctive chemotherapy rarely used
- choice of treatment will depend on stage, patient's age, fitness for anaesthesia and possible disfigurement.

ISSUES TO CONSIDER

- Which other health professionals should be involved in this woman's care?
- In what ways are dentists involved in the recognition of malignant disease? What systemic diseases may be picked up by dentists?

FURTHER INFORMATION

www.emedicine.com/med/topic1132.htm
Information from the emedicine website on the management of head and neck cancer.

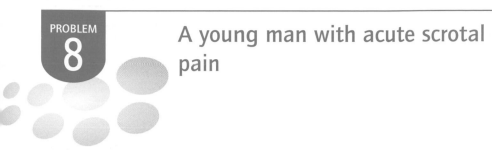

A young man with acute scrotal pain

A 24-year-old man presents to the emergency department with a 2-hour history of pain in the right side of his scrotum. He also has some vague lower abdominal and back pain. The scrotal pain came on rapidly over an hour and is steadily getting worse. He has vomited once. There has been no trauma to the painful area.

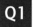

Q1 What other information would you like?

Two years ago he underwent a course of penicillin treatment for what he describes as an 'infection he caught from a girlfriend'. He has had a regular sexual partner for the last 12 months and denies any other sexual contacts. He has no urinary symptoms at present.

On examination he is afebrile. The scrotum looks red and is a little swollen. On the left the testis lies with its long axis in the horizontal plane but feels normal. The right testis is too painful to palpate adequately but a thickened cord can be palpated. There is no associated lymphadenopathy and the rest of the examination is otherwise unremarkable.

Q2 What is the most likely diagnosis? What are the differential diagnoses? What do you do next and why?

An operation is performed. Figure 8.1 shows the operative findings.

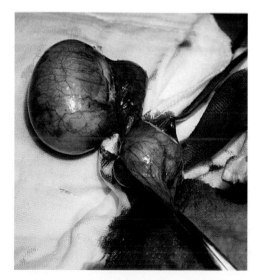

Fig 8.1

Q3 What is the diagnosis and what should be done?

Q4 What are the possible long-term complications of this condition?

ANSWERS

A1 You should obtain details of any urinary or venereal infection. The common mistake is to treat a painful testis as infection without making a definite diagnosis. If the urine has no pus cells or bacteria on Gram staining then a diagnosis of infection should not be sustained. Other important information is a history of any masses associated with the testicle prior to the onset of pain. Inflammatory tumours can also present with acute testicular pain. A history of trauma should be actively sought.

A2 The most likely diagnosis is testicular torsion. Differential diagnoses include infection and the presentation of a testicular tumour, although these are less likely. Your management should be to arrange for immediate surgical exploration of the scrotum as it must be assumed that he has a torsion of the testis until proven otherwise. The abnormal horizontal lie of the left testis strongly supports the diagnosis of torsion. The most expe-

dient, practical and accurate way of proving or disproving the diagnosis is to look at the organ with the naked eye.

A3 The photograph shows a testicle with a twisted spermatic cord. The testicle is dusky but appears viable. The cord should now be untwisted and the testicle observed to ensure that a healthy colour returns. If that is the case, the testicle and its 'normal' partner should both be anchored to the adjacent tunica vaginalis.

A4 The patient was told prior to discharge that both testes were viable and now unlikely to tort, having been sutured to their surrounding tissue. He must seek urgent medical help, should he get a further episode of testicular pain. It is unlikely the patient will suffer any long-term complications related to his torsion. It has been suggested that there is an increased incidence of subfertility in patients who have undergone torsion.

REVISION POINTS

Testicular torsion

- Acute scrotal pain is frequently mismanaged, delaying urgent treatment.
- In adolescents or young adults acute scrotal pain = testicular torsion until proven otherwise.
- Ischaemia >6 hours can result in irreversible damage and loss of the testis.
- Investigation should *never* delay treatment. Testicular torsion is one condition where the surgeon should rely on clinical acumen to make a diagnosis. Ultrasound is almost never helpful in these patients.

- Although the diagnosis is most likely infection in men >40 years, this should never be taken for granted even in this age group.

Differential diagnoses

- Torsion of hydatid of Morgagni or epididymis (esp. <11 years).
- Epididymo-orchitis: usually dysuria, discharge, etc.
- Acute presentation of testicular tumour.
- Trauma.
- Fournier's gangrene: rare life-threatening infection in older men.

continues overleaf

REVISION POINTS — cont'd

Clinical presentation

Acute severe testicular pain often referred to lower abdomen and groin. Vomiting is frequent.

Patient may report previous self-limiting episodes.

Clinical features

- High-lying testicle with thickened cord (early).
- Exquisitely tender with oedematous scrotum (late), may preclude full examination.
- Contralateral testis: look for predisposing anatomical abnormalities, e.g. testicular inversion or partial inversion (testis lies horizontally), prominent mesorchium.

Investigations

Ultrasound of the scrotum and its contents should be undertaken provided they do not delay treatment.

Treatment

Prompt exploration of the scrotum.

Prognosis

Increased incidence of subfertility which may be immune mediated. Most have no long-term effects.

ISSUES TO CONSIDER

- Revise the testicular anatomy.
- How would you start a campaign to publicize testicular cancer in young men and encourage regular self-examination?

FURTHER INFORMATION

Marcozzi D, Soner S. **The non-traumatic acute scrotum**. *Emergency Clinics of North America* 2001;19(3):547–68.

www.emedicine.com/emerg/topic573.htm
Tutorial resource for testicular torsion.

A scrotal swelling in a 19-year-old man

A 19-year-old man presents with a 6-week history of a swelling in the right side of his scrotum. He had noticed a dull ache in the groin and his local doctor had made a diagnosis of epididymo- orchitis and prescribed a course of antibiotics. There has been no change in the discomfort associated with the lump or its size following the course of antibiotics.

 Q1 What further information would you like from the history?

He has no significant past medical history apart from a groin operation at age two. He feels in good health and his review of systems is normal.

Q2 What will you look for on physical examination?

Physical examination is unremarkable apart from the right testis, which is some 3 cm larger than its counterpart. It can be palpated as a distinct entity and is firm and not tender. Both testes are in their normal positions and the right appears to be uniformly enlarged. There is no hydrocele.

Q3 What investigations may be useful at this stage?

The following investigations are made available to you.

Investigation 9.1 Summary of results	
Alpha-fetoprotein	470 KU/l (<11 KU/l)
Beta HCG	91 U/l (not normally detectable)
Chest X-ray	normal
CT chest and abdomen	normal

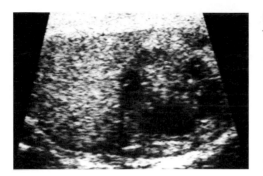

Figure 9.1 shows an ultrasound of the right testis.

Fig 9.1

Q4   What do the above results suggest? What would you like to do now?

The surgeon undertakes an exploration of the right testis through an incision in the groin. On the basis of a frozen section report, a right orchidectomy is performed. Figure 9.2 shows the resected specimen.

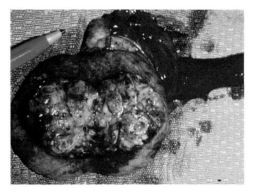

Fig 9.2

Q5   Describe the specimen.

The diagnosis of a malignant testicular tumour was confirmed on frozen section and final histology which showed a teratoma with elements of choriocarcinoma. His tumour markers fall to within normal range.

Q6   How do you plan his subsequent management?

It is decided to follow a plan of close surveillance. The patient is seen regularly and remains well for 12 months with undetectable tumour markers and no disease detected radiologically. Eighteen months after his initial presentation the patient returns to see you with a 2-week history of increasing dyspnoea. He is pale and his haemoglobin is 60 gm/l. His stool tests positive for blood. An endoscopy is performed. A view of the duodenum is shown in Figure 9.3.

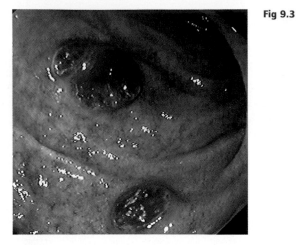

Fig 9.3

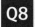 **Q7** Describe the view in the duodenum.

The lesions were biopsied. The diagnosis of metastatic teratoma of the testis is confirmed.

Q8 What do you do next and why?

A CT scan of the abdomen and chest is performed. Two views are shown (Figures 9.4 and 9.5).

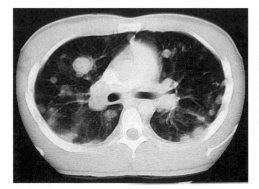

Fig 9.4

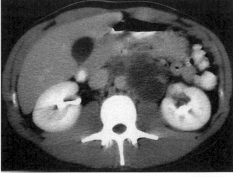

Fig 9.5

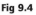 **Q9** What do the scans show?

The patient undergoes a course of cis-platinum-based combination chemotherapy and has a complete remission.

ANSWERS

A1 In any teenager or young man who presents with a swelling in the scrotum it is essential to consider and exclude the diagnosis of testicular cancer. Is there:

- Any pain associated with the swelling?
- Any history of testicular maldescent?
- Any history suggestive of a sexually transmitted disease?
- Any weight loss, sweats or other symptoms suggestive of malignancy?
- Any backache? (enlarged para-aortic lymph nodes).
- Any cough, haemoptysis or dyspnoea? (lung metastases).

A2 The examination will focus on:

- The scrotum and its contents. The three common causes of a swelling in the scrotum are:
  - inguino-scrotal hernia (unable to get above the swelling)
  - epididymal cyst (felt as a distinct entity above the testis)
  - hydrocele (unable to palpate the testis as a distinct entity).
- A general examination to look for evidence of malignancy:
  - weight loss
  - enlarged lymph nodes
  - abdominal masses or hepatomegaly
  - pulmonary signs such as pleural effusions.

A3 Basic investigations should include:

- Full blood count, electrolytes (possible renal impairment due to ureteric obstruction by enlarged para-aortic nodes).
- Liver function tests (liver metastases).
- Blood for tumour markers:
  - alpha-fetoprotein (AFP)
  - human chorionic gonadotrophin (HCG).
- Chest X-ray (pulmonary metastases).
- Ultrasound of the scrotum and contents.

Most germ-cell tumours produce glycopeptides which include alpha-fetoprotein (AFP) and human chorionic gonadotrophin (beta-HCG). Seventy per cent of patients with non-seminomatous germ-cell tumours (NSGCT) will have an elevated

AFP and a similar percentage will produce HCG. A small proportion of patients with pure seminomas will produce HCG. Tumour marker studies must precede any surgical intervention.

Investigations to look for distant spread need to be done:

- CT scan pelvis and abdomen (lymph node or liver involvement).
- CT scan lungs (pulmonary metastases).

A4 The results are virtually diagnostic of a primary testicular neoplasm. The tumour markers are elevated and there is a cystic mass within the right testis. The patient will need a surgical exploration and biopsy. The lesion should not be needled through the scrotum for fear of implantation of tumour into the scrotum and conversion of what could have been a curable orchidectomy into a palliative resection of the scrotum.

A5 There is a 3.5 cm mass in the mid portion of the right testis. The tumour is surrounded by normal seminiferous tissue. There are several cystic areas in an otherwise solid mass. This has the macroscopic appearances of a teratoma.

A6 This patient has stage I disease (confined to the testis), and a management plan of close surveillance is an accepted option. This will involve:

- Monthly measurement of tumour markers. The tumour markers should return to normal if the entire tumour has been removed. This may take several weeks initially as the markers have a long half-life.
- CT scans of chest and abdomen every 3 months for the first 12 months and then at longer intervals for several years.
- If the tumour is likely to recur, the greatest risk is within the first 18 months.

A7 Two raised and ulcerated lesions can be seen. There is blood on the surface of both ulcers.

A8 While he now clearly has stage IV disease, sites of disease need to be fully documented. He

ANSWERS – cont'd

requires a CT scan of his chest and abdomen. His tumour markers need to be repeated. This will be used to help assess his response to further treatment.

A9 The CT scan of the chest shows numerous deposits of tumour through both lung fields. The abdominal view shows enlarged retroperitoneal nodes.

REVISION POINTS

Testicular cancer

Incidence
- 4:100 000 males. Most common cancer in males 18–35.
- More common in whites than blacks.
- Increasing incidence.

Risk factors
Previous maldescent of testes, age 20–40.

Pathology
Seminoma 40%, teratoma 32%, components of both 14%.
- Seminoma: solid, well circumscribed, uniform rounded cells, well differentiated. May contain granulomata.
- Teratoma: haemorrhagic, cystic range of cell types, varying differentiation. May contain yolk sac.

Presentation
- Testicular swelling with discomfort.
- Backache due to enlarged para-aortic nodes.
- Cough, haemoptysis, dyspnoea from lung metastases.

Examination
- Testicular swelling which may have an associated hydrocoele.
- Central abdominal mass due to palpable nodes.
- Pleural effusion.

Royal Marsden staging
I   Limited to testis
II Nodes below diaphragm
III Nodes both sides of diaphragm
IV Distant metastases: L – lungs, H – liver.

Investigations
See above.

Treatment
Stage I tumours
Seminomas respond to a course of radiotherapy to the para-aortic nodes. Teratomas need no further treatment.
Stage II, III or IV tumours
Seminomas will respond to chemotherapy with cisplatin or carboplatin with the possible addition of etoposide. Small volume disease may be treated with radiotherapy alone and radiotherapy will often be given following chemotherapy in other patients.

Teratomas will respond to chemotherapy. Good prognosis tumours will receive 3 x weekly cycles of BEP (bleomycin, etoposide and cisplatin). High-risk patients with extensive disease or very high markers will receive more intensive chemotherapy regimens.

Prognosis
Few patients die from testicular cancer today. Cure is expected in almost all patients with stage I disease and 85% cure for those with more advanced stages.

ISSUES TO CONSIDER

- What long-term risks of chemotherapy do you foresee in patients 'cured' of their testicular cancer?
- This man is keen to have a family. What advice would you give him both before his surgery and before his chemotherapy?
- Why should testicular cancer be more common in patients with maldescent?

FURTHER INFORMATION

www.acor.org/diseases/tc/ An excellent website devoted to testicular cancer. Directed to patients but a good resource for all.

Einhorn L H. **Curing metastatic testicular carcinoma**. *Proceedings of the National Academy of Science USA* 2002;99(7):4592–5.

A 46-year-old woman with a breast lump

A 46-year-old woman presents with a lump in her right breast, which has been there for 2 months. There is no change in the size of the lump during the menstrual cycle, and no discharge from the nipple. She is now mid-cycle. She has had no previous breast problems. Menarche was at the age of 11. There is no family history of breast disease. She is married with two children and has had a tubal ligation.

Q1 What features should you be looking for on examination?

On examination she has an ill-defined 1.5 cm lump in the upper outer quadrant of her right breast. There is no lymph node enlargement or any other abnormal findings on general examination. Her GP has arranged an investigation that is shown in Figure 10.1.

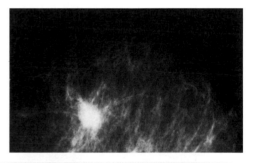

Fig 10.1

Q2 What is this investigation? What abnormal features would you look for? What are the abnormal features in the image?

Her left breast is normal on both clinical examination and mammography.

Q3 What should be done next?

An ultrasound examination confirms that the lump is solid. A fine needle aspiration (FNA) of the lesion is performed.

Q4 What will you do if the FNA shows no malignant cells?

The cytological examination does show malignant cells.

Q5 What will you tell the patient at this stage?

Staging investigations (liver function tests, CT scans, bone scan) do not reveal any evidence of metastatic disease.

Q6 What treatment options are available? What factors influence which are preferred?

This patient undergoes wide local excision and axillary clearance with radiotherapy to the residual right breast for local control. Her tumour is 20 mm in size, grade II on histological assessment and 6 of the 15 axillary nodes identified contain tumour. The tumour is oestrogen and progesterone receptor negative. Consequently she receives adjuvant chemotherapy but no hormonal therapy for systemic control of the disease. The patient is reviewed regularly in the outpatient clinic.

The patient reports no problems until 18 months later when she complains of lower back pain. This has been troubling her for about 4 weeks. The pain is constant and can keep her awake at night. It is exacerbated by movement and can radiate down the back of her left leg. She has lost 4 kg because the pain 'got rid of my appetite'. You perform a plain radiograph of the lumbar spine and then go on to perform the following investigation (Figure 10.2).

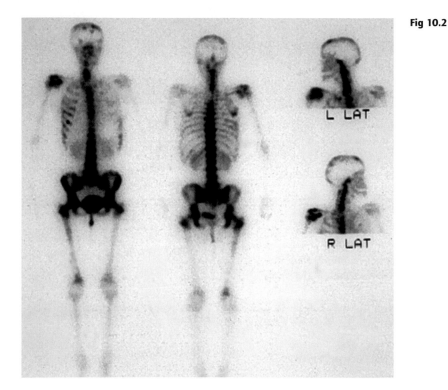

Fig 10.2

Q7 What is this investigation and what does it show? What treatment options are now available?

The plain radiograph of the lumbar showed lytic lesions of L2, L3 and L4 with collapse of the vertebral bodies. With the confirmation of widespread bony metastatic disease on the isotope scan, the patient elected to have a course of radiotherapy to the deposits in her lumbar spine and a course of palliative chemotherapy.

ANSWERS

A1 The discovery of a breast lump will cause much anxiety so breast examination must be undertaken with sensitivity. Explain exactly what you intend to do and the reasons for doing it. Male clinicians need a female chaperone.

Ask the woman to locate the abnormality for you. Start your examination with the normal breast in order to judge 'normality' for this patient. Then assess the lump for size, character, tenderness, mobility and whether or not it is tethered, either to the overlying skin or to the chest wall beneath.

You should examine all areas of both breasts systematically, quadrant by quadrant, noting the character of the underlying breast tissue, looking for further lesions. Finally examine the nipple for discharge, discoloration or inversion.

Examine both axillae and supraclavicular fossae thoroughly for nodal disease. Examine the abdomen and chest looking for evidence of metastatic spread.

Remember the age of the patient only gives a guide as to the likely nature of a breast lump. Fibroadenomas are most common in young women, cysts in women in their 30s and 40s and carcinoma in older patients. You must go on to investigate the lump to rule out a malignancy.

The differential diagnosis of a breast lump includes:
- carcinoma
- fibroadenoma (mobile, 'breast mouse')
- cyst (discrete, smooth outline)
- localized area of thickened benign breast tissue
- abscess (tender, warm, cystic)
- fat necrosis (usually following previous trauma or surgery).

95% of all breast lumps will be one of the first four listed above.

Carcinomas of the breast exhibit a variety of physical signs, depending on the size of the tumour, its site and degree of local infiltration. Look for evidence of attachment to surrounding structures, including the overlying skin, although this is only present in advanced disease.

A2 This is a mammogram. The following features would suggest malignancy:
- a mass of increased density
- an ill-defined mass
- areas of spiculated microcalcification.
- distortion of breast architecture, e.g. thickening of skin over the mass.

The following features are more suggestive of a lesion being benign:
- well-defined lesion
- smooth border.

This woman's mammogram shows:
- fatty involution of breast, consistent with the patient's age
- a 2 cm dense, ill-defined solitary lump with spicules extending into the surrounding tissue in the upper outer quadrant
- no areas of calcification
- no other abnormal tissue.

These features are suggestive of a malignant lesion.

Note: mammography is not likely to be useful in women younger than 35 years of age due to the increased density of the breast tissue compared to older patients.

A3 All patients with a palpable lump require 'triple assessment'. This consists of:
- clinical examination
- radiological assessment (ultrasound or mammography or both)
- pathological assessment.

An ultrasound of the area may be helpful and add further information. Ultrasound is particularly

ANSWERS – cont'd

useful to ascertain whether a lump is cystic or solid. Ultrasonically a carcinoma is likely to distort the normal architecture of the breast, benign lesions will not. Ultrasound can be performed at the same time as mammography in specialist women's health clinics, which have an on-site radiologist to interpret the results immediately.

The patient needs to be kept informed at all times. Remember how anxiety-provoking this process can be.

A fine needle aspiration (FNA) would be the next step. This simple procedure, in which a 23 gauge needle is passed several times through the lump, can be performed in the outpatient clinic. The aspirate is then spread on a microscope slide and examined by an experienced cytopathologist.

A4 A negative FNA does *not* rule out malignancy.

The patient is 46 years old and the mammogram is suggestive of malignancy: in this case a benign FNA is not adequate. The FNA can be repeated, or a core biopsy may be performed (if necessary these can both be performed under radiological guidance). A core biopsy can be performed at the clinic under local anaesthetic. A core of architecturally intact tissue is removed rather than the few loose cells that are retrieved by FNA. If, in cases such as this one, carcinoma cannot be proven by FNA or core biopsy the lump should be removed at open surgical biopsy to exclude malignancy. The sensitivity of FNA and core biopsy is such that only a very few patients should require open surgical biopsy to establish the diagnosis of malignancy.

A5 The diagnosis needs to be given clearly and sympathetically. As with breaking any bad news, the following principles should be observed:
- Break the news in a place that will be free from interruptions.
- It may be helpful to have a close relative or friend present.
- Establish the patient's understanding of their condition so far.
- Give a gentle indication that the news may be bad.
- Use words the patient understands, and avoid ambiguous terms and euphemisms.

- Explain what further tests will be done: for instance, bloods, bone scan, CT scans.
- Outline in broad terms the different treatment options available such as surgery, radiotherapy, hormonal therapy and chemotherapy.
- Remember the two issues that the patient will most likely be concerned about are: 1) will she have to have her breast removed? and 2) is she going to die?
- Try and provide a positive tone to the conversation as much as possible. Reassure her that there are breast-conserving surgical techniques and that it is likely that she can be treated with adjuvant therapy, which can help reduce her risk of metastatic disease. Explain that you will counsel her further once you have the results of the additional studies that will help determine if the cancer has spread. Explain that further decisions can be made once the lump has been removed and you know how many lymph nodes are involved with the cancer.
- Allow for silence and give opportunities to ask questions.
- The patient should be given the opportunity to speak with a trained breast-care nurse following this initial conversation.
- Make arrangements for a prompt follow-up appointment.

A6 Unless the tumour is extensive, surgery will be performed first. Each patient should have either a mastectomy or a wide local excision with an axillary node dissection.

Relative indications for mastectomy are:
- Central tumour behind the nipple.
- Large tumours (>4 cm in diameter – although depends on breast size).
- Patient choice.
- Multifocal tumours.
- Widespread ductal carcinoma in situ.

For smaller, peripheral lesions such as in this case, a wide local excision (breast-conserving surgery) may be performed to remove the tumour with a surrounding core of normal breast tissue.

Even after a wide local excision, a mastectomy may still be required if the margins of resection are not clear on histology.

ANSWERS – cont'd

All patients should have their ipsilateral axillary lymph nodes removed. The reasons for this are first to reduce the chance of recurrence in the axilla and second to help to plan what further (adjuvant) treatment is required for each patient. Currently this is the standard of care. Trials are, however, ongoing to determine the safety of removing only the 'sentinel' lymph node. The procedure involves the injection of a radioactive tracer and blue dye around the tumour. The node to which the lymph from the area of the tumour first drains (sentinel node) is then identified and removed. Theoretically, if this node is negative then no further nodes need be removed, thus sparing the patient the sometimes considerable morbidity associated with a full axillary lymph node clearance. This procedure has not yet been proven to be as safe as an axillary node clearance and so (currently) is only being performed as part of randomized trials.

Further treatment (radiotherapy, chemotherapy and hormonal therapy) should be planned after the results of the surgery are available. All treatment plans should be formulated at a multidisciplinary meeting attended by surgeons, medical oncologists, radiation oncologists, breast-care nurses and geneticists.

Radiotherapy to the residual breast should be considered after all wide local excisions to minimize local recurrence. Radiotherapy to the chest wall and supraclavicular fossa may be necessary for tumours with poor prognostic features on pathology even after mastectomy.

The use of adjuvant chemotherapy is usually reserved for those patients with poor prognostic indicators such as:

- large tumour size
- node positivity
- grade 3 tumours
- extensive lymphovascular invasion.

The decision whether to offer women adjuvant hormonal manipulation depends on the oestrogen receptor status (and to a lesser extent progesterone receptor status) of the tumour. Both overall and disease-free survival is improved in patients with oestrogen receptor positive tumours by reducing oestrogen levels. This can be achieved by:

- blocking oestrogen receptors (tamoxifen)
- reducing oestrogen synthesis (aromatase inhibitors)
- LHRH agonists (goserelin)
- oophorectomy.

A7 This is a bone scan showing multiple areas of increased bone activity in keeping with multiple tumour deposits. The appearances are consistent with bony metastatic disease and with the history of breast carcinoma, this is by far the most likely primary tumour.

A CT scan of the chest and abdomen will establish the presence or absence of further visceral metastatic disease. This will affect treatment recommendations

In the first instance, ensure there are no neurological symptoms and signs to suggest cord compression. Radiotherapy to the lumbar spine is indicated for pain control. While waiting for a response to the radiotherapy, adequate narcotic analgesia and management of narcotic side-effects such as constipation are mandatory. Treatment for her disease is now palliative in intent and the patient must be fully involved in any decisions regarding therapy.

Treatment options include hormonal manipulations versus chemotherapy (particularly for visceral disease) using one of the new agents such as the taxanes. The potential risks and benefits of any such treatment must be weighed with the choice of therapy, and may depend on patient preference.

REVISION POINTS

Breast cancer

Epidemiology
- lifetime risk of approximately 1 in 12
- most common malignancy in females
- 1% of breast cancers occur in males
- peak incidence at 50–70 years
- more common in Western world and in higher socioeconomic groups.

continues overleaf

REVISION POINTS – cont'd

Aetiology
- increased risk if first-degree relative affected
- genetic component, e.g. BRAC-1, BRCA-2
- more common in women with early menarche or late menopause
- artificial menopause before 35, increasing parity, young age at first pregnancy and breast-feeding are all protective.

Pathology
Breast cancers are usually either infiltrating ductal or infiltrating lobular adenocarcinomas. Sometimes the more common, ductal carcinomas have a particular pattern on pathology (e.g. tubular, papillary, mucinous, inflammatory). If malignant cells are present in the ducts or lobules, but have not invaded the basement membrane to become a carcinoma, then this is termed ductal carcinoma in situ (DCIS) or lobular carcinoma in situ (LCIS) respectively. These conditions are a significant risk factor for the development of invasive breast cancer.

Natural history
- primary tumour enlarges and invades local tissue
- dermal lymphatics may become involved leading to 'peau d'orange' appearances
- spread to lymphatics
- distant spread to bone, liver, lung, brain and skin.

Symptoms and signs
- painless breast lump (may be irregular, fixed to skin or muscle)
- discharge from nipple (perhaps bloody)
- nipple retraction
- skin changes (puckering, *peau d'orange*, inflammatory breast can present like an abscess or cellulitis)
- less frequently may present with lymphadenopathy or distant metastases.

Investigations
'Triple assessment' of the lump as discussed in Answers section.

Treatment aims
- immediate local control with optimal cosmetic effect
- limit risk of chest wall recurrence and distant spread
- minimize short- or long-term treatment-related morbidity.

Treatment
Local (surgery/radiotherapy) and systemic (hormonal/chemotherapy). See Answers section.

ISSUES TO CONSIDER

- What impact has breast screening had on the mortality rates for breast cancer? Who should be screened? Who is screened in your system?

- What other public health measures can be taken to reduce the mortality from this disease?

- Do men get breast cancer?

FURTHER INFORMATION

www.cancer.gov An excellent website from the US National Cancer Institute covering many aspects of cancer including consensus statements on the management of breast cancer.

www.cancerscreening.nhs.uk An interesting website covering various aspects of cancer screening including for breast cancer in the UK.

Farndon J R (ed.). **Breast surgery**, 2nd edn. London: Saunders, 2001.

A skin lesion in a 73-year-old man

A 73-year-old retired farmer attends your clinic in the Australian outback complaining of a lump on the back of his hand. He has noticed the lump for about 3 months and it is slowly getting larger. It is not painful and there has been no discharge. Figure 11.1 shows the lesion.

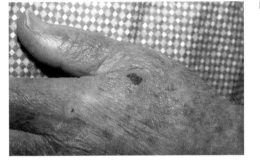

Fig 11.1

 Q1 What are the abnormalities shown in the photograph?

The changes in the skin reflect damage from long-term exposure to sun.

Q2 What should you do next?

The patient says he has several 'sun spots' on his back and arms. They do not bother him. On examination he has many small (less than 2 cm) well-demarcated, brown, scaly lesions on his arms, back and face. Over his left temple there is another lesion. He says this has been present for several years and has not changed at all (Figure 11.2).

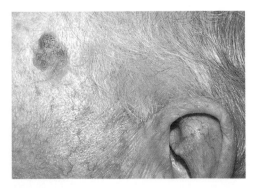

Fig 11.2

Q3 What is this lesion most likely to be? Provide a differential diagnosis.

Your physical examination does not reveal any other significant abnormalities. In particular he has no enlarged nodes in the region draining the left hand.

Q4 How will you manage this patient? What steps can he take to minimize further skin damage in the future?

You arrange to remove the two skin lesions on his hand under local anaesthetic in your clinic.

Q5 What structures might be injured during excision?

The two lesions on the back of the patient's left hand lesion were removed with a 1 cm margin and found to be squamous cell carcinomas. Histologically the tumours were limited to the dermal layers and had not invaded the subcutaneous tissues. They were both completely excised.

ANSWERS

A1 There is a 1 cm raised 'scab' between the thumb and forefinger. The skin is thickened and reddened in the immediate vicinity. This has the characteristics of a squamous cell carcinoma. There is a similar but smaller lesion over the first metacarpo-phalangeal joint. There are a number of other smaller, flatter lesions, which are consistent with solar keratoses. These are the results of chronic sun damage.

A2 Ask the patient if he has any similar lesions elsewhere on his body, or has had other skin lesions removed in the past. Examine him for similar lesions and examine carefully for lymph node enlargement in the axillary and cervical regions on the ipsilateral side.

A3 There is a 2 cm raised, well-circumscribed lesion with a waxy and 'stuck-on' appearance. It has a greasy craggy surface and has the characteristic appearances of a seborrhoeic keratosis (seborrhoeic wart). A differential of this man's skin lesion would include:
- Benign: solar keratosis, keratoacanthoma, seborrhoeic keratosis.
- Malignant: basal cell carcinoma, squamous cell carcinoma, malignant melanoma, Merkel cell tumour.

A4 You should explain to the patient that the lesion on the back of his hand is probably malignant and that you will need to excise it to confirm your diagnosis. You will also want to remove the second, smaller lesion on his hand at the same time. You tell him that these two tumours can almost certainly be treated by local removal and that most such lesions are cured by this method. Since the lesion on his temple has been present unchanged for several years and does not bother him, it can be left alone.

You must counsel him on skin protection, these tumours being most common in fair-skinned people

A N S W E R S – cont'd

who spend time outdoors, particularly in tropical and sub-tropical regions. He should be encouraged to wear a hat, to avoid direct sun exposure particularly between 10 a.m. and 3 p.m. and wear long-sleeved protective clothing. A sunscreen cream with a high block-out for ultraviolet light (sun protection factor SPF 30+, blocking UV-A and UV-B light) should be recommended and used correctly with regular application.

Once you have treated the lesions, you should review him on a regular 3–6-monthly basis indefinitely and encourage him to report the development of any similar lesions.

A5 The specific structures that may be damaged include:

- Nerves: local subcutaneous branches of the radial nerve supplying the back of the hand may be damaged, resulting in minor paraesthesia distal to the site.
- Blood vessels: causing bleeding and bruising.
- Tendons: deep penetration of the lesion or over-zealous excision may expose the underlying extensor tendons or cause tendon injury. Preservation of the fine connective tissue layer covering the tendon is usually possible and preferable.

R E V I S I O N   P O I N T S

Skin cancer and sun-associated skin lesions

Epidemiology

- Skin cancer is the commonest malignancy in white races.
- High incidence in Australia and the southern United States (high population of fair-skinned people particularly of Celtic origin, sunny climate and outdoor lifestyle).

Causes

Long-term exposure to ultraviolet radiation is the single most important factor in the aetiology of these cancers in fair-skinned peoples.

Types of sun damage

Solar (senile) keratosis

- Hyperkeratotic area of skin.
- Usually found on hands, arms, face and neck.
- Lesions are flat, brown and localized. They may crust and have an erythematous base. May have areas of dysplastic change in the deep epidermis and can develop into squamous cell carcinoma.
- Small keratoses should be excised or treated with freeze therapy (CO_2 or liquid nitrogen), while larger, recurrent or multiple ones should be excision biopsied. Other treatments such as topical 5-FU can be used in certain situations.

Seborrhoeic keratosis

- Common benign skin lesions in older people.
- Slightly raised, irregular and can be deeply pigmented with a waxy surface.

- May bleed from repetitive trauma, can be painful, may mimic malignant lesions (e.g. melanoma) or may be unsightly. These are common reasons for excision.

Keratoacanthomas

Can grow rapidly and resemble, both clinically and histologically, a squamous cell carcinoma. The distinguishing feature is that they usually regress as rapidly as they appeared (<6–8 weeks).

Basal cell carcinomas

- The most common skin cancer.
- They may be nodular and raised (most), ulcerated, flat or multifocal in appearance. Classically these have a pearly appearance with fine surface blood vessels.
- They occur most commonly over the face, neck, back and limbs in sun exposed areas.
- Can spread locally and destructively but do not metastasize.

Squamous cell carcinoma

- The second most common skin cancer.
- Found anywhere on the body, but most often in areas with chronic sun exposure often from solar keratoses (although few keratoses progress to malignancy).
- Usually seen in people over 60 years old.
- May occur in areas affected by chronic ulceration (Marjolin's ulcer), following irradiation, burns, chronic venous ulcers or sinuses.

continues overleaf

REVISION POINTS – cont'd

- Presents as a steadily growing painless ulcer with a raised, rolled edge or as a scaly plaque.
- Can be difficult to distinguish from a basal cell carcinoma, and both have similar local behaviour.
- May spread to regional lymph nodes.
- Less than 2% develop metastases. On the other hand, the squamous cell cancers that develop from burns, ulcers or apparently normal skin have a greater propensity to metastasize.

Treatment by local excision with a 1 cm margin of clearance is usually suitable for small basal or squamous cell lesions, with a cure rate of over 95%. Once lymph nodes are involved, these can be treated either by lymph node dissection and/ or radiotherapy, but the prognosis worsens with the presence of metastatic disease.

Melanoma

- Malignancy of pigment cells in the skin and arises from pre-existing naevi in about 60% of cases.
- Can occur anywhere on the skin, including (rarely) the soles of the feet, nailbeds, oral cavity or anal canal.

- Lesions may be superficial spreading (flat), nodular (raised), lentigo maligna (Hutchinson's freckle) or acral lentiginous (nailbeds or soles).
- A change in size, shape or colour usually occurs with malignant change.
- Melanomas are not always pigmented and may be confused with BCC, SCC, Merkel cell tumours, atypical naevi, seborrhoeic keratoses and freckles – all of which may also be pigmented or non-pigmented.

Management

Metastatic disease is lethal. Therefore, early detection is key. Skin lesions suspicious of malignancy should be biopsied – especially if the person is fair-skinned and lives in an area of high ultra-violet radiation intensity. Most individuals will have some moles, freckles or similar skin lesions. If attention is drawn to one of these because of a change in size or pigmentation, or there is bleeding, crusting or itching, it should undergo excision biopsy.

ISSUES TO CONSIDER

- What steps have been taken to heighten public awareness of skin cancer?
- What novel treatments are available for metastatic melanoma?
- What other health risks exist from over-exposure to sunlight?

FURTHER INFORMATION

www.emedicine.com/DERM/topic257.htm A comprehensive electronic tutorial on melanoma. Well referenced with images.

A 27-year-old man with burns

A 27-year-old building worker with burns is brought into the emergency department by ambulance after he and four of his workmates were overcome by superheated steam issuing from a coke furnace close to where they were working.

Q1 While the initial assessment is being made, what key information should be sought?

The patient states he was standing on some scaffolding and was hit by a jet of steam from behind. The steam escaped from a nearby furnace and enveloped him. The steam felt agonizingly hot and was so thick he could not see his workmates for about 15 seconds. He thinks he then passed out, but he knows where he is now.

The ambulance personnel state the accident occurred about 40 minutes earlier.

Q2 Describe the important points of your initial assessment.

There is no evidence of respiratory distress and his blood pressure is 130/75 mm Hg with a pulse rate of 110 bpm. His clothes are removed to allow an accurate assessment to be made of the extent and severity of his injuries. Figures 12.1–12.3 show the injuries sustained.

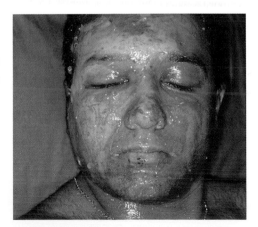

Fig 12.1

Fig 12.2

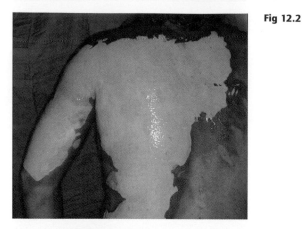

Fig 12.3

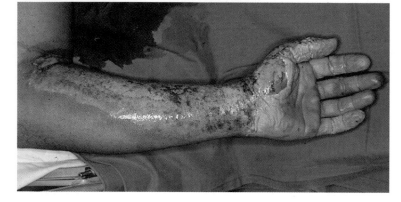

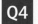 **Q3** Describe the burns and estimate what area of the total body surface they occupy.

He also has internal erythema and swelling of the faucial pillars and the posterior pharyngeal wall. The burns, except those on his arms and back, are painful and tender to touch.

Q4 Describe his management.

The severity of the inhalation or airway injury is uncertain and a careful watch must be kept for the signs of developing respiratory failure. With the inhalation of steam, there is likely to be damage to the upper airway, where increasing oedema of the pharynx and larynx may produce rapid obstruction of the airway.

High-flow oxygen (6 l/min) is being applied by face mask and venous access has been established. One litre isotonic saline is run in rapidly while the initial assessment is under way. A pulse oximeter is attached. The patient is immediately given 2 mg increments of morphine intravenously at 3–5 minute intervals, titrated to control his pain.

A urinary catheter is inserted. Blood is sent off for a complete blood count and electrolytes. He is accurately weighed so that his fluid requirements can be calculated. His arterial blood gases on air are shown below.

Investigation 12.1 Arterial blood gas analysis			
pO_2	75 mm Hg	pH	7.38
pCO_2	39 mm Hg	Calculated bicarbonate	25 mmol/l

Q5 What is your interpretation of these results, and what action do you take?

The inspired oxygen concentration is increased, and the patient is admitted to an intensive care unit for observation. While waiting for transfer you calculate and prescribe fluids for the first 8 hours post burn. The patient weighs 90 kg.

Q6 State what fluids you going to give and describe how you calculate the volume of fluid required by the patient.

In the first 8 hours after admission the patient is given 3 l Hartmann's solution as replacement fluid and 1 l isotonic saline as maintenance fluid. His vital signs remain stable and his respiratory function is not compromised. Four hours after admission his arterial blood gases are repeated and show no deterioration. He is maintained on 6 l/min oxygen. He is prescribed intravenous omeprazole to reduce the risk of gastric stress ulceration.

It is thought that the burns on his face are partial thickness and there are areas of full thick- ness burn on his arms. The burns on the back are also full thickness and appear deeper than those of the arms. The partial thickness burns of the face are treated by saline cleaning, debridement of loose blister skin and application of sterile soft paraffin. The sterile soft paraffin will need repeated application. After assessment as to their depth the remainder of the burns, some super- ficial, some deep dermal and some full thickness, are dressed with silver sulfadiazine.

Q7 Describe the differences between superficial, dermal and full thickness burns. How do these differences affect management?

Five days after his accident, the patient under- went excision of the full thickness burns on his arms and back, which were then covered with split thickness skin grafts. He was discharged from the burns unit 3 weeks after the accident.

ANSWERS

A1 Depending on the severity of the injury, the patient may not be able to provide much information. In any trauma case it is important to interview witnesses and members of the retrieval team to obtain as much information as possible about the nature of events leading up to the injury and what has happened in the time between the injury and arrival in hospital. The following information should be sought:

- the circumstances of the injury, how it occurred, and the likelihood of other associated injuries
- the time that the accident occurred, and hence the time elapsed since injury
- the nature of the burn – chemical, electrical or thermal (fire, steam, gas, etc.)
- nature of the burning agent involved (furniture, steam, petrol, gas, etc.). Some burning substances, such as polyvinyl chloride, can give off toxic fumes (cyanides and hydrogen chlorides), which can cause alveolar and bronchiolar damage
- whether or not the accident occurred in a closed space (more likely to be associated with respiratory problems)
- what clothing the patient was wearing
- pre-existing medical conditions and medications.

A2 The initial assessment (primary survey) will check:

1 Airway. He is able to talk without difficulty, so the airway must be clear.

2 Breathing. There is no immediate evidence of respiratory disease. By the nature of the accident this man is highly likely to have sustained an inhalation injury. You must examine his upper airway carefully. Before doing so, you will want to apply a face mask, give high-flow oxygen (6 l/min) and check his oxygen saturation with a pulse oximeter, and give him pain relief. The following may make you suspect a compromised airway and smoke or thermal injury:

- alteration in the conscious state (hypoxia)
- burns on the face or around the mouth
- singed nasal hair
- sooty sputum

- stridor or hoarseness
- mucosal oedema, haemorrhage or ulceration
- expiratory rhonchi.

3 Circulation. It is highly likely that this patient will have changes to his circulating volume, although these may not be immediately evident. Large burns produce progressive hypovolaemia and hypotension. A burn in an adult of 15% of the total skin area will cause sufficient fluid to be lost to produce hypovolaemic shock. These changes develop secondary to the massive fluid shifts (permeability oedema) that occur. In large burns (>25% of total body area) these changes become widespread and cease to be limited to the burnt area. It is mandatory to establish prompt venous access and commence intravenous fluids.

A secondary survey can now be performed. Particular attention will be paid to the burnt areas:

- estimation of the area of the skin surface burnt
- site of the burns
- depth of the burns.

The area of the body surface burnt will need to be calculated in order to estimate the amount of fluid required in resuscitation. One simple method is to apply the 'rule of nines', in which the head and neck and the two upper limbs each account for 9% of the total body surface area; the front and back of the trunk and the two lower limbs each account for 18% and the genitalia the remaining 1%. Alternatively the area of the patient's hand is equivalent to about 1% of the adult body surface area.

Superheated steam has sufficient specific heat to overwhelm the ability of the respiratory mucosa to remove ingested heat. A burn to the respiratory tract below the larynx may occur in these circumstances. In addition 45% of patients with a facial burn will have inhalation injury.

Other injuries, such as bony trauma sustained when fainting, must be sought.

A3 The patient has burns on his face, involving his cheeks, lips, nose and forehead. The burnt skin on the face has become oedematous and is

ANSWERS – cont'd

weeping. He has a burn extending over the outer aspect of his left arm, arm and shoulder, which is in continuity with a burn on his back. The burn over the back of the left shoulder is a deep scald. The area is white and there is no blistering or surrounding erythema. These are either deep dermal or full thickness burns. There is a separate burn involving his left forearm, thenar eminence and thumb. On the forearm and hand the burns are red and mottled with central areas of white exposed dermis.

The burns on the back occupy about 9% of the total surface skin area. None of the limb burns are circumferential and about 20% of the total body skin area has been burnt.

A4   In addition to the initial measures described in Answer 1, management will include the following:

- Laboratory investigations, including complete blood picture, serum biochemistry and arterial blood gas analysis (including carboxyhaemoglobin concentration). With the severity of his injuries, these will need to be done at least twice daily. Blood should be cross-matched for possible transfusion.
- Initiation of a fluid replacement regimen. The volume of fluid given will be proportional to the area of skin burnt and the weight of the patient.
- Relief of pain. Burns are very painful and narcotics will be required to alleviate this patient's symptoms. This is best provided by an automatic patient-controlled infusion system giving small incremental intravenous doses.
- First aid to the burnt areas. In the emergency department these areas should be covered with a sterile, non-adherent dressing for transfer to a specialist burns unit. Elaborate dressings are not required at this stage.

A5   The patient has suffered a steam injury with facial burns and the hypoxia seen on blood gas analysis suggests that he has a significant inhalation injury. If he deteriorates he may require prompt endotracheal intubation and assisted ventilation. You should increase the concentration of inspired oxygen and arrange his transfer to an intensive care unit. The increasing oedema

associated with a burn injury to the upper airways can lead to rapid respiratory failure.

Intubation in such circumstances can be extremely hazardous and, if necessary, should be performed early before any respiratory obstruction or failure develops. Indications for intubation include:

- hoarseness of voice
- stridor
- laboured breathing.

Swelling of facial and neck tissues and splinting of chest wall movements by thick unyielding burn eschar can exacerbate airway or breathing problems. Escharotomy of chest burns may be required.

In those patients who have inhaled noxious substances, lower airways inflammation, obstruction and oedema which cause respiratory failure may occur after 24 to 48 hours. Estimation of the carboxyhaemoglobin concentration will be a guide to the amount of smoke inhaled. This, and serial blood gas analysis, will give some indication of whether or not ventilation is likely to be required.

Adult respiratory distress syndrome (ARDS) may develop and patients with inhalation injuries are prone to bronchopneumonia. In a seriously burnt patient, the presence of an inhalation injury adds 40% to the mortality. Bronchopneumonia increases this mortality a further 30%. Respiratory complications are now the most common cause of death in fatal burns, and half the deaths are due to pneumonia.

A6   This patient has a major burn and fluid replacement needs in the first 48 hours are likely to be considerable because of:

- widespread 'permeability oedema'
- exudation through the damaged stratum corneum
- increased evaporation of fluids.

Increased capillary permeability (secondary to the release of vasoactive permeability factors as part of the widespread inflammatory response) will lead to considerable fluid shifts out of the intravascular compartment which must be replaced with crystalloid. The losses associated with exudation are protein-rich and may need replacement in the second 24 hours after burning. In the first

ANSWERS – cont'd

24 hours fluid replacement should be Ringer's lactate (Hartmann's solution). The patient will require fluid in volumes proportional to the area of burn (20%) and his body weight (90 kg). There are a number of formulae available to help calculate replacement needs and one suggests the following 24-hour replacement:

- uncomplicated burn: 3 ml Ringer's x kg x % surface area burnt
- complicated burn: 4 ml x kg x % surface area burnt.

This patient might require: 3 x 90 x 20 = 5400 ml/24 hrs. However, as he probably has a pulmonary component to his injuries the effective surface area of burn is larger. This should be treated as a complicated burn and the volume of fluid replacement increased to: 4 x 90 x 20 = 7200 ml/24 hr.

Half of this volume is given over the first 8 hours after the burn injury, and the other half is given over the next 16 hours. These formulae serve only as rough guides to fluid replacement. It is imperative to minimize the risk of hypovolaemia and (pre) renal failure through close monitoring of urine output. This man is likely to require hourly adjustments of his intravenous fluid administration and these should be based on a targeted urine output of 1 ml/kg/hr. Provided a satisfactory urine output is maintained this patient is unlikely to run into electrolyte problems (e.g. hyperkalaemia resulting from burn-related red cell destruction).

A7 Assessment of the depth of the burn is made partially on the nature of the burn and partially on the clinical findings. Burns are more likely to be full thickness if there has been:

- prolonged contact with the injuring agent (e.g. clothing soaked in hot fluid)
- a flammable process
- high intensity of the injurious process (e.g. nuclear radiation).

Partial thickness burns are more likely to be those where a flash or scald is involved.

The injurious agent may produce damage in addition to the burn. Electrical injury is likely to damage not only the skin, but underlying tissues. Clinically, it can be difficult to distinguish full from partial thickness injury. The features outlined in Table 12.1 can provide a guide.

Diagnosis of the depth of the burn will allow a determination of which structures in the skin are damaged and how likely spontaneous healing is to occur (Table 12.2).

Deep (but still partial thickness) burns can heal of their own accord if the epidermal elements present in the hair follicles, sebaceous glands and sweat gland ducts are protected and do not die. These will eventually coalesce and produce an epithelial covering. If the area becomes infected, or dries out, the burn will become deeper and healing will be prolonged. Burns must be covered otherwise infection can supervene. Adherent plastic membrane, hydrocolloid dressings, reconstituted pig skin and similar dressings are suitable coverings. For those superficial dermal burns that become infected, topical antimicrobials such as silver sulfadiazine or silver nitrate are used together with an appropriate antibiotic.

Table 12.1 Guide to burn type

Burn type	Appearance	Colour	Sensation
Superficial	dry and painful	red/erythema	present
Superficial dermal	wet/blisters and painful	white	present
Deep dermal	wet/blisters may be painful	mottled red	present or absent
Full thickness	dry/waxy	yellow-black	absent

ANSWERS – cont'd

In clean wounds, and those where infection has been brought under control, the wound should be excised and a split thickness skin graft applied. This should be performed as soon as possible after admission. The optimal timing for this surgery is between 3 and 5 days post burn. Deeper burns that involve vital structures may need to be covered with a vascularized flap.

Table 12.2 Prognosis for burn type

Burn type	Skin layer burnt	Healing	Treatment
Superficial	epidermis only	spontaneous	nil specific
Superficial dermal	epidermis and superficial dermis	spontaneous	biological dressings
Deep dermal	epidermis and deep dermis	delayed	excision and skin graft
Full thickness	epidermis and deep dermis +/– deeper structures	no healing	excision and skin graft or flap

REVISION POINTS

Burns

Epidemiology
- 1% of the population suffers a burn each year. Of those:
  - 50% will suffer some daily living activity restriction
  - 10% will require admission to hospital. Of these, 10% will have life-threatening burns
- the home is the usual place where burns occur
- 75% of paediatric burns occur in the home.

Risk factors
Those patients requiring hospital admission include:
- burns greater than 10% total body surface area (TBSA)
- burns of special areas:
  - face
  - hands
  - feet
  - genitalia and perineum
  - major joints
- full thickness burns greater than 5% TBSA
- electrical and chemical burns

- burns with an associated inhalation injury
- circumferential burns of the limbs or trunk
- burns in children or the elderly
- burn injury in patients with pre-existing medical disorders which would complicate management, prolong recovery or effect mortality
- any burn patient with associated trauma.

Management
Fluid therapy is an essential part of burn management. The quantity and composition of losses must be calculated with care.

In addition to the management described in the case, the severely burnt patient will require:
- nutritional support to minimize problems associated with catabolism (particularly sepsis)
- early closure of burn wounds to reduce the incidence of infection and reduce morbidity and mortality
- use of silver sulfadiazine cream to reduce burn wound sepsis
- early surgery to full thickness burns to reduce problems related to fibrosis.

ISSUES TO CONSIDER

- What kind of nutritional support is likely to be the most effective in the severely burnt patient?

- What are the organisms that cause most problems in burns units?

- What are new developments in the management of ARDS?

FURTHER INFORMATION

www.burnsurgery.org A comprehensive discourse on many aspects of burns, including emergency management from Harvard Medical School.

Dysphagia in a middle-aged woman

A 55-year-old female presents with a 3-month history of increasing difficulty in swallowing. She is able to swallow liquids but solids are a problem, especially bread and meat. Over the past 3 weeks undigested solid foodstuffs are often regurgitated. There is no pain on swallowing. She is not sure where the food sticks but points to her mid-sternum region. She is concerned that she has lost around 7 kg in weight.

Further questioning reveals that she has suffered occasional heartburn symptoms from her early 20s. She also has a history of coughing at night and this has been worse lately, sometimes being woken from sleep coughing as though she was choking. This has left her feeling hoarse. Her cough is sometimes productive of clear loose sputum but this has never

been bile- or bloodstained. There is no history of angina, shortness of breath, ankle swelling or intermittent claudication. She is not on medication but has sometimes taken 'over the counter' antacid tablets with symptom relief. She continues to smoke 10 cigarettes a day (as she has done for over 30 years) but drinks alcohol only occasionally.

On examination, she is overweight. She is not distressed. She is afebrile and not clinically anaemic or jaundiced. Pulse and blood pressure are within normal limits. There is no cervical lymphadenopathy. Examination of the chest and abdomen are unremarkable. Rectal examination reveals normal coloured stool that is faecal occult blood positive. There is no peripheral oedema and good pulses.

Q1 What are the possible diagnoses?

You arrange some blood tests, the results of which are shown below.

Investigation 13.1 Blood results			
Haemoglobin	102 g/l	White cell count	$5.4 \times 10^9/l$
Platelets	$178 \times 10^9/l$	MCV	71 fl
Sodium	142 mmol/l	Calcium	2.45 mmol/l
Potassium	3.9 mmol/l	Phosphate	1.15 mmol/l
Chloride	102 mmol/l	Total protein	65 g/l
Bicarbonate	27 mmol/l	Albumin	39 g/l
Urea	5.3 mmol/l	Globulins	27 g/l
Creatinine	0.09 mmol/l	Bilirubin	15 μmol/l
Uric acid	0.24 mmol/l	ALT	32 U/l
Glucose	4.4 mmol/l	AST	23 U/l
Cholesterol	3.5 mmol/l	GGT	37 U/l
LDH	212 U/l	ALP	85 U/l

Q2 What do these blood tests reveal?

Q3 What other investigations will help in your management?

A chest X-ray shows a normal mediastinum without lung opacities and nothing to suggest an aspiration pneumonia. The ECG is normal.

The general practitioner had arranged a contrast study before her consultation with you (Figure 13.1).

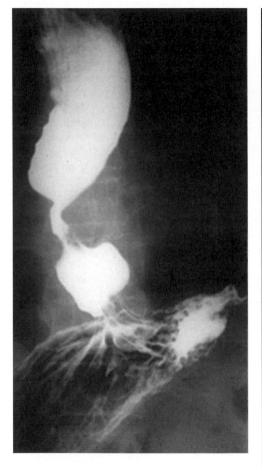

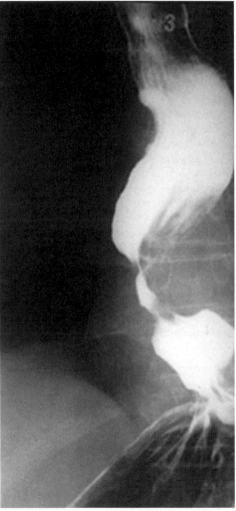

Fig 13.1

Q4 What is the investigation and what does it show?

An endoscopy is performed and this shows a florid oesophagitis, involving the distal third of the oesophagus. There is a stricture that does not allow further passage of the endoscope at 36 cm from the incisor teeth. This is dilated and the endoscopist passes the endoscope down into the stomach. Figure 13.2 is the view in the stomach.

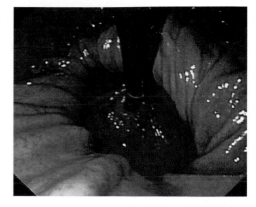

Fig 13.2

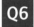 **Q5** What can you see?

The endoscopy reveals a small hiatus hernia below the stricture with the remainder of the examination normal. Biopsies are taken around the area of the dilated stricture and sent for histological examination.

The histology reports a marked inflammatory cell infiltrate consistent with oesophagitis. There is some cellular atypia but in the presence of inflammation this is difficult to interpret. No malignancy is identified.

Q6 What is your management plan for this patient?

At endoscopic follow-up at 6 weeks, the following image is seen with the endoscope at 32 cm from the incisor teeth (Figure 13.3).

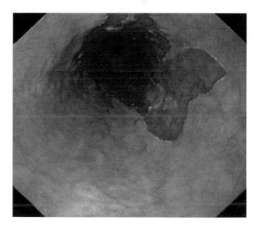

Fig 13.3

 Q7 What is the likely pathological diagnosis? What is your management strategy now?

Biopsies from the lower oesophagus show intestinal metaplasia consistent with a diagnosis of Barrett's oesophagus. The patient is told that she will need regular follow-up indefinitely and a follow-up surveillance endoscopy planned for 5 years' time.

Six months later, the patient returns to the clinic. She is now asymptomatic but continues to take regular omeprazole. She has tried stopping therapy but each time her heartburn returns. She has taken on board the lifestyle changes and has lost more weight and stopped smoking. She is worried that she may have to take the tablets for the rest of her life. She has read the drug information sheet which advises against long-term use.

Q8 What advice would you give the patient? What are the treatment options available for the patient?

ANSWERS

A1 The likely diagnoses are cancer of the oesophagus or cardia or a benign stricture of the oesophagus related to reflux disease. Worrying features here are weight loss although the long history of heartburn supports a peptic stricture. Night cough and the more recent cough with choking sensation are in keeping with reflux and aspiration rather than paroxysmal nocturnal dyspnoea. Patients may also notice wheezing at night with reflux disease.

Extrinsic compression of the oesophagus by malignant lymph nodes or lung cancer is possible. The hoarseness could represent recurrent laryngeal nerve involvement although with malignancy.

Disturbance of motor function of the oesophagus can present with dysphagia. Oesophageal spasm, or corkscrew oesophagus, is typically associated with pain on swallowing. Achalasia typically presents with difficulty swallowing liquids rather than solids. The history in such cases tends to be protracted for months or years.

A2 There is a mild anaemia which is microcytic in keeping with iron deficiency anaemia. The biochemistry is normal. Iron deficiency should be confirmed by checking the ferritin.

A3 The following investigations should be considered:
- Chest X-ray.
- ECG.
- Endoscopy is the investigation of choice. Current guidelines recommend that all patients over the age of 40 years with the onset of new upper gastrointestinal symptoms or a change in the nature of long-standing upper gastrointestinal symptoms should undergo endoscopy.
- Barium swallow/meal is now becoming the investigation of second choice. While it can often suggest the diagnosis, it clearly does not allow biopsy for pathological confirmation. It does have a role in patients with a 'normal' endoscopy with dysphagia to assess oesophageal motility and gastric emptying. In long strictures of the oesophagus, it can serve as a useful roadmap when attempting endoscopic or fluoroscopic dilatation. It may also reveal fistulous connections with the trachea or pleural cavity.

A4 This is a barium swallow. Contrast has outlined the distal oesophagus and proximal stomach with a hold-up in the oesophagus above a stricture. Immediately below the stricture is a small sliding type of hiatus hernia. The stricture looks smooth, but must be biopsied.

A5 The endoscopist has 'retroflexed' the instrument and is looking back up at the cardia. The black-sheathed endoscope can be seen at the top. There is a small (sliding) hiatus hernia in the middle of the picture. The gastric mucosal folds run up through the diaphragm into the hiatus hernia.

A6 The current working diagnosis is a stricture secondary to longstanding gastro-oesophageal reflux disease. Therapy is aimed at preventing reflux and reducing intragastric acidity.

General advice should be given to minimize reflux symptoms and maximize the effect of medical therapy:

ANSWERS – cont'd

- stop smoking
- minimize alcohol intake
- lose weight
- wear looser clothes
- avoid stooping
- avoid chocolate and coffee (these reduce lower oesophageal sphincter tone)
- reduce food intake before going to bed and raise head of the bed.

Many patients will be adequately controlled with such measures along with the occasional antacid medication.

Drug therapy

Antacids and mucosal protecting agents such as gaviscon are effective in many patients in controlling symptoms. In patients with established complications of their reflux disease such as erosions, ulceration, stricture formation or squamous metaplasia) proton pump inhibitors are the drugs of choice. A 1-month course should be given and then further therapy determined on symptoms and response to advice as given above. In cases of stricturing oesophagitis and Barrett's metaplasia, most clinicians would advise long-term treatment. Prokinetic agents such as metoclopramide may be useful in patients with additional motility disorders associated with their reflux.

In view of the cellular atypia noted on the initial biopsies, repeat endoscopy at 6–8 weeks following the initiation of therapy is indicated to assess healing of the oesophagitis, recurrent stricture formation and further biopsies to look for continuing dysplasia.

Although her oesophagitis may be the cause of her iron deficiency anaemia, it cannot be assumed to be so. Further investigations may also be required to exclude other conditions such as coeliac disease or lesions in the colon. A colonoscopy should be considered.

A7 This endoscopic photograph reveals a large tongue of columnar-lined epithelium running up the oesophagus and the endoscopist has measured the squamocolumnar junction at 32 cm. This patient has a Barrett's oesophagus. This is a well-recognized complication of chronic gastro-

oesophageal reflux, occurring in around 10% of patients. The stricture is no longer obvious and the oesophagitis has resolved.

The area of Barrett's oesophagus should be biopsied and carefully examined for evidence of dysplasia. Barrett's oesophagus is considered to be a premalignant disease. Surveillance in such patients is however controversial. There is no good evidence to support the concept that the prevention of acid reflux reverses the metaplasia or changes the malignant risk. If malignancy or high-grade dysplasia is detected, then the mainstay of treatment is surgical resection of the dysplastic segment, an operation with significant morbidity and mortality. Therapeutic strategies to endoscopically locally ablate the dysplastic epithelium are under investigation but are not generally available. Surveillance should thus be undertaken only in those patients considered fit for early surgical intervention. If there is no dysplasia, then 5-yearly endoscopy is reasonable. If dysplasia is detected, then more frequent endoscopy at 3- to 6-month intervals is indicated. Up to one-third of patients with high-grade dysplasia have invasive carcinoma in the resected oesophageal specimen.

A8 The natural history of gastro-oesophageal reflux is for the patient's symptoms to wax and wane. This is complicated by the poor correlation between symptoms and the degree of oesophagitis at endoscopy. Indeed, in some patients with marked symptoms of reflux, the endoscopy is normal. Twenty-four hour ambulatory pH monitoring is useful in these cases to confirm the diagnosis. In the 24-hour period, those who have an oesophageal pH of less than 4 for more than 4.6% of the time are deemed to have significant reflux. Correlation between symptoms and low pH strengthens this diagnosis. While the patient may be able to stop her medication in the future, it is likely she will relapse with time and run the risk of further stricturing.

Proton pump inhibitors (PPIs) have been available for a decade and histamine receptor antagonists almost three decades. These drugs have been used widely throughout the world without any real evidence of any long-term harm.

ANSWERS – cont'd

It was thought that the achlorhydria associated with their use may increase the gastric cancer risk but this has not yet been realized. PPIs produce more effective acid suppression than the histamine receptor antagonists, but are much more expensive and tend to reserved for those with endoscopically proven oesophagitis.

The patient may wish to consider a surgical option. The mainstay of surgery is to repair any hiatal defect and fashion a fundoplication where the fundus of the stomach is wrapped partially or completely around the intra-abdominal part of the distal oesophagus. This can usually be done laparoscopically but occasionally requires an open operation. It is associated with a high satisfaction rate, with most patients having symptoms improved and off medication.

A number of new minimally invasive procedures using the endoscope have been developed and are undergoing evaluation. These are essentially experimental, and their success and long-term prevention of reflux is still unknown.

REVISION POINTS

Gastro-oesophageal reflux disease

This is a common condition. It can mimic the symptoms of upper gastrointestinal malignancy.

All patients over 40 years of age who develop new upper gastrointestinal symptoms should undergo prompt endoscopy. An initial trial of acid suppression may be ill-advised and result in delayed diagnosis of an underlying malignancy.

Management
Management of reflux disease should involve lifestyle changes as well as appropriate levels of acid suppression. Surgery is a successful option for symptom control in a selected proportion of patients.

Barrett's oesophagus
Barrett's oesophagus complicates reflux disease in around 10% of cases. It is a premalignant condition and endoscopic surveillance is indicated in a select group of younger, fitter patients to detect dysplasia/early neoplasia. The effect of reflux control by medication or surgery on the risk of malignancy is unclear.

ISSUES TO CONSIDER

- What is the cost effectiveness of a surveillance programme for carcinoma of the oesophagus? In what circumstances may such a programme be justified?

- What is the role of endoscopy in the management of patients with heartburn?

- What is the link between *Helicobacter pylori* and oesophageal reflux?

FURTHER INFORMATION

www.gerd.com A superb (pharmaceutical company sponsored) website covering all aspects of reflux disease, including links to the 500 most cited articles among many other excellent features.

www.asge.org The website of the American Society for Gastrointestinal Endoscopy includes guidelines on Barrett's oesophagus and the management of the patient with dysphagia.

Vomiting and collapse in an elderly woman

An 81-year-old woman is brought in a moribund condition by ambulance to the emergency department. She lives with her daughter, who has accompanied her. The daughter says her mother woke up that morning feeling ill and declined to get out of bed. One hour later she vomited up a large quantity of bright red blood and collapsed. The daughter immediately called the ambulance. The patient is barely conscious and is covered in blood.

She is pale and sweaty. Her blood pressure is 60/30 mm Hg and her pulse is 130 bpm. She is peripherally cold.

Q1 Describe the initial emergency management of this patient.

You and your team leap into action. Your aggressive resuscitation measures are successful and within 15 minutes her blood pressure has increased to 110/60 mm Hg. You have inserted two large-bore peripheral lines and given 1 litre of a colloid solution as rapidly as possible, followed by 1 litre of isotonic saline over 30 minutes. Her pulse has decreased to 90 bpm. She has not vomited any more blood.

Q2 What are you going to do next?

The daughter tells you that her mother keeps good health, looks after herself, and does her own shopping. She has had no serious illnesses in the past. She has suffered some swelling of the ankles for several years and takes fluid tablets to correct that. The patient has also suffered with indigestion and kept a bottle of antacid at home to relieve her symptoms, but these symptoms have never bothered her unduly.

Two weeks previously the patient went to her doctor complaining of increasing pain in her right hip, worse in the morning and when she started walking. Her local doctor has prescribed some medication for the pain, but the daughter is not sure of the name of the drug. Her mother has smoked about five cigarettes a day until 10 years ago, and she drinks alcohol only occasionally. You rummage in the patient's handbag and find some tablets, which you identify as diclofenac.

The patient remains confused and is unable to give any history. A cardiac monitor shows a pulse rate of 90 bpm in sinus rhythm. You examine her while she is lying flat. The pulse is now of good volume. The blood pressure is still 110/60 mm Hg. The apex beat is not displaced and the two heart sounds are normal. The chest is clear to auscultation. The abdomen is soft with mild epigastric tenderness. There is no guarding or rebound and the bowel sounds are normal. She has mild ankle oedema. Rectal examination reveals foul-smelling, sticky, black tar-like stool. There are no other findings on physical examination that help determine the cause of the bleeding.

A portable chest X-ray is normal and a 12-lead ECG is unremarkable.

The results of some of your investigations are shown below.

Investigation 14.1 Summary of results				
Haemoglobin	86 g/l	White cell count		6.6 x 10⁹/l
RBC	4.39 x 10¹²/l	Neutrophils	57%	60 x 10⁹/l
PCV	0.38	Lymphocytes	27%	2.9 x 10⁹/l
Platelets	239 x 10⁹/l			
Coagulation studies normal				
Sodium	142 mmol/l	Calcium		2.16 mmol/l
Potassium	4.8 mmol/l	Phosphate		1.15 mmol/l
Chloride	106 mmol/l	Total protein		65 g/l
Bicarbonate	27 mmol/l	Albumin		38 g/l
Urea	18.5 mmol/l	Globulins		27 g/l
Creatinine	0.08 mmol/l	Bilirubin		16 µmol/l

You arrange for a central venous catheter to be inserted. Ninety minutes have now elapsed since the patient's arrival and you note that there is only 50 ml urine in the catheter bag. Her central venous pressure is 8 cm water.

Q3 What do you do next? What is the likely diagnosis?

Two units of packed red cells are given and the patient's condition remains stable. The central venous pressure rises to 13 cm and a further 100 ml urine is passed over the next 2 hours.

An endoscopy is performed. The endoscopist reports the patient has a small hiatus hernia, but there is no oesophagitis. There is fresh blood in the stomach and the following views are obtained of the duodenum (Figure 14.1).

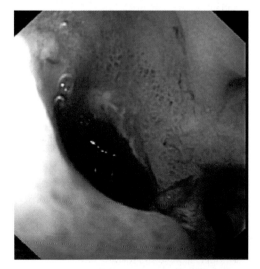

Fig 14.1

Q4 What does Figure 14.1 show and what is the significance of these findings?

What will the endoscopist do now?

A biopsy test for *Helicobacter pylori* is negative. A further unit of red cells is transfused.

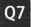 **How should the patient be treated?**

Her haemoglobin after the 3-unit transfusion is 103 g/l. Her observations remain stable over the next 24 hours.

Thirty hours after admission she complains of feeling unwell and vomits 200 ml fresh blood. Her pulse rate has risen to 116 bpm and her blood pressure is 115/60 mm Hg lying. When the woman is sitting up her blood pressure drops to 95/60 mm Hg. Her chest is clear and the abdomen soft. A repeat haemoglobin is 84 g/l.

Q7 **What should be done now?**

In this instance, after joint consultation between the gastroenterologists and surgeons involved in the patient's care, it was decided to undertake a further endoscopic approach to control the bleeding. This proved successful and 6 days later the patient was discharged home.

ANSWERS

A1 Call for help and begin resuscitation. This patient should be resuscitated by a team of experienced doctors and nurses who should be prepared to perform an emergency endotracheal intubation, if it is required. The team will first:
- Ensure that the airway is clear.
- Check the patient's breathing is satisfactory and unhindered.
- Assess the pulse and blood pressure.

After this initial assessment, the resuscitation team will:
- Ensure adequate management of her airway to prevent aspiration. One member of the team will be given responsibility to ensure patency of the airway. Suction equipment must be immediately available. The team must be prepared to intubate the patient if she vomits.
- Apply high-flow oxygen by face mask.
- Insert two large-bore intravenous cannulae and start intravenous fluids (colloid or isotonic saline) running as fast as possible (i.e., the intravenous cannula wide open or under a pressure cuff).
- Collect blood samples for urgent analysis (cross-matching, complete blood picture, coagulation studies and electrolytes).
- Consider giving uncross-matched blood (group O-negative) if bleeding is considered massive, or there is no sign of response to resuscitation in the first 10–15 minutes.
- Insert a urinary catheter, monitor urine output and renal perfusion.
- Make ongoing recordings of her vital signs (particularly blood pressure).

A2 You now have several things to do. First, obtain as much information as you can from the daughter:
- Is there a history of previous ulcer disease?
- Is there a history of liver disease or significant alcohol use?
- Has there been any noted change in bowel function (i.e., seeking evidence of blood loss)?

ANSWERS – cont'd

- Are there any contributing factors: use of ulcerogenic drugs (aspirin or non-steroidal anti-inflammatory drugs (NSAIDs)) or over-anticoagulation?

You should perform a general physical examination and pay close attention to:
- A careful assessment of the patient's circulatory state and respiratory system (possible aspiration).
- Any features that might help determine the underlying cause of the current problem. Within the upper digestive tract, the two most important causes of bleeding are oesophageal varices and peptic ulcer disease. The patient may have stigmata of chronic liver disease. Perform a rectal examination to determine the presence of melaena.

This patient has had a major haematemesis requiring emergency resuscitation. You must warn the Blood Bank that you have an acutely bleeding patient and request urgent matching of 6 units of red cells. Also request that the Bank stay 6 units ahead as units are transfused. Next, contact the gastroenterologist and oesophagogastric surgeon for their immediate assessment. As the patient may require emergency surgery a 12-lead ECG and a (portable) chest X-ray should be performed. The patient may need a central venous line and an arterial line for accurately monitoring fluid status and blood pressure. An anaesthetist should be called and the intensive care unit informed.

A3 The CVP and urine output are both low. This indicates that the patient is still hypovolaemic, and requires further volume resuscitation. Her haemoglobin is also low. Cross-matched blood should be available by this stage, and she should be transfused with at least two units of reconstituted red blood cells.

The high urea in comparison to the creatinine is due to the high blood load in her upper gut and subsequent protein absorption. This urea: creatinine ratio can be helpful in defining the site of obscure gastrointestinal bleeding, although the presence of haematemesis in this woman makes it obvious.

The diagnosis is most likely NSAID-related peptic ulceration. She has had a significant upper gastrointestinal bleed and urgent endoscopy is indicated once she is adequately resuscitated.

A4 The working diagnosis has been confirmed. The endoscopic image shows a 1 cm chronic duodenal ulcer with an adherent clot. This 'stigmata of recent haemorrhage' suggests that this is a 'high-risk' ulcer, meaning that there is a good chance that if left untreated, it will rebleed.

This woman's age, presentation and the recent prescription of NSAIDs make this ulcer likely to be NSAID-induced.

A5 The endoscopist might wash the clot away and look at the base of the ulcer. The presence of a visible vessel would increase concern about the risk of a rebleed. The ulcer can be injected with 1:10 000 adrenaline to reduce the risk of rebleeding. Adrenaline is used because of its vasoconstrictor effects although it is likely that the major haemostatic effects result from tamponade from the fluid injection.

Additional endoscopic methods used in the control of bleeding ulcers include the heater probe, bipolar electrocoagulation, endoscopic clips and argon plasma coagulation.

An antral biopsy can be obtained for a rapid urease test to look for *Helicobacter pylori*.

A6 It is likely the ulcer has developed as a consequence of NSAID use. There is no evidence that the patient has *Helicobacter pylori* – the most common aetiological agent. Treatment consists of:
- Withdrawal of the ulcerogenic drug.
- Promotion of ulcer healing through suppression of gastric acid.

There is now evidence suggesting that proton pump inhibitors (PPIs) prevent ulcer rebleeding and improve outcome after successful endoscopic therapy, although very high intravenous doses are probably required. These drugs promote ulcer healing. Therefore, the standard of care for bleeding peptic ulcers is endoscopic therapy followed by high-dose PPI therapy.

ANSWERS – cont'd

A7 The patient has suffered a substantial rebleed as judged by:

- Fresh blood in the vomitus (more important than the volume).
- Orthostatic hypotension (hypovolaemia).
- The falling haemoglobin.

In the first instance, the patient's condition should be restabilized with resuscitation as done in Answer 1.

There is debate as to whether the patient should now proceed to surgery for operative control of the bleeding duodenal ulcer or whether further endoscopic intervention (e.g. injection sclerotherapy) should be attempted. Elderly patients at high surgical risk may benefit from a repeat therapeutic endoscopy. Conversely, the hypotension and delay in re-establishing haemostasis from repeated unsuccessful endoscopic attempts may have grave consequences. A multidisciplinary approach is important and surgical teams should be involved in the management of bleeding peptic ulcers from the outset.

The Rockall score is an accurate scoring system to predict mortality and rebleeding risk at presentation and following endoscopic therapy. Its use helps risk stratification and the identification of patients likely to require early surgery.

In the longer term, the patient will need up to 3 months of acid suppression with a PPI to allow ulcer healing.

REVISION POINTS

Peptic ulcer disease

Incidence
The incidence of peptic ulcer disease has been decreasing for the last 30–40 years, related to both eradication of *Helicobacter pylori* and availability of potent acid-suppressive medications.

Peptic ulcers remain the most common cause of massive upper gastrointestinal tract bleeding, accounting for about 50 per cent of cases.

Aetiology
- NSAIDs
- *Helicobacter pylori* infection
- hypersecretory syndromes: Zollinger–Ellison syndrome (rare).

Pathogenesis
NSAID-induced ulceration
- NSAID-induced ulcers are often gastric and multiple
- NSAIDs inhibit systemic and mucosal cyclo-oxygenase production, leading to reduced tissue prostaglandin levels and impaired tissue defence. Other factors including polymorphonuclear cells and free radical generation may also be important in the pathogenesis of NSAID ulceration
- high risk of NSAID complications associated with: advanced age, medical co-morbidities,

higher dose, the first 3 months of use, past history of ulcer disease and concomitant steroid use.

Helicobacter pylori-associated ulceration
Infection with *H. pylori* is often found in the majority of peptic ulcers not associated with NSAIDs, although there are increasing reports of NSAID and *H. pylori*-negative ulcers.

The pathogenesis of duodenal ulcer (DU) has been postulated to involve increased duodenal acid load secondary to *H. pylori* gastritis, resulting in gastric metaplasia in the duodenum, inflammation and progression to ulceration.

The association with gastric ulcers (GU) is less clear, but may be related to development of atrophic gastritis and duodeno-gastric reflux.

Why some persons with *H. pylori* infection develop DU and others develop GU is unclear.

Clinical features
- ulcer-type dyspepsia
- 30–50% of patients with NSAID-induced ulcers do not have symptoms.

Management of the acute upper gastrointestinal tract bleed
- rapidly assess the haemodynamic status
- resuscitate
- determine the source of bleeding: endoscopy

continues overleaf

REVISION POINTS – cont'd

- stop the bleeding: endoscopy or surgery
- prevent recurrent bleeding.

Management of NSAID-induced ulcers

- stop NSAID if possible. In case of aspirin, discontinue or change to alternative antiplatelet agent
- commence acid-suppressive medication (PPI or H$_2$-receptor antagonist)
- if NSAID cannot be stopped, then treatment with a PPI is superior to other agents
- the newly introduced selective COX-2 inhibitors are potentially less ulcerogenic than NSAIDs, but ulcers can still occur with these agents.

Diagnosis of *Helicobacter pylori* infection

- rapid urease test (requires endoscopy and biopsy)
- histology
- urea breath test (least inconvenient test)
- serology (evidence of previous, but not necessarily current, infection)
- faecal antigens.

***Helicobacter pylori* eradication therapy**

- Successful eradication of *H. pylori* in *H. pylori*-associated ulcers eliminates recurrence of ulcer disease.

- Most eradication regimens consist of a PPI or ranitidine-bismuth-citrate, plus two antibiotics (usually clarithromycin and amoxicillin), taken for 1 week. Success rates of 80–90% are reported.
- Some studies suggest that eradication of *H. pylori* results in healing of duodenal ulcers even without concomitant acid-suppressive therapy. In practice, however, acid-suppressive medication is given for 4–8 weeks after eradication therapy, particularly for complicated ulcers.

Prognosis

Bleeding stops spontaneously in 80% of bleeding peptic ulcers. The challenge is therefore to identify patients who continue to bleed or develop recurrent bleeding; these patients have significantly higher mortality. Visual assessment of the ulcer base during endoscopy provides clues regarding rebleeding risk. The rate of ulcer rebleeding is minimal if the ulcer has a clean base, but rises dramatically if high-risk stigmata are seen (50% for visible vessel, 90% for active bleeding). After achieving haemostasis with endoscopic intervention, the rate of recurrent bleeding is about 20%, but may be reduced if high-level acid-suppressive therapy is given after endoscopy.

ISSUES TO CONSIDER

- The GP now wants to put this patient on celecoxib for her arthritis. What is your advice?
- How would your management have differed if this patient had bled from a gastric ulcer?
- What is the Rockall score? How does it help your decision-making? What was this woman's Rockall score?
- 'Only eliminate *H. pylori* from those individuals with peptic ulcers.' Is this an appropriate statement?

FURTHER INFORMATION

www.asge.org Website of the American Society of Gastrointestinal Endoscopy. A resource for all things endoscopic.

www.bsg.org.uk/clinical_prac/decision.htm An online Rockall score calculator from the British Society of Gastroenterology.

A 77-year-old man with vomiting

You are asked to assess a 77-year-old man in the emergency department. He has presented with vomiting for several weeks, which has worsened in the last few days.

Q1 What history will help determine the cause of the vomiting?

The patient tells you that he vomits once or twice a day and it is getting worse. It tends to occur in the evenings but is not always related to his evening meal. The vomitus contains clear fluid and partially digested food, sometimes containing food he ate several meals ago. There is no bile and the smell is not particularly offensive. Sometimes prior to vomiting he has mild upper abdominal discomfort but there is usually no warning. There has not been much pain but he has experienced bloating recently. He thinks he might have lost weight in the last few weeks and feels tired and lethargic. His bowel function is normal but less frequent, especially in the last week. He has not had fevers or jaundice.

He is otherwise well and your review of systems is negative. His past history includes a recent chest infection and a myocardial infarction 3 years ago. He underwent a colonic resection for diverticular disease 5 years earlier. His only medication is aspirin and he does not drink or smoke.

Q2 What is the most likely cause of the vomiting and what could be the significance of the recent chest infection?

On examination he looks unwell. His peripheries are warm and well perfused, but there is loss of the normal skin turgor. The pulse rate is 100 bpm and his temperature is 37.4°C. His blood pressure on lying is 140/90 mg Hg and 125/85 mm Hg on sitting. Examination of his cardiorespiratory systems is unremarkable. The upper abdomen looks distended and on palpation it is soft with mild epigastric tenderness. There is nothing else abnormal to find in the abdomen. The bowel sounds are normal and rectal examination is unremarkable.

Q3 What other physical sign might you expect in this patient?

The patient has a marked succussion splash.

Q4 What are you going to do next?

An intravenous cannula is inserted and 1 litre isotonic saline is run in over 2 hours.

Blood is collected for a complete blood picture and electrolytes.

Investigation 15.1 Summary of results			
Haemoglobin	142 g/l	White cell count	10.0 x 10⁹/l
MCV	76 fl	Platelets	270 x 10⁹/l
MCH	29.5 pg		
MCHC	280 g/l		
Sodium	133 mmol/l	Calcium	2.16 mmol/l
Potassium	3.2 mmol/l	Phosphate	1.15 mmol/l
Chloride	85 mmol/l	Total protein	65 g/l
Bicarbonate	27 mmol/l	Albumin	38 g/l
Urea	16 mmol/l	Globulins	27 g/l
Creatinine	0.13 mmol/l	Bilirubin	16 µmol/l
Uric acid	0.31 mmol/l	ALT	30 U/l
Glucose	4.4 mmol/l	AST	29 U/l
Cholesterol	3.5 mmol/l	GGT	45 U/l
LDH	212 U/l	ALP	55 U/l

Q5 What are the abnormalities and how would you interpret these findings?

Chest and abdominal radiographs are performed (Figures 15.1 and 15.2).

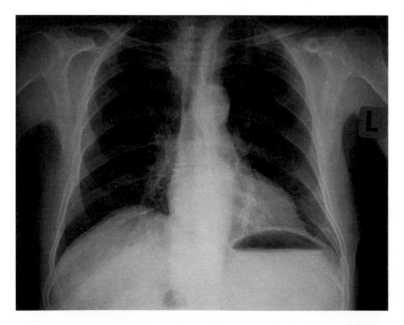

Fig 15.1

Fig 15.2

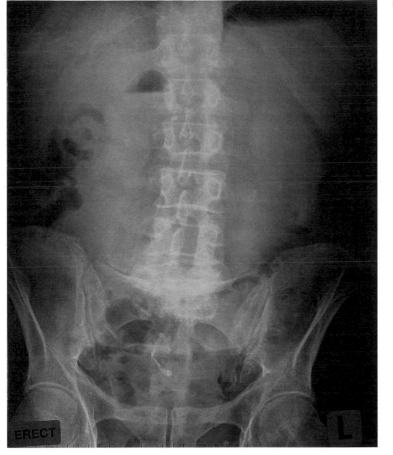

Q6 How would you interpret these radiographs?

Your insertion of a wide bore nasogastric tube is promptly followed by drainage of 2 litres of turbid fluid. Particles of recognizable food are seen in the drainage bag, but no bile.

Q7 How would you manage fluid replacement?

To aid with fluid management, a urinary catheter is inserted and intravenous fluid titrated to achieve an output of at least 30 ml/h. In the first hour after admission the patient is given 500 ml fluid and another 2 l isotonic saline over the following 4 hours.

During the third litre of fluid replacement, the patient's serum electrolytes are repeated (Investigation 15.2).

Investigation 15.2 Serum electrolytes	
Sodium	138 mmol/l
Potassium	3.0 mmol/l
Chloride	104 mmol/l
Urea	8.2 mmol/l
Creatinine	0.11 mmol/l

He has passed 50 ml urine in the last hour and drained a further 1 litre gastric contents. His chest is clear on auscultation.

Q8 What fluids would you prescribe over the next 4 hours?

The patient is monitored in a high-dependency unit and once he is stable an endoscopy is performed (Figure 15.3).

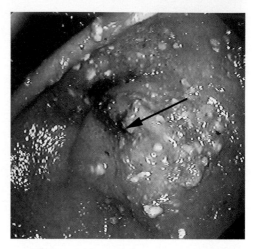

Fig 15.3

This is a view of the antrum, with an arrow pointing to the pylorus.

Q9 What does Figure 15.3 show?

The endoscopist is unable to get her instrument through the pylorus, which appears rigid. She dilates the pylorus with a balloon dilator and takes some blind biopsies through the pylorus. These confirm the diagnosis of adenocarcinoma and a CT scan is performed (Figure 15.4).

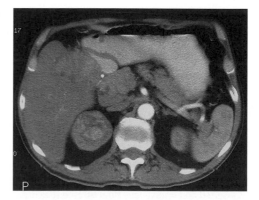

Fig 15.4

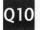**Q10** What does the CT scan show?

This patient had one of the more unusual causes of gastric outlet obstruction. He underwent a laparoscopic gastroenterostomy to bypass the obstructed duodenum.

ANSWERS

A1 To establish the likely cause of his vomiting you will need the following information.

- Details of the vomiting:
  - when it started, how many times a day it occurs and whether the frequency has changed over this period
  - if there is any associated anorexia or nausea
  - if it is projectile
  - what the contents of the vomitus are (e.g. recognizable food, blood, bile. Remember old blood is described as 'coffee-grounds' in appearance)
  - any relationship to food (triggered by food? How long after a meal does it occur?).
- Any associated symptoms, particularly gastrointestinal (dysphagia, pain, distension, bowel change, jaundice, loss of weight).
- Drug history, including alcohol consumption.
- General state of health and past history (e.g. diabetes).

Apart from gastrointestinal causes, you need to consider:

- Central nervous system disorders: raised intracranial pressure deprives the vomiting centre of oxygen and triggers vomiting. Nausea may be absent and the vomiting projectile.
- Medications: these may cause vomiting by irritating the gastrointestinal tract or by acting centrally.
- Infection: especially urinary tract in the elderly.
- Severe pain: vomiting is common in renal colic and myocardial infarction.
- Metabolic disorders including diabetic acidosis, uraemia, Addisonian crisis and thyrotoxicosis. Acidosis and hypokalaemia directly affect the vomiting centre.
- Shock: this causes decreased central oxygenation.
- Vertigo.
- Migraine: this mildly raises intracranial pressure.
- Psychiatric: bulimia, psychosomatic.

A2 From history alone, this patient almost certainly has gastric outlet obstruction. In this setting the stomach will fill to capacity and then empty itself by vomiting, often without warning. As a result there may be no preceding nausea and the vomiting may be projectile. As the stomach is expansile there may not be an obvious relation to food, with vomiting only occurring after several meals. Typically there will be partially digested food but no bile. As the vomiting associated with gastric outlet obstruction can be profuse and abrupt there is always the risk of pulmonary aspiration. The patient's recent chest infection may be a reflection of this complication.

Other gastrointestinal causes should be considered. Oesophageal obstruction usually leads to rapid regurgitation of undigested food and dysphagia is a prominent symptom. Obstruction distal to the stomach will produce a vomitus that contains bile or is faeculent, so described because of its offensive smell and taste, consistency and colour. These patients will usually have other gastrointestinal symptoms (e.g. colicky abdominal pain and distension in small bowel obstruction).

The two most common causes of gastric outlet obstruction in the adult are:

- Malignancy:
  - carcinoma of the antrum
  - extrinsic duodenal compression by pancreatic cancer.
- Chronic duodenal ulceration.

All other causes are rare and include:

- Hypertrophic (adult) pyloric stenosis.
- Pancreatic abnormalities:
  - congenital (annular, heterotopic)
  - pancreatitis +/− pseudocyst.
- Other neoplastic processes:
  - carcinoma of the ampulla of Vater
  - carcinoma of the biliary system
  - duodenal or gastric polyps
  - enlarged lymph nodes
  - functional (adynamic stomach).

This patient's history could be consistent with benign disease or an underlying malignancy.

A3 The classic sign of gastric fullness is the succussion splash, which is elicited by listening over the abdomen while rocking the patient.

ANSWERS – cont'd

Fluid and food is heard 'splashing' in the unemptied stomach. It is always important to explain to the patient what you are about to do beforehand, as this manoeuvre can be disconcerting.

A4 This patient needs resuscitation. He is dehydrated and relatively hypovolaemic, as judged by loss of normal skin turgor and his postural drop in blood pressure. He will require:

- Insertion of an intravenous cannula.
- Rapid infusion of isotonic saline.
- Insertion of a nasogastric tube and gastric aspiration.
- Oxygen by face mask.
- Collection of blood samples for a complete blood picture and biochemistry.
- Radiography of the chest and abdomen.

A5 The red cell indices show microcytosis and hypochromia. Although his haemoglobin is normal, he is dehydrated and haemoconcentrated. Thus, it is likely he has an underlying iron deficiency anaemia.

The urea is disproportionately elevated relative to creatinine and this prerenal impairment is a reflection of dehydration.

The biochemical changes that are sometimes seen in total gastric outlet obstruction and profuse vomiting can be complex. Patients with prolonged gastric outlet obstruction can present with a metabolic alkalosis and a paradoxical aciduria, but such extreme biochemical changes are rare.

In this case, the patient has a mild hyponatraemia accompanied by a hypokalaemia and hypochloraemia. This is a reflection on the profuse and prolonged vomiting directly causing electrolyte loss. In such circumstances, the patient may lose large quantities of hydrogen and chloride ions, with subsequent renal retention of bicarbonate to compensate for the loss of chloride in the vomitus.

A6 The chest radiograph shows a large gastric air bubble under the left diaphragm, with a fluid level. The lung fields are clear and there is no evidence of any pneumonic process. The abdominal radiograph shows a massively dilated stomach,

full of fluid. The greater curve of the stomach can be seen at the level of the iliac crests, and the transverse colon is compressed into the pelvis. The ring of metal staples from his previous surgery can be seen low in the pelvis.

A7 As the patient's primary problem is dehydration, crystalloid fluid is appropriate and isotonic saline should be used rather than dextrose. The patient is dehydrated and will need rapid fluid replacement to maintain renal function and prevent acute tubular necrosis. In the older patient a careful assessment of cardiac function is important to determine the risk of developing cardiac failure with rapid fluid replacement. As this patient has a history of myocardial ischaemia, careful monitoring is necessary. Central venous pressure monitoring may be appropriate.

Commence intravenous fluids at 1 litre over 1–2 hours while monitoring urine output and respiratory function, including saturation. Hourly urine measures are imperative and fluid regimen should be adjusted accordingly. If initial output is low, fluid boluses should be given. Potassium should be replaced but cautiously until urine output is established.

Once fluid deficit has been corrected, fluid rate should be determined by maintenance requirements plus losses. In this setting nasogastric losses may be large and it is preferable to replace the amount separately with 0.45% saline with 1 g (13.9 mmol) potassium per litre.

A8 Your resuscitation with 3 litres fluid has achieved a satisfactory urine output. There is another litre of gastric aspirate to replace and he will need a maintenance regimen prescribed. He has not yet been given any potassium and as you have now shown that his urine function is satisfactory, he needs potassium supplements.

You need to replace the current deficit of fluid and potassium and then prescribe his maintenance (likely between 2–2.5 litres with 180 mmol sodium and 80 mmol potassium). As losses are ongoing the orders will need to be revised regularly. Thus, he could be given isotonic saline at 150 ml/h with added potassium (3 gm per litre of fluid replacement). You should ensure he

ANSWERS – cont'd

maintains a urine output of at least 30 ml/h and recheck cardiopulmonary status and electrolyte measurements frequently.

A9 There are food particles scattered throughout the stomach. As endoscopy is normally performed in the fasted state with the stomach empty of food, this is abnormal. The pylorus is narrowed and there appears to be a mass in this area pushing back into the antrum.

A10 This is a section through the upper part of the abdominal cavity and shows contrast in the stomach. The right lobe of the liver is to the left of Figure 15.4. There is a mass arising from the gallbladder fossa which is compressing the duodenum. There is another mass (of lymph nodes) pressing the duodenum from behind. This is likely to be a carcinoma of the gallbladder, with direct extension into adjacent structures (including the duodenum) and local lymph node spread.

REVISION POINTS

Gastric outlet obstruction

Definition
Obstruction to gastric outflow due to some disease process at the level of the antrum, pylorus or duodenum.

Aetiology
The two important causes are:
- Distal gastric malignancy.
- Duodenal ulcer disease (6–8% of all cases will develop obstruction).

Gastric outlet is seen less frequently because:
- The incidence of distal gastric cancer is declining.
- Duodenal ulcer disease tends to be treated earlier and more effectively (PPIs and *Helicobacter pylori* eradication).

Clinical features
- Profuse vomiting of bile-free vomitus, containing recognizable food, often from meals eaten days earlier.
- May present with severe dehydration, drowsiness and confusion.
- Characteristic finding of a succussion splash.
- Complex biochemical changes which can make resuscitation difficult.

Management
- Resuscitation.
- Rehydration
  - correction of electrolyte imbalances
  - monitoring of urine output
  - large-bore nasogastric tube and nasogastric fluid replacement.
- Identify the underlying cause.

- Treat:
  - the obstruction
  - the underlying cause.

Investigations
- Serum biochemistry.
- Arterial blood gas analysis (metabolic alkalosis is common).
- Radiology
  - plain films (prominent gastric bubble, gastric distension)
  - contrast study (endoscopy preferred, but may not be feasible if the stomach remains full of food)
  - CT to identify structures outside the digestive tract that may be causing compression.
- Endoscopy for
  - precise identification of cause of obstruction
  - biopsy
  - possible dilatation of the narrowed segment.

Treatment
Peptic ulcer disease
- Aggressive medical therapy
  - *H. pylori* eradication
  - acid suppression.

  If still obstructed (after 2 weeks' therapy)
  - endoscopic dilatation (50% success rate) or
  - surgery (pyloroplasty or gastroenterostomy).

Gastric malignancy
- Resection.
- Bypass.

Other treatments depending on the cause.

ISSUES TO CONSIDER

- What electrolyte disturbances would you expect after prolonged vomiting, such as in hyperemesis gravidarum? Remind yourself of acid–base balance and how it is regulated.

- What are the normal daily requirements of potassium and sodium?

- How would a person with small bowel obstruction present, and what are the common causes?

FURTHER INFORMATION

www.emedicine.com/med/topic2713.htm
A textbook approach to the topic of gastric outlet obstruction.

Weight loss in a middle-aged woman

A 53-year-old woman presents with a 3-month history of epigastric pain and 'indigestion'. This is associated with anorexia and occasional vomiting. The vomiting has become more frequent. She has rarely experienced indigestion in the past and since her present symptoms started, she has lost 10 kg in weight. She feels bloated after food and is tired and lethargic.

She used to smoke 20 cigarettes a day but gave up 4 years ago. She drinks 30 gm of alcohol a day and is not on any medication. In the past she has had an appendicectomy and hysterectomy and has had surgery to varicose veins.

On examination she appears to have lost some weight recently but the rest of the physical examination is unremarkable.

Q1 What are the worrying features in the history? What are your differential diagnoses?

You realize that her symptoms warrant investigation, even in the absence of any physical signs, and you go on to arrange some investigations.

Q2 What investigations would you order?

Blood results are as follows.

Investigation 16.1 Summary of results			
Haemoglobin	106 g/l	White cell count	8.3 x 10⁹/l
MCV	77 fl		
MCH	29.5 pg		
MCHC	230 g/l		
Platelets	180 x 10⁹/l		
Sodium	141 mmol/l	Calcium	2.16 mmol/l
Potassium	3.7 mmol/l	Phosphate	1.15 mmol/l
Chloride	104 mmol/l	Total protein	69 g/l
Bicarbonate	29 mmol/l	Albumin	33 g/l
Urea	7.1 mmol/l	Globulins	36 g/l
Creatinine	0.08 mmol/l	Bilirubin	7 μmol/l
Uric acid	0.24 mmol/l	ALT	26 U/l
Glucose	4.4 mmol/l	AST	50 U/l
Cholesterol	3.5 mmol/l	GGT	17 U/l
LDH	127 U/l	ALP	65 U/l

Q3   What do the blood tests show?

A further investigation is performed and a representative film is shown (Figure 16.1).

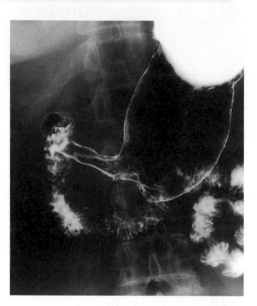

Fig 16.1

Q4   What is this investigation? What does it show?

Based on the radiological findings, the patient is referred for another investigation (Figure 16.2).

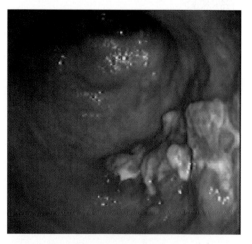

Fig 16.2

Q5   What is this investigation and what does it show?

The lesion is biopsied and confirmed to be a moderately differentiated adenocarcinoma.

Q6   What further investigations are required?

Various imaging investigations are performed and do not show any evidence of tumour dissemination. The tumour appears to be confined to the stomach wall, although there may be some thickening in the immediately adjacent tissues.

Q7   Describe the treatment options available to patients with gastric cancer.

Although it was realized that surgery might not be curative, a surgical approach was recommended. This was because the patient had symptoms of incipient obstruction and investigations had shown a stenosing lesion in the distal stomach. The patient underwent surgery. Figure 16.3 shows the operative view of the upper abdomen.

Fig 16.3

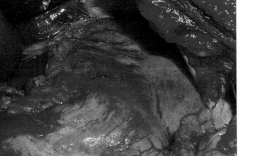

Q8   What can the surgeon see?

A partial gastrectomy is performed and the opened specimen shown in Figure 16.4.

Q9   Describe this operative specimen. What is the prognosis for this malignancy?

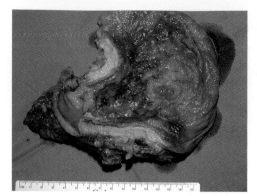

The tumour showed extensive submucosal infiltration by moderately differentiated adenocarcinoma with involvement of the lymph nodes along the left gastric axis. Chemotherapy was discussed with the patient. She declined further treatment and died of disseminated disease 9 months later.

Fig 16.4

ANSWERS

A1 From the history there are several features which point to a diagnosis of gastric malignancy. Indigestion and dyspepsia appearing for the first time in someone over 50 should cause concern and prompt investigation. This patient also has anorexia, vomiting and weight loss, together with suspicious symptoms and risk factors (alcohol and smoking) for gastric cancer.

Other diagnoses to consider include:
● oesophageal cancer
● peptic ulceration
● gallstone disease
● chronic pancreatitis.

A2 Investigations should include:
● complete blood picture (anaemia)
● serum biochemistry (disturbance of liver function with metastatic disease)
● imaging of the upper digestive tract.

A3 The blood results show a mild microcytic anaemia with a low MCV and MCHC. This is typical of iron deficiency anaemia and consistent with bleeding from occult gastrointestinal pathology. The other blood tests are normal.

A4 The contrast study is a barium meal and this shows circumferential narrowing of the distal stomach. The stomach, duodenum and proximal jejunum are lined with contrast, but the antrum will not distend. These appearances are typical of a gastric cancer.

This woman needs an endoscopic examination of her upper gastrointestinal tract. In most circumstances the imaging investigation of choice for a patient with these symptoms would be an endoscopy. However, barium meal examinations are still frequently performed by general practitioners as the initial investigation of upper digestive tract symptoms.

A5 The patient has undergone an endoscopic examination of the upper digestive tract. This shows a tumour extending from the mid body of the stomach to the antrum in the distance.

A6 Further investigations are needed to accurately stage the disease and then determine the best treatment options. These include:

CT scan of the abdomen and chest (with intravenous and oral contrast). These scans (particularly spiral scanners) are capable of providing highly accurate information on:
● the primary tumour (size, position and spread into adjacent tissues)
● presence of metastatic disease in lymph nodes, liver or lungs
● presence of ascites.

The CT is less helpful in the detection of peritoneal deposits. If there is evidence of metastatic disease then no further investigations are required. CT has limitations in detecting nodal disease (N stage) and is not very accurate at assessing the

ANSWERS – cont'd

depth of penetration of tumours through the stomach wall (T stage). CT will generally under-stage both the T and N stage in gastric cancer.

Endoscopic ultrasound scanning (EUS) can give accurate information about depth of penetration of the tumour through the stomach wall and also on the extent of any lymph node involvement. Where available, EUS is a useful adjunct to CT in preoperative staging of gastric cancer.

Staging laparoscopy may be useful in detecting small peritoneal deposits. These are common in gastric cancer and cannot be easily detected by CT or EUS.

A7 The treatment of gastric cancer depends on the:
- histopathology on biopsy
- stage of the disease after investigation
- general state of health of the patient
- need to palliate symptoms related to the primary tumour.

Curative treatment may be considered for:
- early gastric cancers
- gastric lymphomas
- some early stage adenocarcinomas.

Treatment options include:
- endoscopic resection of early gastric cancers
- chemotherapy for lymphomas
- surgical intervention for more advanced adenocarcinomas:
  – radical resection for 'cure'
  – resection or bypass for palliation
- palliative care measures.

Very early and localized cancers that have not invaded the gastric submucosa (early gastric cancer) can be removed endoscopically. These sorts of tumours are rare outside Japan.

In most parts of the world the majority of patients with gastric cancer have incurable disease at the time of presentation. In contrast, gastric cancer is relatively common in Japan where screening programmes are used to detect the disease at a much earlier stage and a high percentage of patients are cured by surgery.

While some individuals can be cured of more advanced cancers, the role of surgery is usually to relieve symptoms and palliate obstruction or bleeding. Improved methods of palliation have decreased the need for surgical intervention. These procedures include endoscopic ablation of the tumour by laser or argon beam coagulation. Self-expanding metal stents can be used to relieve obstruction.

A8 The operative view shows the external sur-face of the stomach in the middle of the picture. The left lobe of the liver is top left and the greater omentum to the bottom of the photograph. The antrum of the stomach is thickened and pale white. There is a ridge which separates this tumour in the antrum from the proximal stomach. The tumour appears to involve the whole circumfer-ence of the antrum.

A9 This is a partial gastrectomy specimen in which about two-thirds of the stomach has been removed. The pylorus is to the left. There is thick-ening of the antrum from tumour infiltration. The mucosa in the proximal stomach looks relatively normal, while that in the antrum is thickened and oedematous on the greater curve distorting the stomach. The pale white area is tumour in the wall of the stomach and the tumour has probably infiltrated at this point (T3).

The prognosis for gastric cancer remains poor with overall 5-year survival of between 10–15% in most Western countries. This reflects the advanced stage of the disease at presentation and the increasing age of the population; many patients with gastric cancer are elderly and frail and not suitable for curative surgical treatment. In Japan the overall 5-year survival is 50% or above. This reflects diagnosis at an earlier stage and more effective surgical treatment.

The incidence of gastric cancer is decreasing dramatically in the West. In developing countries the incidence remains high and is particularly so in Japan, China, East Asia and Latin America. The reason for the fall in incidence in the West is related to environmental factors. *Helicobacter pylori* are associated with gastric cancer. The prevalence of *Helicobacter* in Western commu-

ANSWERS – cont'd

nities has steadily declined as public health and hygiene have improved. This has coincided with the reduction in gastric cancer. Dietary changes with an increase in protein relative to carbohydrate, increasing food hygiene and refrigeration and increasing consumption of fresh fruit and vegetables have probably also decreased the incidence of gastric cancer.

The distribution of gastric cancer in the West is changing. Cancers used to be prevalent in the distal stomach. It is these cancers that are becoming less common whereas, for reasons unknown, the incidence of cancers of the cardia (together with adenocarcinoma of the distal oesophagus) has increased dramatically over the last two decades

In surgical series in the West survival for potentially curative surgery is around 50%. Early gastric cancer (confined to the mucosal layer of the stomach) can be cured by surgery but as the tumour spreads through the gastric wall and involves lymph nodes the likelihood of a cure lessens.

REVISION POINTS

Gastric cancer

Incidence
15–17:100 000 in the Western world
Risk factors
- male sex
- *Helicobacter pylori* infection
- dietary factors (smoked foods, etc.)
- pernicious anaemia
- previous partial gastrectomy
- cigarette smoking and alcohol intake.
Histology
- adenocarcinoma (90%)
- lymphomas (6%)
- gastrointestinal stromal tumours (GIST) (4%).
Presentation
Epigastric pain, indigestion, early satiety, weight loss, vomiting, anaemia, abdominal mass. Patients over 50 with new-onset symptoms should be investigated immediately.
Clinical features
Patients with early disease have no obvious signs but patients with advanced disease are often thin (or even cachetic) and pale. Supraclavicular lymph node enlargement, an epigastric mass or ascites are signs of advanced disease.
Prognosis
The overall prognosis for adenocarcinoma is poor with only 10–15% surviving 5 years.
Investigation
- endoscopy and biopsy for diagnosis
- imaging for staging.
Treatment
- resection for cure (gastrectomy)
- surgery, endoscopic intervention or chemotherapy for palliation.

ISSUES TO CONSIDER

- What are the complications associated with gastric resection?

- Why is gastric cancer more common in Japan? Are there any screening tests or preventative strategies which could be useful?

- How may the changing incidence of *Helicobacter pylori* infection be affecting the changing incidence of proximal and gastric cancers?

FURTHER INFORMATION

www.nci.nih.gov/cancer_information/cancer_type/stomach/ A web page from the National Cancer Institute with links providing current information on many different aspects of gastric cancer.

www.surgical-tutor.org.uk A surgical resource with extensive up-to-date information on gastric cancer.

www.helico.com The website of the Helicobacter Foundation founded by Dr Barry Marshall.

Abdominal pain in a young woman

A 30-year-old woman is referred to your clinic with upper abdominal pain. She has had two episodes of severe pain over the last month. During each episode, the pain was of rapid onset. It started in the epigastrium and radiated to the right upper quadrant. She describes the pain as the worst she has ever experienced. On each occasion she was nauseated but did not vomit. Each attack lasted between 3 and 4 hours and did not abate until her GP administered an intramuscular opiate. Following each attack she was left exhausted for a couple of days but soon returned to her normal daily activities.

Q1 What further information would you like from the patient? What are the possible diagnoses?

On examination she is a well-looking, cheerful lady. She weighs 71 kg and is 172 cm tall. Her abdomen is non-tender and without organomegaly or masses. The rest of your examination is unremarkable.

Q2 What investigations does this patient require?

The GP has already performed the following investigation (Figure 17.1).

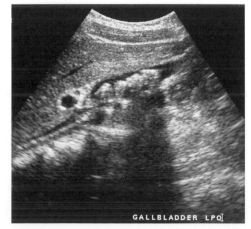

Fig 17.1

GALLBLADDER LPO

Q3 What is this investigation? What does it show?

Urine testing in the clinic does not show any abnormalities. Her liver function tests are unremarkable.

Q4 What advice will you give this woman?

The patient listens to your counsel and agrees to a cholecystectomy. She does not have private medical insurance and is aware that the wait for surgery may be several months.

Three weeks after her visit to your clinic, you are asked to see the patient in the emergency department. She has had further bouts of pain on and off for 2 days and has vomited a number of times. She also reports that her urine has darkened and that her stools are pale. She has not slept well the past 2 nights because of drenching sweats and she reports two violent shivering attacks this morning.

On examination she looks ill and has a temperature of 39.5°. She is flushed and has yellow sclera. Her pulse is 110 bpm and her blood pressure is 110/70 mm Hg. She has dry mucous membranes. Examination of her cardiorespiratory system is unremarkable. Her abdomen is soft and there is no localized area of tenderness.

Q5 What has happened? What investigations will you organize and how will you manage this woman in the emergency department?

The following blood results become available.

Investigation 17.1 Summary of results			
Haemoglobin	145 g/l	White cell count	24.9 x 10^9/l
Platelets	354 x 10^9/l		
Sodium	148 mmol/l	Calcium	2.16 mmol/l
Potassium	4.3 mmol/l	Phosphate	1.15 mmol/l
Chloride	106 mmol/l	Total protein	58 g/l
Bicarbonate	27 mmol/l	Albumin	38 g/l
Urea	15.2 mmol/l	Globulins	20 g/l
Creatinine	0.13 mmol/l	Bilirubin	145 µmol/l
Uric acid	0.24 mmol/l	ALT	118 U/l
Glucose	4.6 mmol/l	AST	123 U/l
Cholesterol	3.5 mmol/l	GGT	397 U/l
LDH	212 U/l	ALP	454 U/l

An ultrasound examination is performed. Figure 17.2 shows a view of the lower part of the common bile duct.

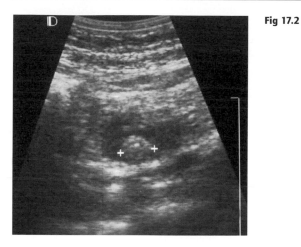

Fig 17.2

 Q6 What does the ultrasound show?

The same investigation shows dilatation of the
intrahepatic biliary system.

Q7 How will these results influence your management? What other results would
you like before proceeding with further investigation?

Her coagulation studies are within normal limits.
She undergoes a further procedure. One image
from this is shown in Figure 17.3.

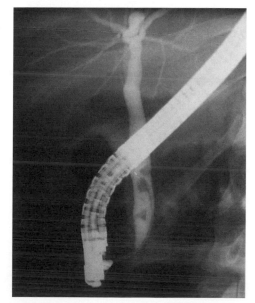

Fig 17.3

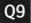 **What is this procedure? What risks would you inform the patient of when seeking consent? What is happening during the procedure?**

Two days after this procedure was performed, the patient feels well and is keen to go home and get back to work. Her jaundice and fever have resolved.

Q9 **What advice would you give this woman now?**

The patient undergoes a laparoscopic cholecystectomy on the next available operating list. The surgery is uneventful and she is discharged home 24 hours after the procedure.

ANSWERS

A1 You would like information on:
- The pain:
  - its nature (constant or colic)
  - radiation (round or through to the back, retrosternal, shoulder, down into abdomen)
  - any relieving or exacerbating features.
- Any associated urinary or gastrointestinal symptoms.
- Any evidence of biliary obstruction during these episodes such as overt jaundice (friends and family may notice), pale stools and dark urine.
- Any past history of gastrointestinal or renal tract problems.

These severe episodes of right upper quadrant pain requiring opiate analgesia are characteristic of biliary colic. The pain will often radiate around the costal margin to the back. Biliary colic results from obstruction of the cystic duct, which typically occurs when a gallstone becomes impacted in Hartmann's pouch. The pain – which is typically unremitting and constant – lasts until the gallstone falls back into the gallbladder and the obstruction is relieved.

Other diagnoses to consider include:
- Myocardial ischaemia or infarction. This woman is very young for an acute cardiac event, but you must remember possible cardiac causes in patients who present with acute epigastric pain.
- Renal stones or ureteric colic. Stones in the renal tract can produce severe upper abdominal and back pain.
- Peptic ulcer disease. The pain is not usually so rapid in onset and is not usually of such severity.
- Oesophageal spasm. Oesophageal pain is usually retrosternal, but this source should always be considered in cases of upper abdominal pain.

A2 The following investigations are required:
- An ultrasound examination of the upper abdomen. The prime objective is to look for gallstones. The examination is performed following a fast, otherwise the gallbladder will be contracted and any stones difficult to see. The thickness of the wall of the gallbladder will also be assessed (thickening may suggest inflammation). The liver parenchyma can be studied and any dilatation of the biliary tree visualized. Renal stones may also be detected, together with any ureteric obstruction.
- Liver function tests looking for evidence of recent or ongoing biliary obstruction.
- Urinalysis to check for haematuria although this is more sensitive for ureteric stones during an acute attack.

ANSWERS – cont'd

A3 This is an image from an ultrasound of the gallbladder showing a thin-walled gallbladder with several echogenic foci which cast acoustic shadows beyond. These are gallstones.

A4 This patient needs the advice that her two episodes of pain were almost certainly biliary in origin.

The ultrasound has confirmed the presence of gallstones and if left untreated, they will most likely give rise to further problems at some time in the future. While gallstones are common and usually asymptomatic, once they do start producing symptoms, the patient will probably face ongoing problems.

Apart from the pain and discomfort caused by these events, there is a significant risk that further episodes will result in serious complications such as biliary obstruction, cholangitis and pancreatitis. Even in the twenty-first century gallstone disease has a significant morbidity and mortality associated with it.

She needs a cholecystectomy. The severity of her symptoms means that this should be done relatively soon. This will almost certainly be undertaken by a laparoscopic approach which, when carried out by experienced laparoscopic surgeons, is safe and minimizes hospital stay and subsequent convalescent time. You must explain to her that if the laparoscopic approach proves difficult or intraoperative complications ensue, the surgeon may need to proceed to an open operation. About 95% of elective cases for gallstone disease will be completed laparoscopically.

If there is any evidence of bile duct obstruction in the history, on ultrasound or on blood testing, the surgeon may choose to organize an endoscopic retrograde cholangiopancreatogram (ERCP) prior to surgery to ensure the bile duct is clear of stones or debris. Alternatively, some surgeons may opt for an intraoperative cholangiogram and laparoscopic exploration of the bile duct in selected cases. In her case, there is nothing to suggest the presence of choledocholithiasis.

A5 She has an obstructed biliary tree causing her jaundice and associated infection within the bile duct (cholangitis). The presence of sweats and rigors indicates that she has a significant bacteraemia. The pale stools and dark urine support your suspicion of biliary obstruction.

Cholangitis can be life threatening. She needs immediate fluid resuscitation, blood cultures and appropriate parenteral antibiotics. Ampicillin is well concentrated in bile and this in combination with a quinolone would be a suitable choice. She needs an urgent ultrasound scan to confirm the presence of biliary obstruction. You should check her complete blood picture, liver function tests, renal function and electrolytes. She will likely need an urgent ERCP to relieve the obstruction and achieve biliary drainage so you should contact the gastroenterologists or biliary surgeons.

If she is unstable she will need admission to a high dependency unit.

A6 The ultrasound reveals a stone at the lower end of the common bile duct. Its diameter is about 8 mm.

A7 The high white cell count is in keeping with her clinical infection. She is dehydrated and has mild renal impairment and therefore needs close attention paid to her fluid balance. Her liver function tests are cholestatic, consistent with biliary obstruction.

You would like to know her INR before proceeding with an ERCP. If a sphincterotomy is performed in the presence of impaired clotting then the risk of significant haemorrhage is greatly increased.

It is important to monitor the results of her blood cultures to ensure that she is on appropriate antibiotic therapy.

A8 This is an endoscopic retrograde cholangiopancreatography (ERCP). The instrument used is a side-viewing video endoscope. There is a specialized channel through which catheters, balloons and other instruments can be inserted into the duodenum. A 'bridge' controlled by the endoscopist allows accurate manipulation of these instruments for cannulation of the common bile duct and pancreatic duct.

In obtaining informed consent for ERCP, you need to explain the rationale for the procedure and its potential risks and benefits. The aim of

ANSWERS – cont'd

the procedure is to decompress the common bile duct and get sepsis under control. The endoscopist may place a stent into the common bile duct and/or may be able to retrieve the stone. The benefit of the ERCP in the present circumstances is that, if successful, the patient may be able to avoid major and hazardous open surgery to her common bile duct. The main risks of ERCP are pancreatitis (1–5%) and haemorrhage (1–2%). Both of these complications can be life threatening and are more common when there is prolonged instrumentation of the biliary tree as in complex cases like these. There is a also a small risk of a retroperitoneal perforation following sphincterotomy and the patient must be informed of these risks in addition to the risks of sedation or anaesthesia needed to carry out the ERCP. In the present circumstances, the potential benefits of ERCP far outweigh the risks.

The image shows opacification of the biliary tree with contrast in the common bile duct and the intrahepatic system. At least two stones can be seen in the common bile duct. A catheter with a balloon tip has been introduced into the common bile duct and the balloon inflated in preparation to extracting the stones. In preparation to removing the calculi, the endoscopist will have made a cut through the sphincter of Oddi using diathermy. This procedure is known as a sphincterotomy.

A9 This woman has had a very serious complication of her gallstone disease. Despite the successful ERCP and sphincterotomy she remains at high risk of further complications. She should have a cholecystectomy at the earliest opportunity, preferably during this admission.

REVISION POINTS

Gallstones

Incidence
- common worldwide (except Africa). Rates vary from 5–36%
- increasing in the Western world possibly due to diet, obesity and an ageing population.

Risk factors
- female sex (3x)
- obesity
- hyperlipidaemia
- diabetes mellitus
- ileal disease
- haemolysis.

Intraductal parasites are an important cause in some parts of the developing world.

Types
- most stones are a mixture of cholesterol and bile pigment. Pure cholesterol or pure bile pigment stones are uncommon but do occur
- most stones in developed countries are predominantly cholesterol
- the exact mechanism of cholesterol stone formation is unknown but may involve mucous

proteins from the gallbladder wall promoting crystal formation
- predominant bile pigment stones are found in patients with haemolysis and parasitic infection.

Clinical presentation
Problems may relate to:
- stones in the gallbladder:
  - biliary colic
  - acute cholecystitis
  - carcinoma (rare)
- stones in the ductal system:
  - jaundice
  - cholangitis
  - acute pancreatitis
- stones in the small intestine:
  - gallstone ileus (rare).

The vast majority of gallstones are asymptomatic. 15% of patients with gallstones will also have duct stones. Stones in the common bile duct tend to produce symptoms. What is sometimes labelled 'chronic cholecystitis' is more likely to represent

continues overleaf

REVISION POINTS – cont'd

something within the spectrum of functional gut disorders and the gallstones found on investigation of these patients are merely coincidental.

Imaging studies
- gallstones:
  - abdominal ultrasonography (90% sensitivity)
- duct stones:
  - abdominal ultrasonography (50% sensitivity)
  - ERCP
  - transhepatic cholangiography
  - magnetic resonance cholangiopancreatography (MRCP).

Treatment
- Laparoscopic cholecystectomy.

A balance must be reached between the risk of surgery and the potential benefit to the patient.

The patient must be fully involved in the decision-making process. Treatment should be recommended for patients who have developed symptomatic gallstones.

In acute cholecystitis, initial treatment should be conservative with pain relief, intravenous rehydration and, if not settling, antibiotics. Cholecystectomy should then be performed at the earliest opportunity.

- Ductal calculi should be managed initially with ERCP or in selected cases, transhepatic cholangiography or laparoscopic bile duct exploration.
- Dissolution therapy with urso- or chenodeoxycholic acid is suitable only for a very small proportion of patients with small stones and has largely been superseded by laparoscopic cholecystectomy.

ISSUES TO CONSIDER

- What are the constituents of normal bile? How do alterations in the balance of these constituents predispose to gallstone formation?

- What other conditions may mimic the pain of gallstone disease?

- Are there any circumstances where patients with asymptomatic gallstones should be advised to have a cholecystectomy?

FURTHER INFORMATION

www.laparoscopy.com An interesting website with information and links to many aspects of laparoscopic surgery including the history of the technique.

www.gastro.org/public/brochures/gallstones. html Up-to-date information on gallstones with a patient slant from the American Gastroenterological Society.

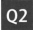

PROBLEM

18

A man with acute upper abdominal pain

A 56-year-old salesman is admitted with an 18-hour history of severe upper abdominal pain, which started in the epigastrium, went through to the back and gradually increased in severity. The pain is constant and is associated with anorexia, nausea and vomiting. His bowels have been normal and he has no other symptoms. The previous day he had been at a wedding and he tells you he 'really cut the rug'. On further questioning you establish that this involved consuming considerable amounts of alcohol. He drinks regularly and gets through a bottle of whisky every week. He also tells you that he drinks 'a little more' on weekends and you note that 'the weekend starts on Thursday'. He does not smoke and is on no medications. There is no other past history of note. On examination he looks ill. He is apyrexial but looks dehydrated. His pulse rate is 110 and regular and his blood pressure is 160/ 90 mm Hg. Cardiorespiratory examination is unremarkable. His abdomen is distended and he is tender in the epigastrium. There are no masses and the bowel sounds are normal.

Q1 Briefly discuss the differential diagnoses.

After your initial history and examination you cannot be sure of the diagnosis and order some investigations.

Q2 What are the initial investigations you require, and what are you seeking with each investigation?

The patient's ECG, chest X-ray and plain abdominal X-ray are normal. The blood tests are shown in Investigation 18.1.

Investigation 18.1 Summary of results			
Haemoglobin	178 g/l	White cell count	14.3 x 10⁹/l
Platelets	324 x 10⁹/l		
Sodium	143 mmol/l	Calcium	2.1 mmol/l
Potassium	3.2 mmol/l	Phosphate	1.2 mmol/l
Chloride	101 mmol/l	Total protein	62 g/l
Bicarbonate	28 mmol/l	Albumin	35 g/l
Urea	7.1 mmol/l	Globulins	27 g/l
Creatinine	0.12 mmol/l	Bilirubin	18 μmol/l
Uric acid	0.24 mmol/l	ALT	29 U/l
Glucose	11.0 mmol/l	AST	44 U/l
Cholesterol	3.5 mmol/l	GGT	110 U/l
Amylase	1875 U/l	ALP	54 U/l
LDH	212 U/l		

Q3 What do these results tell you? What is the likely diagnosis? What other investigations would you like?

The arterial blood gas analysis on inspired room-air shows the following values.

Investigation 18.2 Arterial blood gas analysis			
pO₂	64 mm Hg	pCO₂	36 mm Hg
pH	7.42	Calculated bicarbonate	30 mmol/l

Q4 How would you manage this patient?

Initially, the patient is nursed in the high dependency unit and his condition gradually improves.

Q5 What is the likely underlying cause of his pancreatitis? What investigations should be performed to help you decide this? What is the next stage in his management?

An abdominal ultrasound scan shows a normal biliary tree with no gallstones.

Although the patient's general condition improves, his abdominal pain does not settle and a CT scan is arranged (Figure 18.1).

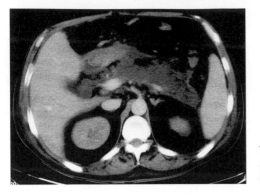

Fig 18.1

Two weeks later a fullness is noticed in his epigastrium. Results of biochemical and haematological investigations now show:

Investigation 18.3 Summary of results			
Haemoglobin	150 g/l	White cell count	8.2 x 10⁹/l
Platelets	540 x 10⁹/l		
Sodium	138 mmol/l	Calcium	2.1 mmol/l
Potassium	3.5 mmol/l	Phosphate	1.2 mmol/l
Chloride	103 mmol/l	Total protein	58 g/l
Bicarbonate	26 mmol/l	Albumin	32 g/l
Urea	5.2 mmol/l	Globulins	26 g/l
Creatinine	0.08 mmol/l	Bilirubin	18 μmol/l
Uric acid	0.24 mmol/l	ALT	29 U/l
Glucose	6.4 mmol/l	AST	42 U/l
Cholesterol	3.5 mmol/l	GGT	93 U/l
Amylase	700 U/l	ALP	63 U/l
LDH	212 U/l		

A repeat CT examination of his upper abdomen is performed (Figure 18.2).

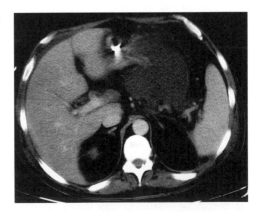

Fig 18.2

 Q6 What do the CT scans show? How have they changed? What do the blood tests add?

Q7 How should this problem be managed?

Six weeks after his discharge a repeat ultrasound showed a normal biliary tract again, with no evidence of gallstones, but there was persistence of the pseudocyst. Percutaneous radiological drainage was attempted, but this failed, and the patient went on to surgical drainage. At laparotomy a cystogastrostomy was performed, following which the patient made an uneventful recovery and the pseudocyst resolved. The serum amylase returned to normal.

Q8 What else needs to be done in this patient's management?

ANSWERS

A1 The likely diagnoses to explain this man's illness include acute pancreatitis, perforated peptic ulcer, acute cholecystitis and myocardial infarction. Progressive upper abdominal pain and vomiting in a heavy drinker, particularly after a binge, makes acute pancreatitis the most probable diagnosis. A perforated peptic ulcer is less likely as the onset is typically sudden and the patient would almost certainly have a rigid abdomen. Acute cholecystitis is also less likely, but gallstone disease is common in developed countries and must always be considered. Similarly, the possibility of myocardial infarction, particularly an inferior infarct, must always be borne in mind in cases of epigastric pain and vomiting.

Other possible diagnoses include ischaemic gut, strangulated bowel and intestinal obstruction. Intestinal ischaemia is always a difficult diagnosis to make. It is most often seen in patients with severe vascular disease, or occasionally atrial fibrillation, and vomiting is not usually a major component of the illness.

A2 At an early stage you are going to require the following investigations:
- ECG: to exclude acute myocardial infarction
- serum amylase: hyperamylasaemia of acute pancreatitis
- erect chest X-ray: possible gas under the diaphragm
- complete blood count: look for evidence of inflammation (elevated white cell count)

- serum biochemistry: possible electrolyte disturbance secondary to vomiting.

A3 This patient has acute pancreatitis. The elevated blood sugar level and the white cell count are in keeping with pancreatitis. The creatinine and haemoglobin values are raised, reflecting dehydration. A hyperamylasaemia of this degree is virtually diagnostic of acute pancreatitis, but lesser elevations may be associated with several other acute intra-abdominal conditions including acute cholecystitis and ischaemic gut. The degree of hyperamylasaemia does not correlate with the severity of the pancreatitis. His chest X-ray is normal, but there is often a small sympathetic left pleural effusion.

A full biochemical screen is required for estimation of liver enzymes and calcium. Also required is arterial blood gas analysis to detect any hypoxia, which is common in acute pancreatitis. The GGT is slightly elevated and this is suggestive of alcohol abuse as the underlying cause of his acute pancreatitis.

A4 The patient needs to be resuscitated and given intravenous fluids. Commence with an infusion of isotonic saline. He is dehydrated now and over the next few days may continue to lose large volumes of fluid, as the acute inflammatory condition will promote fluid accumulation around the swollen pancreas and within the paralysed loops of intestine. He may need many

ANSWERS – cont'd

litres of intravenous fluid and will require insertion of a central venous catheter to facilitate fluid replacement and medications and also to monitor his central venous pressure.

A nasogastric tube is inserted and put on free drainage to relieve vomiting and he is kept fasted to rest the gut. He requires opiate analgesia. His hypoxia should be treated with, e.g., nasal cannulae 2–4 l/min with monitoring by pulse oximeter.

The patient will also need regular monitoring of electrolytes, including calcium, blood sugar, and white cell count. A degree of hypocalcaemia and hyperglycaemia is common, and usually these problems will correct themselves as the patient's condition improves. In severe attacks of acute pancreatitis, the patient may require intravenous supplements of calcium.

Given his alcohol use it would be reasonable to give intravenous thiamine.

The severity of this patient's illness suggests that the patient may be best managed in an intensive care unit and these arrangements should be made early.

Consideration needs to be given to starting parenteral nutrition.

A5 Provided the patient's condition does not deteriorate, ultrasonography is performed as a semi-urgent measure to look for gallstones as a possible cause. In this case, provided the ultrasound scan is normal, as there is a history of alcohol abuse, it is reasonable to assume that alcohol is the likely cause of his pancreatitis. If the patient's condition worsens, a CT scan will be required to assess the perfusion of the pancreas.

A6 Figure 18.1 shows a severely oedematous pancreas – a phlegmon. He then has a persistent hyperamylasaemia and a non-tender mass in his upper abdomen both of which suggest the development of a pancreatic pseudocyst. Figure 18.2 shows a collapsed stomach with a large loculated cyst behind it (in the region of the body of the pancreas). The patient has no evidence of sepsis, either clinically or haematologically. This is a pancreatic pseudocyst as opposed to a pancreatic abscess.

A7 About 20% of pancreatic pseudocysts resolve spontaneously within 6 weeks. So long as the patient remains well, no active intervention is needed. If the cyst does not resolve, it will need to be drained. In the first instance, percutaneous needle aspiration and drainage can be attempted. If this does not succeed, some form of internal drainage, either into the stomach or jejunum, may be required.

A8 This illness has been caused by abuse of alcohol. The patient needs to be counselled to stop drinking alcohol – ideally, he should stop altogether. Often this requires ongoing counselling and groups such as Alcoholics Anonymous can be extremely valuable.

REVISION POINTS

Acute pancreatitis

Causes
Gallstones, alcohol, iatrogenic (ERCP/surgery), viral illness (e.g. mumps), hypercalcaemia, hyperlipidaemia, drugs, idiopathic.

Presentation
Upper abdominal pain, nausea, vomiting and anorexia.

Investigations
Initial:
- ECG to exclude cardiac cause

- erect CXR to exclude visceral perforation
- serum amylase to confirm diagnosis.

Subsequent:
- ultrasound to look for gallstones as a cause
- CT scan to assess pancreatic perfusion.

Treatment
- supportive (i.e. resuscitation) analgesia, assess severity, determine cause
- rarely surgery (delayed cholecystectomy for gallstones, laparotomy and necrosectomy if dead pancreas).

continues overleaf

REVISION POINTS – cont'd

Prediction of severity
- Ranson's criteria: (3 or more = severe–30% mortality)
- on admission
  - age >55 years
  - white cell count >16 x 10^9/l
  - blood glucose >12 mmol/l
  - serum LDH >350 U/l
  - serum AST >250 U/l
- changes at 48 hours
  - fall in haematocrit >10%
  - fluid requirement >6 l
  - calcium <2.0 mmol/l
  - arterial pO_2 <60 mm Hg
  - blood urea >10 mmol/l
  - base deficit >4 mmol/l.

Complications
Usually none, occasionally respiratory/renal failure, coagulopathy, prolonged ileus, upper GI tract haemorrhage, pancreatic abscess/necrosis, pseudocyst.

Prognosis
Usually benign and resolves spontaneously, overall mortality 10%, death usually due to haemorrhagic/necrotizing pancreatitis (mortality 70–90%).

ISSUES TO CONSIDER

- What are the chances of this man developing chronic pancreatitis?
- What would you advise him to do about his drinking? Should he give up altogether?
- What is the risk of pancreatitis following an ERCP?

FURTHER INFORMATION

www.emedicine.com/EMERG/topic354.htm
A comprehensive discourse on pancreatitis from the emedicine series.

A woman with acute upper abdominal pain

A 45-year-old woman comes into the emergency department with right upper quadrant and flank pain. 'I feel ill,' she tells you, 'I've had this pain for about 5 hours and it's made me throw up. I thought I had gastro, but it won't stop. Can you give me something?'

The patient describes spasms of severe pain lasting 10 minutes with moderate pain in between. The pain is much worse than 'when I bust my leg last year'. Her symptoms have been associated with episodes of nausea and uncontrolled vomiting She has mild hypertension and smokes 25 cigarettes a day. Apart from her fractured femur, her last presentation to hospital was 17 years ago for the birth of her fourth child.

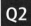 **Q1** What are the differential diagnoses and likely causes for her illness?

She does not suffer with dyspepsia, is not on any medications, and drinks 'only a couple of beers a day, doc'.

The patient looks unwell and is in pain. She has a temperature of 37.5°C and is dehydrated. Her blood pressure is 140/90 mm Hg and her pulse rate is 100 bpm. Examination of her cardiorespiratory system is unremarkable. Her abdomen is soft and there is no evidence of peritonitis. You think the most likely diagnosis at this stage is biliary colic.

You insert an intravenous cannula into an arm vein and put up 1 litre isotonic saline to run in over 1 hour.

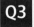 **Q2** What do you do next and why?

Blood is taken for serum troponin estimation and an ECG is performed (Figure 19.1).

Q3 What does the ECG show?

You note the result of the ECG and plan the next step.

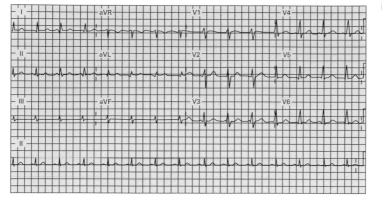

Fig 19.1

Q4   What will you do next?

While you were arranging the next investigations, the serum troponin estimation is faxed through to you. It is normal.

The chest X-ray is unremarkable and there is no free gas under the diaphragm. The abdominal X-ray is shown in Figure 19.2.

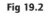

Fig 19.2

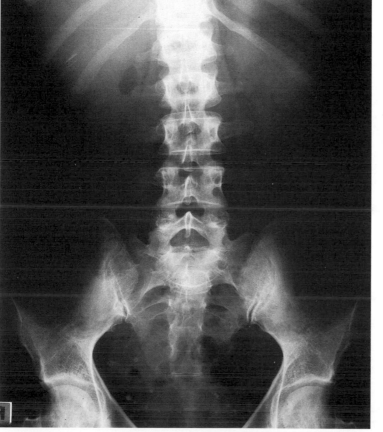

Q5 How do you go about interpreting this X-ray and what abnormalities does it show?

None of your investigations have helped. The beta HCG is negative and the white cell count is at the upper margin of normal. The serum lipase is normal and her biochemistry unremarkable. Puzzled, you turn to the urinalysis. It reveals a large amount of blood and a few leucocytes.

Q6 What are you going to do next and why?

Another investigation is arranged. Two of the films are shown (Figures 19.3 and 19.4).

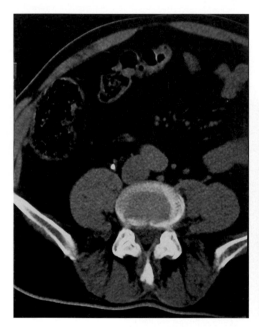

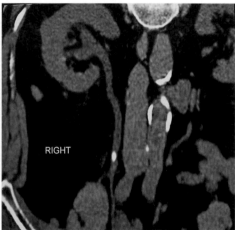

RIGHT

Fig 19.3

Fig 19.4

Q7 What do the films show and what should you look for on the scan?

Now you have the diagnosis.

Q8 How will you manage this patient in the acute setting?

After 4 hours the pain has not improved and you decide to admit the patient. While you are making arrangements for this, you give some thought to that stone travelling down the ureter.

Where in the renal tract do calculi typically become impacted?

Your patient asks if you can perform surgery to 'get rid of this stone'.

 In what circumstances would the urologist consider urgent intervention?

Q11 What are the management options of nephrolithiasis?

The patient passed her stone spontaneously 24 hours after admission and was back at her work 3 days later.

The patient did not give a personal or family history of stone disease. Her serum calcium was normal and urine culture was sterile. You give her advice to stay well hydrated as well as instructions concerning her diet to prevent further stone formation.

ANSWERS

A1 There are several ways of constructing your list of possible aetiologies:
- 'common things occur commonly', i.e. starting with the most common diagnosis consistent with the presentation (used by experienced clinicians)
- anatomical location of symptoms
- the pathological process (i.e. the 'surgical sieve').

The patient is describing episodes of colicky pain. This suggests that the primary underlying pathological process is obstruction rather than inflammation. Common causes would include:
- biliary disease (i.e. biliary 'colic')
- renal colic
- small bowel obstruction.

If you consider the anatomical location, the possibilities include:
- intra-abdominal
- gastrointestinal tract
  - peptic ulcer disease
  - hepatitis
  - biliary obstruction, cholecystitis
  - pancreatitis
  - diverticulitis
  - appendicitis
  - bowel obstruction

- urinary
  - renal (stone)
  - ureter (stone)
- chest
  - pulmonary: pneumonia
  - cardiac: infarct, ischaemia
  - oesophagus: oesophagitis, spasm.

The pathological approach is to categorize the process according to whether it may be congenital or acquired.

If acquired: obstruction of hollow viscus, which may be the result of:
- trauma
- neoplastic
- inflammatory
- metabolic
- infectious
- degenerative
- iatrogenic
- factitious.

A2 This woman has acute onset of upper abdominal pain. The most sinister of all the possible diagnoses you have considered is myocardial disease. This patient needs an ECG.

ANSWERS – cont'd

A3 The ECG is normal.

A4 The following investigations are required:
- complete blood picture
- serum biochemistry (electrolytes, liver function tests)
- serum lipase (or amylase)
- urine analysis
- chest and abdominal radiographs.

A leucocytosis, raised liver enzymes and abnormal lipase may all help towards a diagnosis, but will not necessarily be conclusive. It is also wise to perform a serum beta-HCG estimation on any woman of childbearing age who presents to the emergency department with acute abdominal pain.

A 'dipstick' test is used to measure pH and to look for protein, blood, sugar, ketones, nitrates and leucocytes. Urine can be sent to the laboratory for examination for cells, casts and bacteria and for culture.

A5 A systematic examination of a plain abdominal X-ray should be performed in the following order:
- *Bony structures*. Look for fractures, degenerative problems and metastatic deposits.
- *Soft tissues*. In a thin patient the psoas muscles and the kidneys can be visualized.
- *Gas patterns*. Gas is normally found in the stomach, colon and rectum. Gas in the small bowel is suggestive of intestinal obstruction. Gas outside the intestine is pathological. Abnormal sites include the liver (infection or biliary–enteric communication), bladder (infection or colovesical fistula) or peritoneum (intestinal perforation). When the patient sits up, free gas in the peritoneum will accumulate under the diaphragm and is best seen on the chest X-ray.
- *Calcification*. This may be due to degeneration, chronic infection (TB), stone formation or rarely, tumours. Some important sites and causes include: vascular calcification (aorta, splenic artery and pelvic veins), lymph nodes (TB), renal tract (stones).

In Figure 19.2 the bony structures appear normal. The renal outlines and psoas shadows are normal. There is a paucity of gas and it is appropriately distributed. There are small areas of calcification in the pelvis. Most of these are probably phleboliths. The tooth-shaped structure in the right side of the pelvis is probably within an ovarian dermoid.

A6 This woman appears to be in severe pain, she has blood in her urine, and a number of opacities in her pelvis, many of which may be phleboliths; there is the possibility of a ureteric stone. She needs further investigation and a high-resolution, non-contrast helical (spiral) CT scan of the abdomen is warranted, looking for renal and ureteric calculi.

A7 The spiral CT scan shows a stone in the right ureter. In the axial film the stone is visible as a white opacity immediately anterior to the right psoas muscle. In the sagittal section, the stone can be clearly seen within the ureter. There is some proximal dilatation of the ureter.

In patients with ureteric colic, look for the following changes:
- primary changes
  - stone
  - dilatation of the affected ureter
  - hydronephrosis
- secondary changes
  - peri-renal stranding
  - peri-ureteric stranding.

A8 The patient requires analgesia. Renal colic can be excruciatingly painful. As you are confident she has ureteric colic an opiate is appropriate. Parenteral NSAIDs (e.g. ketorolac or toradol) have also been shown to be as effective as narcotics in reducing symptoms of ureteric colic. NSAIDs can also be given rectally, e.g. indometacin suppositories. These can be considered if there is suspicion of drug-seeking behaviour. Remember, NSAIDs can have adverse effects and should be avoided with older patients, dehydration or patients with renal impairment or asthma.

Intravenous antiemetics should be given to stop vomiting. You have already started fluid replacement and this will need to be modified

ANSWERS – cont'd

depending on further losses (vomiting). She will also require maintenance fluids (approximately 100 ml/h).

Instructions must be given to collect and strain all urine specimens to look for a stone.

Inform the patient that she has a stone which is 'like a small piece of gravel which is passing from the kidney down to the bladder'. Reassure her that the pain will stop when the stone has passed. Tell her that although this is very painful it is usually not dangerous as most stones will pass by themselves. Tell her that for the moment you will keep her under observation and give her painkillers. You should appreciate that patients who have received narcotics and even intravenous antiemetics often do not remember anything you say and the information may need to be repeated. Also, even if the stone passes soon, she will not be able to drive home due to the after-effects of the medication. Get the nursing staff to contact a friend or relative.

A9 There are three locations in the renal tract where stones typically become impacted. They are:
- the junction of the renal pelvis and ureter (PUJ)
- where the ureters cross the pelvic brim
- at the junction of the ureter and the bladder (VUJ).

A10 Surgical intervention for renal tract stone disease is undertaken in the following circumstances.
- absolute indications
  - worsening renal function
  - urinary infection unresponsive to antibiotics
  - sepsis from an obstructed kidney
- relative indications
  - patient unable to pass a large stone

- persistent pain
- pregnancy
- solitary kidney
- diabetes
- evidence of damage to the urinary tract with extravasation of urine.

The position and size of the stone must be considered in planning management of this patient. Stones smaller than 4 mm have a 90% chance of passing spontaneously, while larger stones of greater than 6 mm will only pass without intervention in 20% of cases. Calculi in the proximal ureter are less likely to pass than those in the distal ureter.

A11 Renal tract stones may be managed by several techniques:
- extracorporeal shock wave lithotripsy (ESWL)
  - high pressure shock waves result in fragmentation of stones
  - non-invasive treatment of choice of upper ureteric and renal calculi
- ureteroscopy (flexible or rigid)
  - traditionally used for lower and mid ureteric stones but now with the flexible ureteroscope and holmium laser it is commonly used throughout the collecting system
- percutaneous nephrolithotomy (PCNL)
  - used for large stone burden or those unresponsive to ESWL
- open surgery
  - now rarely performed
  - used if endourologic procedures failed or to correct underlying anatomical abnormality
- chemolysis
  - cystine, struvite and uric acid stones may be dissolved by modifying the urine
  - used less commonly due to the development of ESWL and improvements in endourology.

REVISION POINTS

Stones

Composition
- calcium oxalate 45%
- calcium phosphate 10%

- mixed calcium oxalate and calcium phosphate 15%
- magnesium ammonium phosphate 10%
  - struvite/infective stone

continues overleaf

REVISION POINTS – cont'd

- uric acid 15%
- cystine 2%
- other 3%
  - xanthine, silicates and drug metabolites.

The majority of stones can be seen on a plain X-ray except uric acid, xanthine and pure cystine stones.

Epidemiology

- annual incidence of nephrolithiasis is 200:100 000
- males have 3 times the incidence of females: lifetime incidence 7–10% males, 2–3% females
- calcium stones are the most common form of stones in males
- infective (struvite) stones are the most common in females.

Evaluation following first episode of renal colic

- medical history:
  - systemic disease causing metabolic abnormality
  - previous stones and family history
  - medication
  - occupation
- serum chemistry including calcium:
  - if calcium elevated, measure parathyroid hormone

- stone analysis if available
- uric acid
- mid-stream urine:
  - urine culture
  - urine pH
  - crystalluria
- identify if other stones present:
  - spiral CT scan.

Additional evaluation for recurrent stone formers

In recurrent stone formers a 24-hour urine should also be performed, measuring calcium, oxalate, magnesium, citrate, creatinine, sodium, uric acid and citrate.

A spot cystine should be performed.

These patients should be sent for specialist assessment.

Principles of prevention

- high fluid intake (encourage patients to have urine the colour of 'gin' and not 'whisky')
- restrict animal protein consumption
- low sodium diet
- avoid stone-provoking medication
- specific medical therapy dependent on results of previous investigations.

ISSUES TO CONSIDER

- What specific dietary advice would you give to patients to avoid recurrent stones?
- What organisms are likely to be involved in an infection caused by an obstructed kidney? How do you manage pyelonephritis?

FURTHER INFORMATION

www.emedicine.com/emerg/topic621.htm
A website on imaging in patients with acute abdominal pain.

A 67-year-old woman with acute lower abdominal pain

A 67-year-old woman presents to the emergency department with severe lower abdominal pain. The pain is constant in nature and maximal in the left side of the abdomen. The pain has been gradually increasing over 48 hours, and she has passed several loose stools over the last 24 hours. Over the last 3 years she has suffered occasional bouts of mild intermittent left-sided abdominal pain. Her past history is otherwise unremarkable except for an appendicectomy 20 years previously. Her bowel function is normally constipated and she takes a variety of laxatives.

On examination she is flushed and looks unwell. She has a temperature of 38.4°C, a pulse of 115 bpm and a blood pressure of 130/95 mm Hg. Her abdomen is not distended, and there are no signs of peritonism. You are able to palpate a tender, non-pulsatile mass in the left iliac fossa. The mass measures 10 cm in maximum diameter. Rectal examination reveals soft brown-coloured stool.

Q1 What is the likely diagnosis and what investigations are you going to undertake?

Her abdominal X-ray is normal, and her blood picture is shown below.

Investigation 20.1 Summary of results			
Haemoglobin	127 g/l	White cell count	16.3 x 10⁹/l
Platelets	289 x 10⁹/l		
Sodium	138 mmol/l	Calcium	2.14 mmol/l
Potassium	3.8 mmol/l	Phosphate	1.17 mmol/l
Chloride	106 mmol/l	Total protein	66 g/l
Bicarbonate	27 mmol/l	Albumin	39 g/l
Urea	6.8 mmol/l	Globulins	27 g/l
Creatinine	0.12 mmol/l	Bilirubin	22 μmol/l
Uric acid	0.24 mmol/l	ALT	22 U/l
Glucose	5.3 mmol/l	AST	34 U/l
Cholesterol	3.4 mmol/l	GGT	43 U/l
LDH	212 U/l	ALP	87 U/l
Lipase	33 U/l		

Q2 How do these tests help you and what is your management plan?

The patient is started on antibiotic therapy. Oral intake is prohibited except for ice-chips and she is given intravenous fluids. She is given pethidine for analgesia.

Six months previously her general practitioner had arranged for the patient to have some X-rays performed for investigation of her prior bouts of abdominal pain. Two representative images are shown in Figures 20.1 and 20.2.

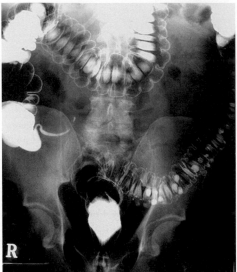

Fig 20.1

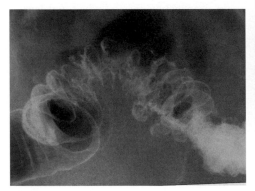

Fig 20.2

Q3 What is this investigation and what does it show?

As a result of this investigation, she underwent a further test (Figure 20.3).

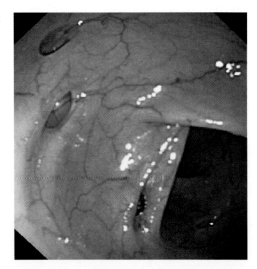

Fig 20.3

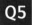

Q4   What is the investigation and what is shown?

Over the next 2 days the patient's condition worsened and her abdomen becomes more tender with signs of peritonitis.

Q5   What would you like to do now?

It is decided to undertake an exploratory laparotomy. She is found to have a mass in the sigmoid colon and a purulent exudate in the lower half of the peritoneal cavity amounting to 300 ml turbid fluid. The diseased region of the sigmoid colon is resected and the proximal end brought to the skin surface as an end colostomy and the distal end closed (the so-called Hartmann's procedure).

Histological examination of the specimen confirms the presence of a pericolic abscess secondary to diverticular disease. There is no evidence of malignancy. The patient makes an uneventful postoperative recovery.

Q6   What information and advice will the patient need on discharge?

ANSWERS

A1 She almost certainly has diverticulitis complicated by a pericolic abscess. Differential diagnoses include infective colitis, urinary tract infection and a perforated sigmoid carcinoma.

You should take blood and secure intravenous access. Blood tests should be sent for culture, full blood count, electrolytes and amylase. Bedside urinalysis should be performed. Urine and stool should be sent for microscopy and culture. If she were of childbearing age she would need a pregnancy test.

An erect chest X-ray is needed to exclude air under the diaphragm, which would indicate bowel perforation.

A supine abdominal X-ray is usually normal in diverticular disease, but is necessary to exclude other causes of abdominal pain (e.g. dilated loops of intestine in acute obstruction).

A2 The raised white cell count is consistent with an infective cause. A normal lipase rules out pancreatitis, which would be a very unlikely diagnosis with this presentation.

Treatment should be with intravenous fluids and antibiotics. Antibiotic therapy should be targeted at sepsis secondary to faecal organisms. A suitable regimen would be a broad-spectrum cephalosporin plus metronidazole. Local guidelines for antibiotic use should be consulted.

Oral intake should be stopped and she may require a nasogastric tube if persistent vomiting is a feature.

Opiate analgesia is often necessary in the acute stages of the illness

A senior surgeon should be consulted.

A3 These films are from a double-contrast barium enema series. Figure 20.2 is a close-up view of the sigmoid region.

There is extensive diverticular disease seen in the colon, particularly in the sigmoid colon. The appendix has been outlined with barium.

A4 The investigation is a flexible sigmoidoscopy. It enables a closer examination of the sigmoid colon, and an opportunity to take biopsies if

ANSWERS – cont'd

there is still any doubt as to the aetiology of the stricture. On this endoscopic view, several diverticulae can be seen: one is plugged by a faecal pellet. There is no evidence of malignancy.

A5 Most cases of pericolic abscess formation can be treated expectantly and will settle on conservative management.

If there is any doubt about the diagnosis, ultrasound examination may be undertaken to look for a fluid- and gas-filled cavity. Alternatively, a CT scan can also provide further useful information. It is not wise to perform a barium enema at this stage as the introduction of air and contrast under pressure could result in perforation of the abscess.

The patient's temperature, vital signs and abdomen must be kept under regular review for evidence of progression or free perforation.

In the majority of instances the abscess will discharge spontaneously into the colon. Provided the condition settles spontaneously, the preferred further investigation will be a colonoscopy performed when the patient has fully recovered.

If the pain and tenderness persist or worsen, operative intervention may be required.

If there is any doubt about the cause of the pericolic abscess, the patient may require flexible sigmoidoscopy or colonoscopy. Most cases of pericolic abscess formation result from diverticular disease, but are occasionally due to malignancy or Crohn's disease.

A6 The patient will need advice and information as follows:
- How to manage her stoma, with ongoing support from stomal therapy nursing services.
- Reassurance that bowel continuity can be restored.
- How to make arrangements for follow-up in the surgical clinic.
- Reassurance that any consideration of further surgery will be left until she has made a full recovery from this illness and the inflammatory process has resolved (this may be in 3–6 months' time).
- Advice on maintaining a high-fibre diet to try and minimize further problems related to her diverticular disease.

REVISION POINTS

Diverticular disease

Epidemiology
Common disorder of the large bowel in Western communities. Probably caused by chronic lack of non-digestible material (fibre) in the diet. High prevalence in societies which consume low-residue diets and virtually unknown in communities which depend on high-roughage foodstuffs. In the developed world it has been estimated that 10% of individuals have developed diverticulosis by the age of 40, and 70% have the condition by the age of 80.

Nomenclature
- Diverticulum: saccular, full-thickness protrusion of the bowel wall.
- Diverticula: plural of diverticulum.

- Diverticulosis: merely the presence of diverticula, and may be asymptomatic.
- Diverticular disease: symptomatic diverticulosis.
- Diverticulitis: inflammation of one or more diverticula.

Pathogenesis
The colonic lumen has pre-existing weak points situated where nutrient blood vessels penetrate through to the mucosa from the serosal surface. Increased intraluminal pressure may lead to herniation of the mucosa through the circular muscle and serosa leading to diverticula formation.

Distribution
May occur in any part of the colon but most often seen in the sigmoid.

continues overleaf

REVISION POINTS — cont'd

Clinical features

Asymptomatic in the majority. Problems may be acute or chronic. The most common symptom is chronic constipation with mild left iliac fossa pain. These patients can be helped with bulk laxatives and stool-softening agents.

Complications

Acute complications include inflammation, abscess formation, perforation, fistula, haemorrhage and, occasionally, total luminal obstruction.

Treatment

- Gut rest, antibiotics and analgesics.
- Abscess formation may be due to obstruction of the diverticulum and bacterial overgrowth within it. Usually the abscess discharges into the colon but when perforation and peritonitis occur, there is a very high mortality.
- Chronic inflammatory change may produce fistula formation, e.g. into bladder leading to recurrent urinary tract infection and pneumaturia, or vagina leading to faeculent discharge.
- Treatment is via faecal stream diversion and closure of fistula.
- Haemorrhage results from a small abscess eroding into an artery in the bowel wall, leading to brisk rectal bleeding. Normally this stops spontaneously.
- Stricture formation is common, but frank intestinal obstruction relatively rare.

ISSUES TO CONSIDER

- What laxatives are commonly used in the treatment of troublesome diverticular disease? What classes of laxatives exist and in what situations should they be used?
- Discuss the differential diagnoses of strictures within the colon. What clinical and radiological features may help distinguish them? What investigations are mandatory?
- What dietary advice would you give to a patient requesting a high-fibre diet? Is there a link between dietary fibre and colonic carcinoma?

FURTHER INFORMATION

Farrell R J, Farrell J J, Morrin M M. **Diverticular disease in the elderly**. *Gastroenterological Clinics of North America* 30(2);2001:475–96.

www.digestivedisorders.org.uk/Leaflets/divertnew.html Useful information source for sufferers.

www2.gastrojournal.org Website of the journal *Gastroenterology* with links to policy statements including on the link between dietary fibre and cancer.

A 49-year-old man with abdominal pain and vomiting

A 49-year-old labourer presents with a 2-day history of abdominal pain and bilious vomiting. He describes his pain as peri-umbilical and colicky. He has been anorexic for the last day. He reports his bowels have not moved for 3 days which is very unusual for him and he has not passed any wind for 24 hours. In addition he has noticed a dull ache in his lower abdomen on the right for several weeks but he has been able to work.

On physical examination the patient appears dehydrated and unwell. His pulse is 95 bpm and his blood pressure 150/90 mm Hg. Cardiorespiratory examination is unremarkable. His abdomen is distended and tympanic but soft to palpation. A scar is noted from a prior appendicectomy as a child. Rectal examination reveals an empty vault with no masses, occult blood is negative. Both groins and the genitalia are normal.

Q1 What is your preliminary diagnosis for this patient and what are most common causes of this problem?

Q2 What investigations would you like to order?

The results of the investigations are shown below and in Figures 21.1 and 21.2.

Investigation 21.1 Summary of results			
Haemoglobin	160 g/l	White cell count	8.6 x 10⁹/l
PCV	0.53		
Platelets	379 x 10⁹/l		
Sodium	145 mmol/l	Calcium	2.16 mmol/l
Potassium	4.6 mmol/l	Phosphate	1.15 mmol/l
Chloride	105 mmol/l	Total protein	62 g/l
Bicarbonate	27 mmol/l	Albumin	35 g/l
Urea	6.1 mmol/l	Globulins	27 g/l
Creatinine	0.09 mmol/l	Bilirubin	16 µmol/l
Uric acid	0.24 mmol/l	ALT	28 U/l
Glucose	4.6 mmol/l	AST	24 U/l
Cholesterol	4.5 mmol/l	GGT	17 U/l
LDH	212 U/l	ALP	51 U/l

Fig 21.1

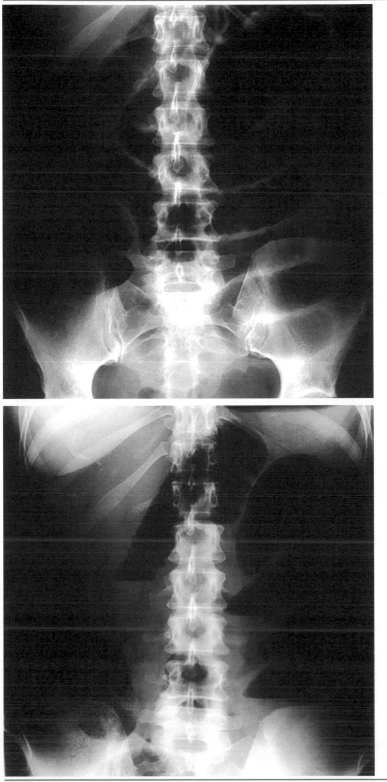

Fig 21.2

Q3 What is your interpretation of the investigations?

The results of the investigations support your clinical diagnosis.

Q4 What is your initial management plan for this patient?

Over the next 24 hours, the patient's pain settles and his abdomen becomes less distended. He is adequately hydrated and his electrolytes are normal. His nasogastric tube drainage remains high (>1 1/8 h). You persist with conservative management, but the obstruction does not settle. A decision is made to perform an exploratory laparotomy. Figure 21.3 shows the operative findings.

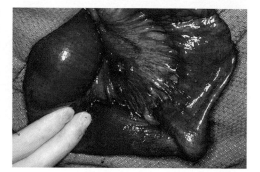

Fig 21.3

Q5 What does Figure 21.3 show?

The patient undergoes a limited small bowel resection. While you wait for the histopathology report, more details are sought from the patient. He reports having a mole removed from his back years ago. Its original appearance is shown in Figure 21.4.

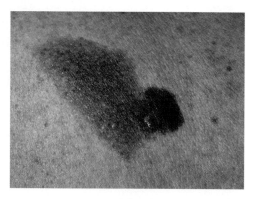

Fig 21.4

Q6 Describe this lesion. What is the diagnosis?

You receive the pathology report for this specimen and the diagnosis is confirmed. The lesion is reported to have invaded into the reticular dermis with a maximum depth of invasion of 1.34 mm.

The lesion was reported to have been completely excised.

Q7   What is the significance of the pathology report?

The pathology report from the resected small bowel identified a deposit of melanoma at the apex of the intussusception. The enlarged lymph node in the mesentery contained malignant melanoma.

Q8   How should this patient be managed now?

A further investigation is performed (Figure 21.5).

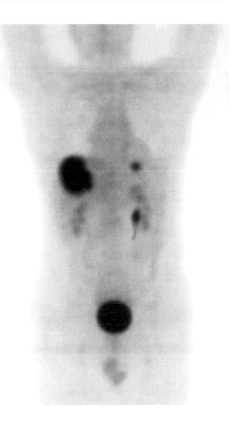

Fig 21.5

Q9   What is the investigation and what does it show?

The patient was referred to medical oncology for follow-up, was entered on a Phase I experimental study and died 6 months later of extensive metastatic disease.

ANSWERS

A1 The patient's presentation is consistent with small bowel obstruction. Since vomiting is a major feature for this patient, his obstruction is likely to be in the proximal bowel. The most common cause of small bowel obstruction in the developed world is surgical adhesions. The next most common cause is an abdominal wall hernia. Rarer causes include neoplasms and intussusception. Large bowel obstruction may be the result of volvulus, neoplasia or diverticular disease. This patient's prior appendicectomy suggests adhesive obstruction.

A2 A complete blood count and serum electrolytes will help assess the patient's degree of dehydration. Abdominal X-rays will confirm your diagnosis of a bowel obstruction.

A3 An elevated haematocrit (PCV) and blood urea confirm the patient's dehydration. The upright and supine abdominal films show dilated loops of small bowel and air-fluid levels. No gas is seen in the colon or rectum confirming the diagnosis of a small bowel obstruction. There is evidence of thickening of the bowel wall which suggests oedema and possibly bowel ischaemia. Bowel ischaemia is a devastating complication of bowel obstruction leading to perforation and peritonitis. Also of note: no gas overlies the hernial orifices, nor is there gas in the biliary tree, which would suggest a rare cause of small bowel obstruction – gallstone ileus.

A4 Intravenous rehydration with an isotonic solution supplemented with potassium and intestinal decompression with a nasogastric tube are the mainstays of initial therapy. Intravenous fluids administered should also take into account any loss through nasogastric decompression. Analgesia is prescribed for the patient's pain. Repeat abdominal examinations will alert the managing physician to any changes that would alter the conservative plan. These changes include a change in the nature of the pain (colicky to constant), localized tenderness and tachycardia. In addition, the patient's need for analgesics might increase.

A5 The small bowel. The bowel on the left of the photograph is dilated and that on the right is collapsed. The cause of the obstruction is an intussusception, seen to the bottom of the photograph. There is a black node in the mesentery.

Intussusception in the adult is rare, accounting for less than 5% of all cases. An intussusception has a lead point, and in most adult cases this is a tumour (benign or malignant).

A6 A brown-black lesion with an irregular margin is noted. In one area there is a raised black patch with a nodular appearance. The appearance is consistent with a malignant melanoma.

A7 Depth of invasion of a malignant melanoma strongly correlates with its metastatic potential. Thickness greater than 0.76 mm is associated with a 30% incidence of local recurrence or metastatic disease. Greater depths of invasion carry an even more grim prognosis. Delineation of depth of invasion by dermal level is the Clark grading system. For reticular dermal invasion, 5-year survival is less than 70%. Preference now is the direct measurement in millimetres of the depth of invasion (Breslow thickness).

A8 This is a well-recognized clinical scenario: an isolated deposit of melanoma giving rise to symptoms several years after treatment of the primary lesion. On reflection, this patient was at significant risk of developing recurrent disease. The digestive tract is a relatively common site for secondary deposition of melanoma.

It would now be reasonable to look for other evidence of metastatic disease. Some form of radiological investigation may be helpful.

A9 Figure 21.5 is a composite image from positron emission tomography (PET). The photograph is a whole body projection image (a series of superimposed coronal views to give a 3-D effect). There is a large area of increased activity in the right lobe of the liver and a smaller area in the plane of the left hemi-diaphragm, which could represent a deposit in the spleen. There is also a faint focus above the left pole of the kidney, which might represent a deposit in the pancreas. The distribution of tracer elsewhere is physiological.

REVISION POINTS

Small bowel obstruction

- Most cases in developed countries are due to adhesions.
- No temporal relationship between date of original operation and onset of obstruction.
- 80% of these cases will resolve spontaneously.
- 30% of patients will have recurrent episodes of obstruction.
- Conservative management unless the patient shows evidence of bowel ischaemia (change in nature and severity of pain, localized tenderness, fever, tachycardia, leucocytosis).
- Abdominal wall hernias are the commonest cause of obstruction in developing countries.
- Hernias should be treated by prompt surgical correction.

Malignant melanoma

- Increasing incidence over last 50 years (18:100 000 in USA).
- Prevalent in areas of high UV exposure, e.g. Australia and southern USA.
- Risk factors include fair skin, atypical mole/dysplastic naevus syndrome, blistering sunburn, immunosuppression, family history of melanoma.
- ABCD of melanoma: any pigmented skin lesion must be regarded with suspicion and biopsied if there is:
  Asymmetrical growth
  Border irregularity
  Colour variegation
  Diameter greater than 6 mm.

Some melanomas can be totally devoid of pigment and difficult to recognize. Any lesion that is increasing in size, changes colour, crusts, becomes itchy or in any way bothers the patient should be removed and examined.

Tumour thickness (depth) is the most important histopathologic determinate in the management of melanoma. Thickness greater than 0.76 mm is associated with a 30% incidence of local recurrence or metastatic disease. Tumours greater than 4 mm in thickness have greater than 60% chance of distant disease.

Surgical excision is the mainstay of initial therapy with depth of invasion determining surgical margins. Lesions with less than 1 mm depth of invasion require a 1 cm margin. Lesions between 1–2 mm in depth, 2 cm is necessary, and a 2–3 cm margin is required for lesions greater than 2 mm depth of invasion.

Lymph node dissection should be considered for patients with a high risk of occult disease and/or clinically positive nodes.

The results of therapy for metastatic disease are dismal and the choices are between chemotherapy, palliative supportive care and experimental therapy. The fact that metastatic disease is lethal has led to the investigation of therapies such as biologic response modifiers and vaccines at presentation for patients with advanced local disease who are at high risk for future metastases.

Prevention and early detection are of the utmost importance through increased community and medical awareness of:

- Dangers of UV radiation exposure.
- Early excision of suspicious skin lesions.

ISSUES TO CONSIDER

- Are any therapies now available to reduce the risk of recurrence in patients with melanoma?
- What metabolic upset might you expect in cases of prolonged and severe small intestinal obstruction?
- What are the major causes of intestinal obstruction in developing countries?

FURTHER INFORMATION

www.emedicine.com/EMERG/topic66.htm Another excellent chapter from emedicine.

www.radiology.co.uk/srs-x/ An educational resource from the Scottish Radiological Society with lots of cases including some intestinal obstruction.

Jaundice in an older woman

A frail 83-year-old woman is referred with a 3-week history of jaundice. She has noticed that her urine has become dark and her stools pale. She has been feeling generally unwell for some weeks and has lost her appetite. She has lost 5 kg in the past 2 months.

Q1 What further information would you like from the history and why?

There is no other helpful information from the history. On examination she looks unwell, is apyrexial and is obviously jaundiced. The rest of the examination is unremarkable. She has no stigmata of chronic liver disease and your clinical suspicions are that the patient has an extrahepatic cause for her jaundice. You arrange some blood tests, the results of which are shown below.

Investigation 22.1 Summary of results

Haemoglobin	132 g/l	White cell count	5.5 x 10⁹/l
Platelets	299 x 10⁹/l		
Sodium	138 mmol/l	Calcium	2.39 mmol/l
Potassium	3.6 mmol/l	Phosphate	1.15 mmol/l
Chloride	100 mmol/l	Total protein	65 g/l
Bicarbonate	27 mmol/l	Albumin	38 g/l
Urea	4.6 mmol/l	Globulins	27 g/l
Creatinine	0.12 mmol/l	Bilirubin	85 µmol/l
Uric acid	0.24 mmol/l	ALT	78 U/l
Glucose	4.4 mmol/l	AST	91 U/l
Cholesterol	3.5 mmol/l	GGT	356 U/l
LDH	212 U/l	ALP	457 U/l

Q2 Interpret these results. What further investigations may help you formulate the diagnosis?

You arrange an ultrasound of the upper abdomen. It shows dilatation of the extrahepatic bile duct to the level of the ampulla. The common bile duct is estimated to be 1.3 cm at maximum diameter. No cause for the obstruction is shown.

You then organize another investigation for your patient. An X-ray taken during this procedure is shown in Figure 22.1.

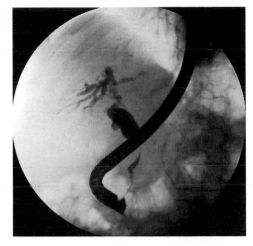

Fig 22.1

Q3 What investigation has been performed? What does it show?

You note the appearance (Figure 22.1).

Q4 What further investigations can be performed? What treatment options are open to you?

In view of the patient's age and frailty a stent was inserted to relieve the obstruction and to palliate her symptoms.

Figure 22.2 shows the metallic (expandable mesh) stent in position across the malignant stricture. The stent has only just been deployed and will continue to expand over the next 24 hours.

Her jaundice resolves slowly over the following week and she regains enough strength to be discharged to the care of her daughters.

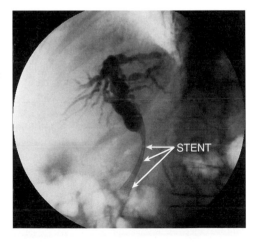

Fig 22.2

ANSWERS

A1 When taking a history from an acutely jaundiced patient there are several enquiries that may help you reach a diagnosis before any test results are available.

- Is the patient generally unwell? Has she lost any weight? Many patients with malignant biliary obstruction, for instance, will report ill health and weight loss preceding the onset of jaundice.

ANSWERS – cont'd

● Has the patient experienced any pain? What is its nature? The patient with common bile duct gallstones will often report classical biliary colic with episodes of nausea, vomiting and, if cholangitis develops, fevers and rigors. They may even report previous episodes of jaundice or a history of gallstones. Patients with pancreatic cancer characteristically have intractable epigastric pain, which radiates through to the back.

● Has the patient any risk factors for viral hepatitis? A recent diarrhoeal illness, bathing in polluted waters or foreign travel to developing countries may suggest hepatitis A. A past history of blood transfusion or intravenous drug abuse puts the patient at risk from hepatitis B and C, although the latter rarely presents acutely with jaundice. For the same reasons, although unlikely to be relevant in this woman, it may be prudent to enquire about a patient's sexual history.

● An alcohol history and a thorough drug history are essential. Remember that most prescription drugs have the potential for hepatotoxicity. Of particular importance is any history of recent antibiotic exposure. Clavulanic acid, for instance, may cause a cholestatic hepatitis, especially in the elderly.

● Has the patient any other medical conditions? For instance, congestive cardiac failure can present as jaundice and abdominal pain in the elderly.

A2 This woman's blood tests suggest a cholestatic cause for her jaundice. The raised alkaline phosphatase and gamma GT in comparison with the mild elevation of the transaminases support cholestasis. Her pale stools and dark urine suggest that there is an obstruction to the flow of bile and therefore it is likely that she has an extrahepatic obstruction.

Her electrolytes and renal function tests are normal. Her normal complete blood picture makes cholangitis (infection within the biliary tree, usually secondary to calculus obstruction of the biliary tree) unlikely.

A serum albumin may be useful. A depressed level suggests either poor synthetic liver function or a chronic inflammatory process. A prothrombin time (PT) is also useful. Patients with chronic biliary obstruction may be deficient in vitamin K, a fat soluble vitamin that requires bile for absorption. Therefore, they may have a prolonged PT. Patients with severe disturbance of liver function secondary to parenchymal disease may be unable to synthesize clotting factors effectively, also leading to a prolonged PT and APTT.

An ultrasound of the upper abdomen is essential. It may show dilatation of the intra- and extrahepatic bile ducts. Gallstones may be seen within the gallbladder or bile ducts. A pancreatic carcinoma may show up as a mass in the head of the pancreas. The investigation may also reveal abnormalities of the liver parenchyma or the presence of metastatic disease.

A3 This is an ERCP (Endoscopic Retrograde Cholangiopancreatogram). The endoscope lies across the middle of the film. Contrast has filled the common bile duct, the common hepatic duct and both left and right intrahepatic ducts. The radiograph shows that the common bile duct is dilated. There is a long strictured segment at the lower end of the common bile duct and there are no filling defects seen within the biliary tree. This appearance is characteristic of a carcinoma of the head of the pancreas.

A4 The first priority in this case is to achieve decompression of the biliary tree and thereby relieve the jaundice.

This can be achieved during the ERCP by insertion of a stent across the obstruction. Stents are normally plastic tubes of varying length and diameter. In some cases, expandable metallic stents are used. Occasionally, decompression of the biliary system cannot be achieved endoscopically and a PTC (Percutaneous Transhepatic Cholangiogram) must be performed.

Further imaging of the pancreas will help confirm the diagnosis as well as provide information on possible operability. Note also that:

● CT scanning is widely used.
● MR scanning and the use of endoscopic ultrasound are on the increase.
● The diagnosis can be confirmed histologically by biopsy.

A N S W E R S – cont'd

- In practice, a pancreatic biopsy is often not performed because in frail patients or those with advanced disease, histological confirmation is unlikely to alter the treatment or prognosis.

In a few patients operative resection may be appropriate. The 'Whipples' procedure, however, still only has a 5-year survival of 10–20% in those with tumours <3 cm in size. The much rarer tumours of the ampulla of Vater have a far better prognosis with a 5-year survival of 40% following resection. Chemotherapy is largely unsuc-

cessful, although some novel trial regimens have achieved modest success in recent years.

In reality, most pancreatic tumours are treated with palliative measures. Adequate analgesia and the early involvement of palliative care teams are often the most important elements of management. The median survival following diagnosis of pancreatic carcinoma is 11–13 weeks. Occasionally stents may block and/or become infected (cholangitis). This may then necessitate replacement, although such complications are less common with the metallic stents.

R E V I S I O N   P O I N T S

Pancreatic carcinoma

Incidence
9:100 000 in the Western world (estimated).
Risk factors
- male sex
- smoking
- poor diet probably plays a role.
Histology
Most tumours (c. 90%) arise from ductal epithelium and are therefore adenocarcinomas. The remainder are mostly of neuroendocrine origin.
Presentation
- abdominal pain
- anorexia
- weight loss (often profound)
- painless jaundice
- diabetes (rarely).

Clinical features
The patient is often gaunt, jaundiced and cachectic. In advanced disease there may be ascites and local lymphadenopathy. In patients with biliary obstruction, the gallbladder may be distended and palpable. If painless, this is unlikely to be due to gallstones (Courvoisier's law).
Prognosis
Adenocarcinomas have a very poor prognosis with only 2–5% surviving 5 years.
Investigation and treatment
See Answer 4. Novel treatments include aggressive chemotherapeutic regimens and photodynamic therapy. The involvement of palliative care teams early in the course of the illness is paramount.

ISSUES TO CONSIDER

- Expandable stents have many uses in medicine. Where else are they used and what is their role in the conditions in which they are used?

- What are other common causes of jaundice and how would you differentiate them?

- What debilitating symptoms may this woman experience and how can they best be treated?

- What is a 'Whipples' procedure?

FURTHER INFORMATION

www.asge.org The website of the American Society of Gastrointestinal Endoscopy with clinical updates and guidelines including the treatment of obstructive jaundice.

www.EndoAtlas.com An excellent website featuring an atlas of over 700 high-quality endoscopic images.

www.cancerlinks.com/pancreas.html
A useful starting place on the web for information on carcinoma of the pancreas.

A young man with profuse diarrhoea

A 26-year-old teacher attends your general practice surgery with a 3-day history of diarrhoea. He feels unwell and has eaten little since the diarrhoea started. His bowels have been loose but not watery and contain some mucus. There is no visible blood in the stool. He has had loose motions every 2 to 3 hours, which persist even at night. He also describes some cramp-like abdominal pain, which is eased when he opens his bowels. His general health has been good and he has had no previous illnesses of note. He is not on any medications. He had a similar episode of diarrhoea 3 months ago, which he attributed to over-indulgence at a local Chinese restaurant. Ten days previously he returned from a holiday in Bali.

Q1 What are the likely causes of the diarrhoea?

The physical examination is unremarkable, and in particular the abdominal examination is normal. Rectal examination reveals soft stool and sigmoidoscopy shows a mild inflammation of the rectal mucosa. You arrange for stool microscopy and cultures to be performed, with a request to look for amoebae, red cells and white blood cells (pus). You advise him to rest at home, drink plenty of fluids and return to see you if the diarrhoea does not settle within 3 days, or if it worsens. You also tell him you will contact him if the stool samples detect any infection that needs to be treated.

The patient's symptoms do not improve and the diarrhoea worsens. The stools become blood-stained. He returns 2 days later to see you. On examination he looks unwell, is dehydrated and has a temperature of 38.5°C. He has a tachycardia of 110 beats/min. He has generalized abdominal tenderness. Repeat sigmoidoscopic examination reveals marked erythema and oedema of the rectal mucosa with contact bleeding. You biopsy the mucosa.

Q2 What other key points are needed from the history?

While you are arranging his admission to hospital, you send blood samples for haematological and biochemical analysis, blood culture and blood grouping. At the same time you organize an X-ray of his abdomen.

Q3 How do you continue his management?

He begins to feel better after intravenous fluid replacement and you now have the results of the blood tests. They are shown below. The stool cultures sent off 3 days previously are negative, but you send off a further stool sample for examination, and include a request for ova, cysts and parasites. The abdominal X-rays are normal.

Investigation 23.1 Summary of results			
Haemoglobin	115 g/l	White cell count	15.6 x 10⁹/l
MCV	80 fl	Neutrophils 70%	10.9 x 10⁹/l
Platelets	395 x 10⁹/l		
Sodium	134 mmol/l	Calcium	2.40 mmol/l
Potassium	2.7 mmol/l	Phosphate	0.90 mmol/l
Chloride	99 mmol/l	Total protein	62 g/l
Bicarbonate	20 mmol/l	Albumin	35 g/l
Urea	16.8 mmol/l	Globulins	27 g/l
Creatinine	0.14 mmol/l	Bilirubin	16 µmol/l
Uric acid	0.24 mmol/l	ALT	44 U/l
Glucose	4.4 mmol/l	AST	32 U/l
Cholesterol	3.5 mmol/l	GGT	45 U/l
LDH	212 U/l	ALP	54 U/l

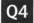 **Q4** Question 4 What is your interpretation of the blood results?

The following day the patient continues to have severe diarrhoea. Blood cultures and stool microscopy are both negative for significant pathogens, but you decide to commence him on antibiotics as a precaution against an infective diarrhoea. You start him on oral ciprofloxacin and metronidazole. You wonder if there might be another cause for the patient's illness and urgently contact the histopathologist for the result of the rectal biopsy. What she has seen is shown in Figure 23.1.

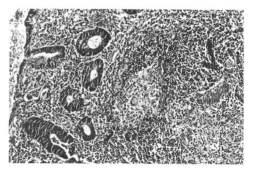

Fig 23.1

Q5 What does Figure 23.1 show, and how is this going to alter your management?

After 24 hours of fluid replacement and antibiotics he is still ill, with a temperature of 38.2°C and a tachycardia, and has profuse bloody diarrhoea. His latest results are shown in Investigation 23.2.

Investigation 23.2 Summary of further results

Haemoglobin	98 g/l	White cell count		18.5 x 10⁹/l
MCV	80 fl	Neutrophils	72%	13.3 x 10⁹/l
Platelets	420 x 10⁹/l			
Sodium	136 mmol/l	Calcium		2.40 mmol/l
Potassium	2.2 mmol/l	Phosphate		0.90 mmol/l
Chloride	99 mmol/l	Total protein		54 g/l
Bicarbonate	20 mmol/l	Albumin		28 g/l
Urea	9.8 mmol/l	Globulins		26 g/l
Creatinine	0.12 mmol/l	Bilirubin		18 µmol/l
Uric acid	0.24 mmol/l	ALT		42 U/l
Glucose	4.0 mmol/l	AST		35 U/l
Cholesterol	3.5 mmol/l	GGT		25 U/l
LDH	194 U/l	ALP		44 U/l

The White cell count value is expressed as $18.5 \times 10^9/l$, Neutrophils as $13.3 \times 10^9/l$, Platelets as $420 \times 10^9/l$.

Q6 What is the significance of these results and what action do you take now?

The patient is started on high-dose intravenous hydrocortisone, and central intravenous access is inserted to facilitate administration of high volumes of fluids, more rapid correction of his hypokalaemia, multiple intravenous drugs and total parenteral nutrition (TPN). He is dehydrated and hypokalaemic despite initial therapy. Initially he is given 2 litres intravenous normal saline over 1 hour. Subsequently, he requires 5 litres intravenous fluids per day to maintain a normal state of hydration. To replace the hypokalaemia, he is given 100 mmol potassium chloride (KCl) over 5 hours, and is then maintained on 20 mmol KCl per litre of maintenance fluid with repeat electrolyte checks every 8 hours. His haemoglobin stabilizes at 79 g/l and therefore a transfusion is withheld, but the haemoglobin concentration is checked every 8 hours. The antibiotics are stopped. A further investigation is performed (Figure 23.2).

Fig 23.2

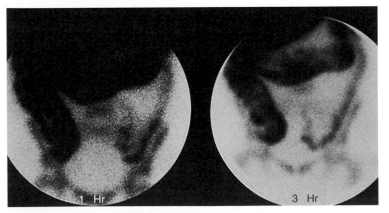

Q7 What is this investigation and what does it show?

The patient is seen in joint consultation by the gastroenterologists and the surgeons, who agree that the intensive medical therapy currently being undertaken is the appropriate treatment. Over the next 6 days his temperature and tachycardia settle, and his abdominal pain subsides. His bowel actions gradually diminish to four per day, with little bloodstaining. His intravenous hydrocortisone is changed to oral prednisolone. Oral fluids and then food are reintroduced. Ten days later the patient is ready to leave hospital on prednisolone and mesalazine, which contains the active 5-aminosalicylic acid moiety of sulfasalazine. The steroids will be tapered off over the next 2 months if he remains in remission. Mesalazine is continued as it has value in maintaining remission.

Two months after his discharge he has ceased the prednisolone and has undergone a small bowel barium follow-through examination, and a colonoscopy in order to delineate the distribution of the disease. These demonstrate that the disease has a patchy distribution involving most of the colon. The small bowel is unaffected. The colonoscopy shows the colitis to be in remission. His haematological and biochemical measurements are now normal.

Six months later the patient is readmitted with a further episode of acute colitis. He has stopped taking his medication. He has had bloody diarrhoea for 6 days and has been opening his bowels every 2 hours. He is dehydrated, pyrexial and tachycardic. He is once again anaemic, with hypokalaemia and hypoalbuminaemia. He is rehydrated with intravenous fluids and potassium replacement and again started on intravenous

hydrocortisone. Stool samples are sent for culture, but these are negative. TPN is given. On this occasion his response to intensive medical treatment is not so rapid. After 5 days his condition has remained unchanged with a low-grade fever, tachycardia and frequent bloody stools. He develops some abdominal tenderness and an X-ray is performed (Figure 23.3).

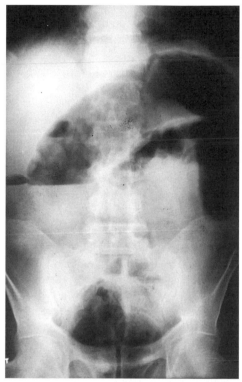

Fig 23.3

Q8 What does the X-ray show?

The patient has not shown any significant improvement in his condition and in view of the radiological findings, an operation is advised. The patient undergoes a sub-total colectomy, with formation of an ileostomy and closure of the rectal stump. Part of the operative specimen is shown (Figure 23.4).

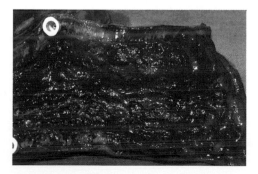

Fig 23.4

Q9 What does Figure 23.4 show?

After this procedure the patient made an uneventful postoperative recovery and was in good health 6 months later.

ANSWERS

A1 The most likely causes of acute diarrhoea in a young man are either an infective gastroenteritis or inflammatory bowel disease.

Viral infections are a common cause of diarrhoea. These infections are usually mild, self-limiting and cause little systemic upset. Rotavirus and adenovirus are commonly implicated.

Bacteria such as *Campylobacter* spp., *Salmonella* spp. and *Staphylococcus aureus* are often implicated in food poisoning. These infections are mostly self-limiting, but may cause systemic symptoms, and occasionally require treatment with antibiotics.

'Traveller's diarrhoea' may be caused by a wide range of viral, bacterial and parasitic organisms. Common infectious agents include *Entamoeba histolytica*, and *Giardia lamblia*. Treatment will vary considerably dependent upon the organism involved. Identification of the causative organism is usually made by stool microscopy, although occasionally other methods are required, e.g. serological testing for amoebic fluorescent antibody titre (*Entamoeba histolytica*), duodenal aspirate (*Giardia lamblia*).

A2 Questions must be asked about the following:
- Any recent travel (this may give clues to a particular infective organism).
- Other medical conditions, use of prescription medications and any history of recreational drug use.
- Risk of immunocompromise, e.g. HIV infection.
- Sexual habits. Homosexuals may develop colitis secondary to gonorrhoea, lymphogranuloma venereum or *Chlamydia trachomatis*, which may resemble the colitis of inflammatory bowel disease. Similarly, individuals immuno-

compromised with the acquired immunodeficiency syndrome (AIDS) may develop diarrhoea as part of the syndrome or secondary to infection with agents such as cytomegalovirus (CMV) and *Cryptosporidium*.
- Recent antibiotics usage, which may be responsible for a *Clostridium difficile* colonization, resulting in pseudomembranous colitis.

A3 He now requires admission to hospital. The most pressing need is for intravenous rehydration. The quantity and rate of fluid replacement will depend on his degree of dehydration and electrolyte disturbance. From your clinical assessment he has lost at least 2 litres of fluid from his extracellular space. You can afford to give him 2 litres isotonic ('normal') saline rapidly (over 4 hours). He will also require potassium replacement, which will be guided by the severity of the hypokalaemia on the biochemical screen. Substantial potassium loss will continue for as long as the diarrhoea persists.

He should have further stool samples sent for urgent microscopy and culture, and blood tests should be sent for routine biochemistry and haematology.

You are still uncertain of the cause of his illness, although a viral gastroenteritis is unlikely in view of the severity and duration of his illness. Such illnesses are usually mild and self-limiting with little or no systemic upset. He could still have infectious gastroenteritis, and *Campylobacter*, Salmonella and Shigella can all cause severe diarrhoea with fever, vomiting and prostration. All of these organisms are distinct possibilities. Bearing in mind his recent return from the tropics, amoebiasis must also be considered and stool examined for ova and parasites. Acute Staphylococcal food poisoning can produce a

A N S W E R S – cont'd

severe illness with diarrhoea and gastrointestinal upset. Vomiting is usually prominent, however, and the illness usually occurs within a few hours of eating the contaminated food. In these cases the illness is due to the ingestion of a preformed toxin. This patient should be treated as if the diarrhoea is infective in origin, until proven otherwise.

Most instances of infectious diarrhoea will be self-limiting and the patient will be satisfactorily treated with fluid replacement alone. In severe cases due to bacteria, antibiotics may be required. The results of the stool culture will determine which antimicrobial agent is used.

You must consider the possibility of inflammatory bowel disease. Often there is nothing specific in the patient's history or examination findings that indicate an inflammatory colitis. The endoscopic findings are consistent with either a severe infectious colitis or an inflammatory colitis.

All antidiarrhoeal agents should be stopped as they may precipitate colonic dilatation in patients with colitis. They also render interpretation of a stool chart meaningless.

A4 Despite his dehydration, he has a low haemoglobin, and anaemia is a common finding in severe colitis, although non-specific.

The elevated white cell count supports a diagnosis of infection or inflammation, but again is non-specific.

The electrolyte changes show hyponatraemia, hyporchloraemia, hypokalaemia and reduced bicarbonate, consistent with prolonged diarrhoea.

A5 There is an intense submucosal inflammatory cell infiltrate, and several granulomas are seen. It now appears that your patient may have Crohn's disease and is suffering a severe episode of colitis.

You will now have to consider starting him on high-dose intravenous steroids. He may still have infective diarrhoea, which can sometimes be difficult to distinguish histologically from Crohn's disease. It is vital that you exclude an infectious cause for the diarrhoea before you use steroids, as steroids may exacerbate infectious diarrhoea.

You continue your close monitoring of the patient and repeat the biochemical and haematological investigations, and continue fluid replacement as required.

A6 He is still toxic and dehydrated; his anaemia has progressed and he has marked hypokalaemia and hypoalbuminaemia. He needs to be aggressively rehydrated and central intravenous access achieved to facilitate administration of high volumes of fluids, more rapid correction of his hypokalaemia, multiple intravenous drugs and total parenteral nutrition (TPN). From the information given it is unclear if he needs a blood transfusion. This needs to be a clinical decision. He has microcytosis suggestive of iron deficiency and he is also likely to have a component of chronic disease. As he is young and otherwise fit he will tolerate moderately severe anaemia and his tachycardia may be primarily from dehydration. If he has frank bloody diarrhoea and his haemoglobin drops rapidly he may need to be treated as an acute gastrointestinal haemorrhage and thus transfused. He needs to be carefully monitored with frequent monitoring of his vital signs (e.g. at least every 2 hours) and electrolyte and haemoglobin checks (e.g. every 8 hours).

The patient should be started on high-dose intravenous hydrocortisone. A suitable regimen would be intravenous hydrocortisone 100 mg, 6-hourly.

He should be made nil by mouth except for ice-chips. The rationale for TPN is to maintain nutritional replacement in a patient who is unlikely to be taking much by mouth over the next few weeks. Resting the bowel can induce remission in Crohn's disease.

He must be monitored closely for two complications of acute severe colitis, namely acute colonic dilatation and perforation of the colon. Acute dilatation may lead to perforation, but perforation can occur without obvious radiological dilatation of the colon. Perforation in a patient with acute colitis has a mortality rate that approaches 50%. The monitoring will consist of close observation of the patient's vital signs, regular palpation of his abdomen and daily abdominal radiographs.

ANSWERS – cont'd

A7 This investigation is a 99ᵐTechnetium-labelled white cell scan.

The scan involves removing approximately 50 ml of the patient's blood, labelling their leucocytes, and reinjecting the cells into the patient. The white cells accumulate in areas of inflammation and show up as 'hotspots' on the resultant gamma scan.

There are two scans, which have been taken 1 and 3 hours after the injection of autologous-labelled leucocytes. The cells have accumulated within the ascending, transverse and, to a lesser extent, in the descending colon. These findings are not specific for Crohn's disease, but in the clinical setting are likely to represent areas of Crohn's disease activity.

A labelled white cell scan gives an indication of disease distribution, and will show disease activity in both the small and large bowel. Steroid treatment can cause false negative results. This technique is not able to highlight areas of quiescent Crohn's disease.

A8 This shows a grossly dilated loop of transverse colon. The colon should be less than 6 cm in diameter when viewed on a standard X-ray. The colon is in imminent danger of perforation. Some mucosal thickening can be seen in the descending and sigmoid colon.

The condition seen with these changes, together with the patient's condition, is referred to as 'toxic megacolon'.

A9 The mucosa is abnormal, with oedema, haemorrhage, slough and ulceration. There is no normal mucosa visible.

REVISION POINTS

Investigation and management of diarrhoea

Aetiology
- Infective: viral, bacterial, parasitic.
- Inflammatory: Crohn's, ulcerative colitis.
- Drugs: e.g. proton pump inhibitors, antibiotics.
- Surgical: e.g. post-gastrectomy, short bowel syndrome.
- Malabsorption: e.g. bacterial overgrowth, coeliac disease.
- Neoplasia: e.g. carcinoma of colon.
- Miscellaneous: thyrotoxicosis, laxative abuse, amyloidosis.

Investigation
History-taking will give the most clues, and guide investigations.
- Stool:
  - microscopy and culture
  - *Clostridium difficile* toxin
  - quantitative stool collection
  - 3-day faecal fat estimation.
- Urine:
  - laxative screen
  - 5-HIAA for carcinoid

  - VMA for phaeochromocytoma.
- Blood:
  - coeliac serology
  - thyroid function
  - CRP/ESR.
- Other:
  - flexible sigmoidoscopy and rectal biopsy
  - duodenal biopsy
  - small bowel barium radiology
  - breath tests
  - pancreatic function tests.

Treatment
Direct at underlying cause.

Crohn's disease

Incidence
- 6:100 000 in the Western world.
- Striking variation in racial and geographical distribution.

Risk factors
- Higher rates in Caucasians.
- Lower rates in Asia, Africa and South America.
- Genetic and environmental factors are both implicated.

continues overleaf

REVISION POINTS – cont'd

- Higher rates than would be expected are seen among smokers.

Histology

- Inflammatory changes involving the full thickness of the bowel wall.
- Non-caseating granulomas, lymphoid hyperplasia.
- Acute and chronic inflammatory cell infiltration.
- Any part of GI tract from mouth to anus may be involved.

Presentation

- Abdominal pain.
- Diarrhoea.
- Weight loss.

Clinical features

- Colicky abdominal pain/subacute obstruction.

- Sequelae of malabsorption and chronic diarrhoea (e.g. low vitamin B12, calcium, Fe, Mg).
- Fistulating disease.
- Extraintestinal features include arthritis, episcleritis, erythema nodosum and gallstones.

Diagnosis

- Histological diagnosis obtained by endoscopy is gold standard.
- Barium radiology and white cell scanning are useful.

Treatment

- Corticosteroids/5-aminosalicylic acid derivatives/azathioprine/methotrexate/anti-TNF-alpha antibodies (infliximab).
- Surgical resection of affected areas.
- Bowel rest (elemental diet/TPN).
- Omeprazole for gastric and duodenal Crohn's.

ISSUES TO CONSIDER

- What measures are advisable to avoid infectious diarrhoea when travelling to tropical countries?
- What problems do you foresee in a 26-year-old man following an ileostomy? How could these be addressed?
- Does he need any long-term medication to prevent disease recurrence or is he now 'cured'?

FURTHER INFORMATION

Rampton D S. **Management of Crohn's disease**. *British Medical Journal* 1999;319:1480–85.

www.nacc.org.uk UK-based IBD resource for patients and clinicians.

Rectal bleeding in a 65-year-old woman

A 65-year-old woman is referred with a 3-week history of rectal bleeding. She has noticed bright red blood on the toilet paper. The bleeding is associated with defaecation and is not mixed with the stool. Over the last 4 months she has suffered increasing constipation. She has a good appetite, her diet has not altered recently, and her weight is stable. Her general health is good and she has had no major illnesses in the past. She describes troubles with 'haemorrhoids' 10 years previously, and had some injection treatment for them. She smokes 20 cigarettes a day and is not taking any medications.

On examination she looks well and there is no obvious evidence of recent weight loss. Her cardiorespiratory system is normal. On abdominal examination there are no abnormal findings. A rectal examination is performed which shows she has two anal skin tags and some prolapsed internal haemorrhoids.

Q1 What should be done next?

A sigmoidoscopic examination to 20 cm is normal. Proctoscopy confirms the presence of large internal haemorrhoids, which bleed easily on contact.

Q2 What is the likely explanation for the bleeding? What is the next step?

You explain to the patient that while the bleeding is most likely to be due to her haemorrhoids, a complete investigation of the large bowel is indicated. You arrange a colonoscopy. A lesion is found (Figure 24.1).

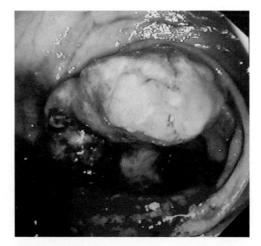

Fig 24.1

Q3 What does Figure 24.1 show?

The tumour is situated about 25 cm from the anal verge. Otherwise the colonoscopy was normal to the caecum. The biopsy shows moderately differentiated adenocarcinoma confirmed.

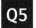 **Q4** What should you do after the colonoscopy and why?

Her haemoglobin is 120 g/l, her liver function tests and biochemistry are normal. A chest X-ray and ultrasound of the liver are also normal.

Q5 How would you counsel this patient?

At operation a carcinoma of the sigmoid colon is found and a high anterior resection is performed. There is no evidence of adjacent or distant spread of the tumour. Apart from the tumour, there was nothing else abnormal in the resected specimen of bowel. There was no indication to perform a defunctioning ileostomy and she makes a good recovery. The histology is confirmed and the carcinoma involves the muscularis propria and extends into the pericolic fat. There is no perineural, vascular or lymph node involvement.

 Q6 What further advice is the patient going to require?

The patient understands that you will keep her under surveillance. She would like to know what this will involve.

Q7 What is the aim of the follow-up programme? What kind of surveillance will you employ?

The patient wants to know if any of her children are at risk for developing this cancer.

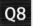 **Q8** What is your counsel?

You explain to the patient that the risk to her children is slightly greater than it would be for the general population. Table 24.1 shows the risks.

Table 24.1 Risk factors in colorectal cancer	
Family history	Risk
Category 1 One first-degree or second-degree relative with colorectal cancer diagnosed at 55 or over	Up to 2 fold
Category 2 One first-degree relative with colorectal cancer diagnosed under 55 Two first-degree or second-degree relatives on the same side of the family with colorectal cancer diagnosed at any age	3 to 6 fold
Category 3 Proven or suspected HNPCC (hereditary non-polyposis colorectal cancer) Suspected or proven FAP (familial adenomatous polyposis) Somebody in family in whom the presence of a high-risk mutation in the APC (adenomatous polyposis coli) or one of the mismatch repair (MMR) genes has been identified	1 in 2 lifetime

The patient's son is with her. He understands that he is at slightly increased risk and would like to know what screening you would recommend for him. He is aged 42.

Q9 What is your advice to the son?

You advise him that if he is symptom free, he does not need any surveillance at this stage. If he does have symptoms, they should be investigated as appropriate. In patients over the age of 40 who have a positive occult blood test, it is recommended they have a colonoscopy. Similarly, you explain to him that any patient over the age of 40 who presents with new rectal bleeding needs investigation. As a guiding rule, any patient over the age of 40 who presents with an iron deficiency anaemia needs a full colonic investigation.

The son has heard that 'polyps in the bowel usually turn to cancer'.

Q10 What kinds of polyps occur in the large bowel and what is their malignant potential?

The patient remains in good health and is kept under regular surveillance.

ANSWERS

A1 The patient has two symptoms that cause concern: increasing constipation and rectal blood loss. You should ask further questions that may indicate why she is constipated. There are many possibilities in addition to colonic pathology, such as dietary changes, use of narcotic analgesia (codeine) or development of hypothyroidism. You should enquire about a personal history of polyps and family history of colon cancer. In the absence of an obvious cause for her constipation, such as recent use of a codeine-containing compound, this patient will require examination of all of her large bowel. A sigmoidoscopy may be performed as part of the general physical examination and might clarify matters and identify a source for the bleeding in the anal canal or lower rectum. Even if the patient does have internal haemorrhoids, which may be the cause of the bleeding, she must be investigated further. Haemorrhoids are extremely common, but it is important to inspect the rest of the large intestine and so not overlook a tumour.

A2 The most likely cause of her bleeding is internal haemorrhoids, but it is essential to exclude a more sinister cause for the blood loss, especially as she has recently become constipated for no obvious reason. Cancer of the colon is relatively common in this age group and often presents with these symptoms. Despite the haemorrhoids, she must have a colonoscopy. In the absence of other symptoms and the visualization of a bleeding haemorrhoid it would be reasonable to treat the haemorrhoids and only investigate further if the symptoms persist. If a colonoscopy was not available (uncommon) then a barium enema would be satisfactory but does not allow any diagnostic or therapeutic manoeuvres such as biopsy and snaring of polyps to be undertaken.

A3 This lesion has the typical appearance of a polypoidal adenocarcinoma. There is some blood clot at the base of the tumour where it has ulcerated. It is almost circumferential and about 3 cm in length.

A4 As part of the work-up, the following investigations are required:

- Complete blood picture, serum biochemistry and serum CEA (carcino-embryonic antigen).
- Chest X-ray.
- Ultrasound of the liver.

Iron deficiency anaemia is common in cases of colorectal cancer and must be excluded. The patient may have secondary spread of her disease. Colorectal cancers tend to spread to the liver, but metastatic deposits can also be found in lung and bone. A chest X-ray, liver enzymes and an ultrasound examination may not affect the decision-making of how to manage the primary tumour, but will give an indication of possible spread of the disease.

In cases such as this the entire large bowel must be examined. This patient had a negative colonoscopy other than the lesion visualized. However, co-existent disease is often present and patients may have polyps or other primary tumours. Synchronous tumours occur in 5% of patients and polyps may be found in up to 20% of cases. The discovery of polyps or another tumour will influence the extent of surgical resection required.

A5 You should explain the diagnosis and management to the patient, who needs to understand that she has a cancer of the colon, although at this stage there is no evidence that the disease has spread outside the bowel. Explain that she requires surgery to prevent total obstruction of the colon and attempt to cure her of the disease.

You must explain to the patient in simple language (and be prepared to repeat things several times) what the operation will involve and the risks and benefits of the proposed treatment. You must explain that:

- The surgery will be done under general anaesthetic.
- She is likely to be in hospital for at least 7 days.
- The bowel will need to be prepared for operation, i.e. empty it of its faecal contents. To do this she will need to drink a solution which will induce diarrhoea and empty her bowel.

A N S W E R S – cont'd

- She will be placed on antibiotics to reduce the risk of infection.
- The surgeon will look to see if there is evidence of tumour spread outside the bowel.
- The surgeon will cut out the tumour and adjacent colon and then ideally will join the two ends back together.
- If this were not possible she would require a colostomy or ileostomy. This is when a piece of the bowel is brought out through the abdominal wall to drain into a bag.
- Given the site of her tumour and that the operation is not an emergency, she is unlikely to require a colostomy.
- Should such procedure be necessary, the colostomy or ileostomy will be temporary and only required for about 12 weeks.

Risks including infection, anastomotic leakage and operative mortality must be discussed. You can emphasize that these should be kept in perspective, as the patient has little alternative as, untreated, she will develop complete intestinal obstruction.

Remember that fears of being left with a colostomy are common and these concerns must be fully addressed. However, with modern stapling techniques and the realization that the incidence of local recurrence is no greater with a 2 cm margin of clearance than a 5 cm margin, fewer patients now undergo total excision of the rectum with the formation of a permanent colostomy. Most patients with carcinoma of the rectum do not need complete excision of the rectum and anus. Fifty years ago, only 15% of all rectal cancers were treated with a restorative procedure, whereas that figure currently exceeds 65%. Temporary or defunctioning colostomies are still fashioned, but it is unlikely that the case discussed in this problem would require one. Colostomies (or defunctioning ileostomies) may be required after a difficult dissection deep in the pelvis or after emergency surgery for perforated or obstructed colon. The aim of a colostomy or ileostomy in such circumstances is to reduce the risk of anastomotic leakage, or in the event of established peritoneal contamination, to prevent further soiling.

Surgery remains important in incurable metastatic disease when the primary tumour is producing troublesome symptoms such as bleeding, obstruction or tenesmus.

A6 This patient must be given a prognosis. Her tumour has been staged as a stage B and she will have an approximate 60% 5-year survival rate. Expressed simply to the patient, she could be told that all the cancer has been removed, she has a good chance of cure, but will be monitored to look for recurrence of her disease or development of polyps which might develop into a new cancer. The surveillance will require repeated colonoscopy.

Although chemotherapy has no role in the initial treatment of colorectal cancer, it is well accepted that adjuvant chemotherapy will improve survival for patients with Duke's stage C cancers.

A7 The aim of any cancer follow-up programme is threefold and is to detect:
- Local recurrence.
- Metastatic disease.
- New primary tumours.

Surveillance strategies
- Estimation of carcino-embryonic antigen (CEA) is of most value if the levels were elevated prior to surgery and then returned to normal following resection of the tumour. Of more value is detection of blood in the stool.
- The faecal human haemoglobin (FHH) test detects bleeding distal to the terminal ileum. Other tests (e.g. haematest) are less specific and may detect blood in the stool that could have originated anywhere in the gastrointestinal tract. These tests are simple to perform and cause minimum inconvenience to the patient. They are highly sensitive, although not specific. In other words, most cases of occult bleeding will be detected, although the bleeding may be from a benign cause. In patients such as the one described in this case, faecal occult blood testing should be performed every 12 months.
- Colonoscopic follow-up would be recommended every 3 years if there were no other polyps at initial colonoscopy.

ANSWERS – cont'd

A8 The cause of colorectal cancer is unknown, but diet is likely to play an important role. In certain instances there may be a genetic predisposition to cancer (e.g. familial adenomatous polyposis), or the patient may have a condition such as ulcerative colitis that places them at high risk. It is also apparent that first-degree relatives have a two-to-threefold increase in risk of developing colorectal cancer. People also at increased risk of developing colorectal cancer are those who have a past history of the disease. However, in most cases no obvious risk factor exists and the cancer is thought to arise from a pre-existing adenoma.

In this instance no particular risk factors can be identified and the patient should be counselled that her children would be at slightly increased risk over the general population. Use of the chart indicated in the text can be helpful.

A9 On the assumption that he has no digestive tract symptoms (particularly rectal bleeding), then nothing needs to be done until he reaches the age of 50. The following guidelines should be applied. These recommendations for screening of first-degree relatives of patients with colorectal cancer follow the NH and MRC Guidelines (Table 24.2).

A10 An adenoma is one of four types of polyps that can be found in the colon and rectum. Apart from neoplastic lesions, there are three benign groups which include hyperplastic and inflammatory polyps and hamartomas. All adenomas have malignant potential. Adenomas may be tubular (often pedunculated), villous (usually sessile) or tubulovillous and can be found in any part of the bowel. As with cancers, the most common site for adenomas is the distal colon and rectum. The larger the polyp, the greater the chance of it being malignant. 50% of all polyps greater than 2.0 cm contain a focus of malignancy.

Table 24.2 Screening guidelines for colorectal cancer

Screening guidelines	Recommendation
Category 1	Faecal occult blood testing (FOBT) annually from age 50 Sigmoidoscopy (preferably flexible) every 5 years from age 50
Category 2	Colonoscopy every 5 years starting age 50 or 10 years younger than the index case FOBT annually
Category 3	Careful surveillance which needs to be tailored to the subgroup Consideration for genetic testing

REVISION POINTS

Colorectal cancer

Epidemiology
- One of the most common cancers in developed countries.
- Increasing in incidence (probably a reflection of increasing proportion of older people in the population).

Risk factors
- Diet.
- Genetic predisposition (e.g. familial adenomatous polyposis).
- Ulcerative colitis.
- Family history (see below).
- A past history of colorectal cancer.
- Pre-existing adenoma.

continues overleaf

REVISION POINTS – cont'd

Symptoms

Will vary with site of tumour.

- Rectum/sigmoid colon (60% of colorectal cancers):
  - change in bowel habit
  - rectal bleeding
  - tenesmus
  - mucorrhoea.
- Right-sided neoplasms:
  - tiredness and lethargy (secondary to an anaemia).

Surveillance

- The case for surveillance of the general population has yet to be made.
- Mass screening (FOBT) is not justified.
- 'Average risk' individuals: FOBT for those aged over 50.
- Individuals with a family history of colorectal cancer: see Answer 9.
- Screening of 'at-risk' groups:
  - inflammatory bowel disease
  - familial adenomatous polyps
  - adenomatous polyps
  - previous colorectal cancer.

Regular colonoscopy is recommended for the above groups.

Rectal bleeding

- Will usually be from a benign lesion (e.g. haemorrhoids).
- If bleeding cannot be seen coming from this source, the rest of the bowel must be examined to exclude malignancy.

Change in bowel habit

Important causes of constipation include:

- Change in diet.
- Irritable bowel syndrome.
- Diverticular disease.
- Medications.
- Malignancy.

ISSUES TO CONSIDER

- Colorectal cancer is virtually unknown amongst the indigenous population of southern Africa – why might this be so?
- If you found a 30-year-old patient with multiple colonic polyps, how would you set about devising a plan of management?

FURTHER INFORMATION

Guidelines for the prevention, early detection and management of Colorectal Cancer (CRC) National Health and Medical Research Council, Canberra 1999.

www.noah-health.org/english/illness/cancer/colorectalcancer.html A patient-orientated website on colorectal cancer, with many links covering most aspects of the disease.

www.gastrolab.net/lc20.htm Endoscopic images presented in an MCQ fashion.

A 42-year-old man with haematuria

A 42-year-old man presents with a 1-week history of passing blood in his urine. It is intermittent and is not associated with any pain. His health is otherwise good and there are no other symptoms of note. On examination he looks fit and well and his pulse rate is 70 and regular. His blood pressure is 140/80 mm Hg. The rest of the physical examination is unremarkable.

Q1 What are the most likely causes of his symptoms?

There is no other information from the history to help throw any light on the underlying aetiology of the haematuria.

Q2 What further information from the patient's history may help you decide the site of urinary tract bleeding?

The patient describes the blood as being plum-coloured and present in the entire urinary stream. He has not passed any clots.

Q3 What are you going to do next and why?

Urinalysis shows 3+ (c. 250 red cells/µl) of blood, but no protein. Microscopy of a sample of urine shows red cells with normal morphology but no other cells, casts or bacteria. There is no significant growth on culture. His haemoglobin is 143 g/l and serum biochemistry is normal. An intravenous urogram is performed and one of the films is shown in Figure 25.1.

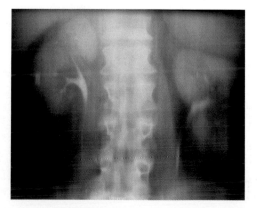

Fig 25.1

Q4 What does Figure 25.1 show?

The radiologist reports that the intravenous urogram (IVU) shows a mass in the right kidney.

Q5 What do you do next and why?

The following investigation is performed (Figure 25.2).

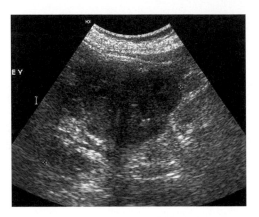

Fig 25.2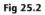

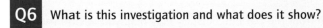

Q6 What is this investigation and what does it show?

A chest X-ray is normal.

Q7 What do you do next and why?

A scan of the abdomen is performed and two of the images are shown (Figures 25.3 and 25.4).

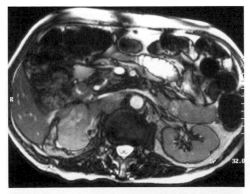

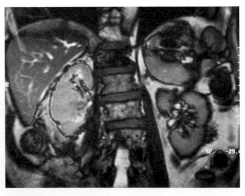

Fig 25.3   **Fig 25.4**

Q8 What kind of investigation is this and what do the images show?

Based on your history, examination and results of the investigations, you decide that the patient has a neoplasm of his right kidney with no evidence of spread.

Q9 How will you counsel the patient?

The patient underwent a radical right nephrectomy (excision of kidney, ipsilateral adrenal, proximal half of the ureter with renal hilar and regional lymph nodes). The patient made an uneventful postoperative recovery and returned home for follow-up.

ANSWERS

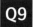 **A1** In a 42-year-old man the most important causes of painless haematuria to consider are:
- carcinoma of the bladder
- carcinoma of the kidney.

Other conditions include:
- infection (usually painful)
- prostatic hypertrophy (older men)
- stones (usually associated with pain).

Depending on the patient's origins and general state of health, it may be necessary to consider:
- chronic infection (e.g. tuberculosis or schistosomiasis)
- primary renal disease (e.g. IgA nephropathy and analgesic nephropathy). IgA nephropathy is associated with dysmorphic erythrocytes and red cell casts indicating a glomerular (medical) cause for the haematuria. Proteinuria may also be present
- coagulation disorders (particularly over-anticoagulation with warfarin)
- haemorrhagic cystitis (e.g. a post-transplant complication in bone marrow transplant patients).

A2 A more precise description of the blood in the urine can help determine the site of origin of the blood loss:
- when bleeding occurs from the bladder,

ureters or kidneys, the blood is usually well mixed throughout the urine and the patient sees dark and/or blood-coloured urine
- when the bleeding is from the prostate, bladder neck or urethra, it may be independent of micturition or seen at the beginning or end of voiding
- elongated clots suggest bleeding from above the bladder, while clots that form in the bladder tend to be larger and more rounded in appearance.

A3 Investigations should include:
- urinalysis:
  - dipstick analysis (red cells, protein, nitrites, glucose)
  - microscopy (red and white blood cells, red cell morphology, casts, bacteria)
  - culture (Note: If positive, must treat before any cystoscopy)
- complete blood picture and coagulation studies
- biochemistry: renal and liver function studies as well as bone parameters: calcium, phosphate and alkaline phosphatase. Elevation of the latter may suggest the presence of underlying cancer and metastatic disease
- imaging studies. In the first instance an intravenous urogram (IVU) is performed to look at anatomy and function of the upper tracts while helping to exclude pathology both in

ANSWERS – cont'd

the upper tracts and the bladder (e.g. urothelial tumour or calculi). A tumour in the renal parenchyma may if large enough or strategically placed show up as a space-occupying lesion which may produce displacement of the pelvicalyceal system

- if the IVU shows a renal filling defect, further evaluation is required to delineate if the renal lesion is cystic, solid or indeterminate. Simple cysts are common and present in up to 50% of the population aged over 40 years and as such of no clinical significance unless they cause obstruction by virtue of their size or position. If the IVU is normal then endoscopic (cystoscopy) evaluation of the lower urinary tract is needed as the problem may lie in the bladder.

A4 Both kidneys function, with contrast in the renal parenchyma and pelvicalyceal systems. The left kidney appears normal.

The right kidney contains a filling defect in the middle of the organ. It is causing some distortion of the pelvicalyceal system.

A5 The mass may be solid or cystic. An ultrasound examination rapidly, simply and accurately differentiates between the two.

A6 Figure 25.2 is an ultrasound examination of his right kidney which shows the normal renal parenchyma and the adjacent mass. The mass is solid and is almost certainly a neoplasm.

A7 Since the patient is likely to have a renal neoplasm, you want to know if there is any evidence of local or distant spread. Such staging will help determine treatment.

This tumour is almost certainly a renal cell carcinoma and can spread by the bloodstream to the lungs and liver (commonly) and to bone (infrequently). The primary tumour may invade adjacent structures, spread to regional lymph nodes or extend into the renal vein and inferior vena cava.

A chest X-ray is usually sufficient to exclude pulmonary metastases and a bone scan is only indicated if bony deposits are suspected on

clinical grounds (bone pain or elevated alkaline phosphatase of bony origin).

A rapid-phase helical CT scan of the abdomen and pelvis pre- and post-contrast will:

- define the primary tumour (size and position within the kidney)
- show the relationship of the tumour to surrounding structures
- identify any lymph node enlargement
- show any renal vein or IVC involvement (MR scanning is better for this)
- allow an accurate assessment of other intra- and retroperitoneal organs and structures including the bones for detection of secondary spread or other pathology.

An MR scan may be performed in place of a CT. In addition to showing good definition of the primary tumour and its relationship to adjacent structure, the MR scan provides an accurate assessment of any spread into the renal vein (or IVC).

A8 These are magnetic resonance scans. Figure 25.3 is a transverse scan and shows the neoplasm in the middle of the right kidney. The renal vein is seen and there is no evidence of extension of tumour into the vein.

Figure 25.4 is a coronal view which has focused on the right kidney. The tumour has displaced the pelvicalyceal system inferomedially and superiorly.

A9 You will explain to him that he has a greater than 90% chance of a cancer involving his right kidney and that the tests have shown no obvious disease spread.

You should tell the patient that surgery to remove the diseased kidney, adjacent fat, lymph nodes and adrenal gland offers an excellent chance of cure. It is important to stress that other treatments including chemotherapy or radiation therapy are not effective in this type of cancer.

Explain what the surgery will involve and how long you anticipate he will be in hospital.

Finally, you must also tell him that he will maintain normal renal function after the operation as he has a healthy left kidney.

REVISION POINTS

Renal cell carcinoma

Incidence
- 4.6:100 000 (female)
- 10:100 000 (male)
- incidence rises with age.

Risk factors
- smoking
- obesity
- hypertension
- adult renal polycystic disease
- acquired renal cystic disease in dialysis patients
- horseshoe kidneys
- familial glomerulonephropathy
- Von Hipple–Lindau disease
- tuberous sclerosis.

Classification
- conventional (non-papillary)
- papillary
- chromophobe
- collecting duct carcinoma.

Presentation
- 60% are found incidentally on ultrasound or CT
- anaemia
- hypertension
- pyrexia
- polycythaemia
- the classic triad of haematuria, flank pain and a mass is rare

- 10% of patients will have haematological or biochemical abnormalities (e.g.anaemia, polycythaemia, hypercalcaemia).

Treatment
- primarily surgical
- metastatic disease is difficult to treat as the cancer is relatively insensitive to chemotherapy
- immunomodulatory approaches are currently being investigated. As there may be a graft-versus-malignancy effect, one approach currently undergoing Phase I studies for relatively fit patients is haematopoietic stem cell transplantation using non-myeloablative preparative regimens.

Prognosis
See Table 25.1.

Table 25.1 Prognosis in renal cell carcinoma

Stage	5-year survival (percentage)*
Confined to kidney	85–95%
Renal vein/IVC involvement	70%
Perinephric fat invasion	50%
Lymph node spread	30%
Distant metastases	5%

*20% of patients have metastatic spread at the time of presentation

---

ISSUES TO CONSIDER

- How would your management of this patient differ if he had presented with a bony deposit and pathological fracture rather than disease confined to the kidney?

- What are the hereditary forms of renal cell carcinoma and how do they differ in their presentation?

FURTHER INFORMATION

www.emedicine.com/MED/topic2002.htm A succinct description of renal neoplasms and their management.

www.surgical-tutor.org.uk There are sections in this website on the investigation of patients presenting with haematuria and the management of renal cell cancers.

merck.praxis.md/bpm/bpm.asp?page=BPM01N P04 A comprehensive and well-reviewed site covering the management of haematuria.

A 70-year-old man with a painful hip

A 70-year-old retired chartered accountant presents with a 1-month history of increasing pain in his right hip. The pain radiates into his groin and to the lateral aspect of his thigh. The pain is worse on walking and is eased by rest. He now limps as he walks and has difficulty in rising out of a chair. When you saw him 2 weeks ago you prescribed a non-steroidal anti-inflammatory drug, but this has not relieved his symptoms. The patient has had no significant illnesses in the past, but he does get short of breath on exertion. He smoked 20 cigarettes a day until 10 years ago. He describes a 'smoker's cough' and produces a small quantity of clear sputum each day. The patient says his general health seems to have deteriorated over the last couple of years but, apart from fatigue, he is unable to be more specific. He has no cardiovascular nor gastrointestinal symp-

toms. He gets up twice every night to void and says that his urinary stream is not as forceful as it used to be and he sometimes has difficulty starting. He is on no other medications and drinks 10–20 grams of alcohol each day.

On examination he looks older than his years. His cardiorespiratory system is unremarkable. His abdomen is normal and in particular his bladder is not palpable. On rectal examination his prostate does not appear to be enlarged, although the median sulcus cannot be felt. The gland feels firm. His left hip has a full range of movement, but on the right there is loss of internal rotation, with an inability to abduct or fully extend the hip. You notice that when the patient puts his weight on the left leg with his right leg flexed, the pelvis tilts up on the right side and when he stands on the right leg, the pelvis drops towards the left side.

 Q1 What is your interpretation of the locomotor signs?

The only other abnormal finding is an area of tenderness over the lateral aspect of his right 5th rib.

 Q2 What investigations would you like to do and why?

You perform the following investigations.

The chest X-ray shows mild emphysematous change throughout both lung fields. There is no focal lung lesion. The X-ray of the pelvis shows several sclerotic areas in the pelvis including one close to and eroding into the right acetabulum.

Investigation 26.1 Summary of results			
Haemoglobin	105 g/l	White cell count	6.5 x 10⁹/l
MCV	88 fl		
MCH	29.5 pg		
MCHC	300 g/l		
Platelets	120 x 10⁹/l		
Sodium	139 mmol/l	Calcium	2.30 mmol/l
Potassium	4.4 mmol/l	Phosphate	1.05 mmol/l
Chloride	106 mmol/l	Total protein	62 g/l
Bicarbonate	27 mmol/l	Albumin	35 g/l
Urea	6.1 mmol/l	Globulins	27 g/l
Creatinine	0.10 mmol/l	Bilirubin	16 μmol/l
Uric acid	0.24 mmol/l	ALT	28 U/l
Glucose	4.4 mmol/l	AST	43 U/l
Cholesterol	3.5 mmol/l	GGT	22 U/l
LDH	212 U/l	ALP	456 U/l
PSA	46.0 ng/ml		

 Comment on the results. What is the most likely diagnosis? What would you like to do next?

Your investigation is shown in Figure 26.1.

 What is this investigation? Describe the abnormalities shown.

The patient goes on to have a transrectal prostatic biopsy performed. The histology shows a prostatic adenocarcinoma.

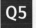 **What are you going to tell the patient and what are the treatment options available to him?**

Fig 26.1

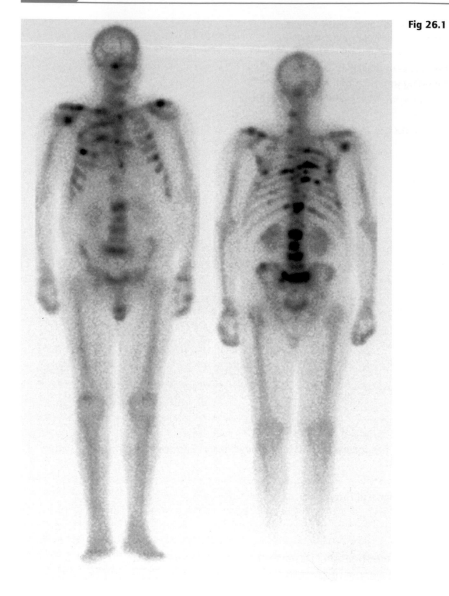

ANSWERS

A1 This is called a positive Trendelenburg's sign. Normally the adductors will contract to lift the pelvis up on the unsupported side. This shifts the weight from the unsupported limb on to the supported one. In this instance, pain prevents the adductors from contracting and the pelvis falls away from the affected hip.

A2 The following investigations should be considered:
- Hip and pelvic radiographs looking for evidence of bone pathology or degenerative joint disease.
- Complete blood picture looking for anaemia which would indicate systemic disease such as underlying malignancy, and biochemistry including renal function, calcium and total protein and alkaline phosphatase (ALP). Remember myeloma may present with anaemia, hypercalcaemia, renal failure and elevated total protein. Bone metastases may elevate ALP and also cause hypercalcaemia.
- A chest radiograph should be performed in view of his smoking history. He may have a primary lung cancer which has metastasized to bone.
- In view of his abnormal-feeling prostate and urinary symptoms, a serum prostate specific antigen (PSA) needs checking.

A3 Significant findings are:
- Normochromic normocytic anaemia and thrombocytopenia which may suggest bone marrow involvement. However, haematinics should still be checked.
- Markedly raised alkaline phosphatase suggests bony disease. A raised alkaline phosphatase may also be of liver origin and may suggest infiltrative liver pathology. Other liver function tests should be checked.
- Raised serum prostate specific antigen (PSA).

Since the chest radiograph shows no evidence of primary lung carcinoma, the PSA is raised and the prostate is clinically abnormal, the most likely diagnosis is metastatic carcinoma of the prostate. The pelvic radiograph showing sclerotic bony lesions further supports this diagnosis. Prostatic carcinoma is one of the few malignancies that produces sclerotic rather than lytic bony metastases.

A4 This is a bone scan. It shows widespread areas of increased isotope uptake throughout the whole skeleton. The posterior view shows intense areas of uptake in the lumbar vertebrae and ribs, typical of metastatic prostatic cancer deposits.

A5 The patient needs to be told the diagnosis sensitively and given time to assimilate the news as well as ask questions. He needs to be told that he has cancer of the prostate gland and it has spread to his bones. His hip pain is likely to be due to a tumour deposit and will need some treatment for the pain. He should be told that you will not be able to cure him of the cancer but may be able to slow its progress. Moreover, you should emphasize that you will be able to affectively treat symptoms from the disease paying particular attention to pain control. The anaemia and urinary symptoms may also need treating at some stage.

You should emphasize that pain control is very important and will be achieved initially with long-acting slow-release oral morphine with rapid-acting morphine for breakthrough pain. As his disease is treated you can emphasize that his need for painkillers will hopefully decrease. Allied health professionals such as oncology nurses should be involved in his care from the outset.

He should be counselled concerning the several forms of treatment available:
- Radiotherapy to the hip to control his bone pain.
- Hormone therapy, e.g. antiandrogen drugs or gonadotrophin releasing hormone (GnRH) antagonists.
- Orchidectomy.

REVISION POINTS

Prostate cancer

Incidence
19:100 000 (UK data).

Risk factors
- age
- family history
- Western diet
- heavy metal exposure (cadmium).

Pathology
- most commonly develops around periphery of gland 70% with 10% central
- remainder are in transient zone
- 85% are diffuse multifocal tumours
- microscopically adenocarcinoma.

Natural history
- local growth: infiltration of gland and surrounding tissues
- lymph node metastases are not often prominent in this disease
- spread predominantly bloodborne especially to vertebrae
- spread to lung and liver are uncommon but recognized.

Symptoms
- often asymptomatic and incidental finding at autopsy
- prostatic outflow obstruction: frequency, poor stream, terminal dribble
- bone pain or cord compression due to bone metastases
- symptoms relating to hypercalcaemia
- general symptoms due to malignancy, e.g. malaise, anorexia, weight loss, etc.

Signs
- palpable tumour: hard nodule, loss of midline sulcus
- bony tenderness if bone metastases
- neurological signs if cord compression.

Investigations
- blood counts, Ca, PSA, renal function
- CT scan may identify local invasion and lymph node enlargement
- plain radiographs and isotope bone scan to identify bone metastases
- histological diagnosis via transurethral resection or transrectal biopsy.

Treatment
- radical prostatectomy or radical radiotherapy if cancer localized to prostate gland
- hormone therapy will achieve 70–80% response
- first-line treatment for metastatic disease would be cyproterone acetate or a gonadotrophin-releasing hormone (GnRH) agonist
- permanent androgen deprivation (orchidectomy) may be offered to responders with the alternative of continuing medical treatment.

ISSUES TO CONSIDER

- What are the arguments for and against screening for carcinoma of the prostate?
- What role does PSA have in the screening of men for prostatic carcinoma? What are its limitations? What other measures should be taken to make screening techniques more effective?
- What other malignancies produce sclerotic bony metastases? What non-malignant conditions lead to areas of bony sclerosis?
- What is the mechanism of action of the various drug treatments for prostatic carcinoma?
- What new therapies do you know of and what approach is favoured in your hospital?

FURTHER INFORMATION

www.urologychannel.com A patient-based website with interesting and useful information on prostate carcinoma and other urological conditions.

Acute back pain in a 75-year-old man

You are asked to see a 75-year-old retired electrician who has been brought into the emergency department with an 18-hour history of increasing back pain. He tells you that the pain came on gradually and now goes down into his left groin and thigh. The pain is constant, getting worse. He has never had this pain before. He does not think the pain was precipitated by anything and nothing seems to ease it. In particular, there is no history of trauma, and walking or exertion do not affect it. There are no other associated symptoms.

Eight months ago he suffered a myocardial infarction and since that time has suffered with moderate angina on effort. He takes isosorbide dinitrate 10 mg three times a day for the angina and uses nitrate skin patches at night. He used to smoke 20 cigarettes a day, but ceased after his heart attack. He drinks 20 gm of alcohol at the weekends. He suffers occasional episodes of indigestion for which he takes an over-the-counter antacid preparation.

The review of systems is otherwise unremarkable apart from symptoms of increasing bladder neck outflow obstruction, which have been worse over the last 2 years. He gets up twice every night to void and says he feels that he can never empty his bladder properly. He has not passed urine since the pain started.

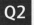

Q1 What diagnoses go through your mind?

On examination he is thin and in pain. His blood pressure is 140/90 mm Hg and he has a regular pulse rate of 100 bpm. His jugular venous pressure is not elevated and his apex beat is displaced 2 cm lateral to the mid-axillary line and is felt in the fifth interspace. Both heart sounds are normal with no added sounds. His chest is resonant and breath sounds are vesicular. He has a tender mass in the abdomen which feels like it is 6–7 cm in diameter and situated at the level of the umbilicus. The mass

is pulsatile. There is dullness to percussion in the suprapubic region extending four fingerbreadths above the pubis. Both femoral pulses are of good volume and pedal pulses are palpable. His legs are neurologically normal and the straight-leg raise and sciatic stretch tests are negative. The patient's previous X-rays are available.

The patient recently had an abdominal ultrasound for his urinary frequency (Figures 27.1 and 27.2).

Q2 What does the investigation show?

The ultrasound findings confirm your clinical suspicions.

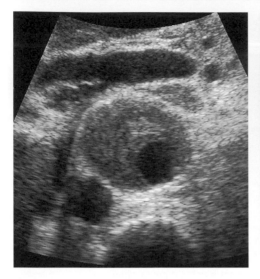

Fig 27.1

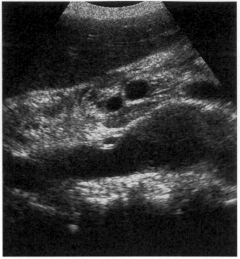

Fig 27.2

Q3 What is your next action?

Q4 What further investigations may be indicated?

As this patient is haemodynamically stable, a further investigation is performed expeditiously. Two of the images are shown (Figures 27.3 and 27.4).

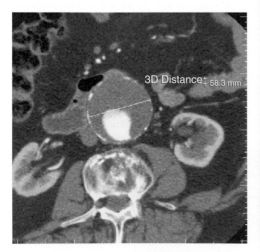

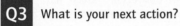

Fig 27.3

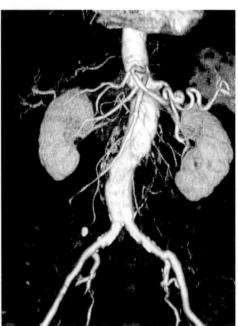

Fig 27.4

Q5 What type of images are these and what do they show? How do these findings affect your management?

The patient and his family are informed of the diagnosis and the likely outcome if surgery is not undertaken promptly. The aneurysm is in imminent danger of rupture, with a subsequent high mortality. Surgery also has its risks, particularly in this patient with known cardiac disease.

The cardiologists and anaesthesiologists are asked to review the patient, and prepare him for emergency surgery. At surgery, the aneurysm is repaired using a dacron tube graft. Following the procedure he is transferred to the intensive care unit.

Q6 What complications may follow an aortic aneurysm repair?

The patient makes an uneventful recovery and is home 10 days after the procedure.

ANSWERS

A1 Acute pain in the back, radiating to the groin, in an elderly male with known atheromatous disease must make you consider a leaking or stretching abdominal aortic aneurysm. This is the diagnosis that needs to be excluded. Other conditions include:
- aortic dissection
- acute pancreatitis
- ureteric colic
- urinary retention.

This is unlikely to be a musculoskeletal problem (e.g. herniated disc), as the pain is not aggravated by movement.

A2 The ultrasound shows a large fusiform abdominal aortic aneurysm. The image in Figure 27.1 shows the aneurysm in transverse section and in Figure 27.2 the aorta in longitudinal view. Some thrombus is shown in the wall. The measurement of aneurysm size is taken on the transverse image and is the maximum anteroposterior or transverse diameter. The length of the aneurysm is not important from a management point of view.

A3 This man has an abdominal aortic aneurysm, which is symptomatic and may now be leaking or about to leak. This is a vascular emergency. Your priority is to insert a wide-bore intravenous catheter, collect blood for electrolytes,

full blood count and grouping together with cross-matching and coagulation screens. You must alert the surgeons immediately. Also attach a cardiac monitor and insert a urinary catheter to monitor urine output. Notify the patient's relatives.

A4 The need for further investigations will hinge on whether the patient is haemodynamically stable. If not, further investigations will only delay definitive management. In that case, the patient should go directly to the operating theatre.

As the patient is haemodynamically stable, the surgeons may request a CT scan of the aorta to assess the size of the aneurysm, its relationship to the renal arteries, whether it has leaked and to exclude any other cause of intra-abdominal pain.

A5 Figure 27.3 shows a standard transverse cut through the aneurysm sac. Contrast has been administered and the non-enhancing contents of the aneurysm sac represent laminated thrombus. It is these images which provide the surgeon with vital information regarding the presence or absence of a leak. This shows a 5.8 cm abdominal aortic aneurysm which had not leaked. The pain is presumably due to expansion and stretching of the aneurysm.

Figure 27.4 is a spiral CT angiogram reconstruction. The reconstruction gives the surgeon

ANSWERS – cont'd

useful information regarding patency/stenoses of renal and iliac arteries, vessel tortuosity and relationship of the aneurysm to the renal arteries. The renal arteries are patent and the iliac vessels are not aneurysmal.

The transverse cuts give the essential diagnostic information regarding size of the aneurysm sac and the presence or absence of leaking blood. The laminated thrombus in the sac does not show up on CTA reconstructions. The spiral CT reconstruction is essential in the elective situation if endoluminal repair of the aneurysm is being considered.

A6 The majority of the morbidity and mortality (2–15%) associated with elective abdominal aortic aneurysm repair is due to pre-existing cardiac disease. The risk of a peri- or early postoperative myocardial infarction in this man will be high.

Other possible complications include:
- cerebrovascular event
- acute thrombotic/embolic events leading to:
  – renal failure
  – bowel infarction
  – critical lower limb ischaemia
- graft infection.

REVISION POINTS

Abdominal aortic aneurysms (AAA)

Incidence
- 5% of males over 65 years of age
- less common in women
- occur in 10–15% of claudicants.

Risk factors
- smoking
- hypertension
- hyperlipidaemia
- genetic predisposition (e.g. Ehlers–Danlos syndrome type IV).

Note: diabetes not a risk factor.

Pathology
- degenerative process involving all layers of aortic wall
- appears to be caused by increased activity of matrix metalloproteinases (extracellular matrix-degrading enzymes which break down collagen and elastin in the aortic wall). These enzymes seem to be activated by aortic endothelial injury caused by smoking, hypertension or hyperlipidaemia: i.e. aneurysms are not caused by atherosclerosis, although atherosclerosis may co-exist.

Clinical features
- most frequently asymptomatic
- may present with abdominal, back or loin to groin pain (if stretching, leaking or ruptured)
- collapse or cardiac arrest may occur in acute rupture.

Natural history
- aneurysms less than 5–5.5 cm in diameter rarely rupture (1–2% per year)
- rupture rate increases exponentially with increasing size over 5.5 cm.

Management
- AAA less than 5 cm in diameter should be treated with aggressive control of risk factors and 6-monthly ultrasound surveillance, unless there is rapid increase in size or development of symptoms, e.g. abdominal or back pain
- AAA over 5 cm can be considered for repair if risks of surgery (mainly cardiorespiratory) are less than risk of rupture
- open repair is the gold standard
- endoluminal stent graft repair can be considered in elderly or high-risk patients.

ISSUES TO CONSIDER

- How might a thoracic aortic aneurysm present?

- How would you diagnose and manage a dissecting aneurysm?

- Why do symptomatic patients develop groin and testicular pain?

FURTHER INFORMATION

www.scvir.org/patient/aaa/ A website from the Society for Cardiovascular and Interventional Radiology. Patient directed but with good information about endoluminal treatments.

www.postgradmed.com/issues/1999/ 08_99/gorski.htm A good overview from the *Postgraduate Medical Journal.*

www.NEJM.com Long-term outcomes of immediate repair compared with surveillance of small abdominal aortic aneurysms. *New England Journal of Medicine* 2002;346:1145–52.

A 59-year-old man with calf pain

A 59-year-old man presents with a 4-month history of pain in the right calf. The pain occurs only on walking and presents as a cramp-like discomfort, which comes on after he walks about 100 metres. The pain eases off when he stops walking, and he is still able to make his way to the local shops, although he is now reluctant to do so.

Q1 What is the likely cause of his symptoms and what other information would you like from the history?

Three years previously he suffered a myocardial infarction and since then has been on enteric-coated aspirin. He takes no other medications apart from a salbutamol inhaler which was pre-scribed by his general practitioner for 'when he gets a bit tight'. In the past he has had an appen-dectomy and a prostatectomy. He smokes 20 cigarettes a day and drinks 20 gm of alcohol a day. He is 170 cm tall and weighs 75 kg.

Q2 What will be the important points to look for on examination and what investigations will you perform?

His blood pressure is 150/85 mm Hg and his heart rate is 84 and regular. Examination of his heart is unremarkable. He has a bruit over his right carotid artery. His chest is resonant with decreased breath sounds and a prolonged expi-ration, but no added sounds. Abdominal exami-nation is normal. His femoral pulses are palpa-ble, as are the more distal pulses in his left leg. His right popliteal pulse is not palpable and neither are the right pedal pulses. Both legs are of similar temperature and there are no other signs of limb ischaemia.

Q3 What is an ankle–brachial index measurement and what is its significance?

His ankle–brachial index is 0.5 on the right and 0.8 on the left. His lipid profile is reported as being marginally raised and a random blood sugar is within normal limits. His serum biochemistry is unremarkable.

Q4 How would you explain his condition to him, and what is your advice at this point?

Twelve months later he comes back to see you. He had managed to continue his daily walks down to the local shops until 2 months ago, but despite your advice he has continued to smoke. His pain has worsened recently and now comes on at about 20 metres. He now finds these symptoms interfere with his lifestyle. Most recently he has been woken at night by pain in his leg, which he relieves by dangling the leg over the edge of the bed.

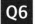 **Q5** What has happened and what do you do now?

Your examination of his cardiorespiratory system does not reveal any new findings. His abdomen is soft, there are no pulsatile masses and both femoral pulses are palpable. His legs and feet are cool to the touch, and the right foot is colder than the left. The toes on his right foot are dusky and there is sluggish capillary return to his big toe. When the leg is lowered over the side of the examination couch it assumes a reddish purple colour, and when the leg is elevated the foot becomes pale. His popliteal and pedal pulses cannot be palpated on either leg. His Doppler pressures are measured and he has an ankle–brachial index of 0.3 on the right and 0.7 on the left.

On your advice he agrees to see a vascular surgeon, who recommends that angiography be performed. The aortogram and bilateral femoral angiograms are shown in Figure 28.1. The unsubtracted film is on the left and the subtracted film on the right. These are AP views with the patient's right leg on the left side of Figure 28.1.

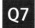 **Q6** What does the angiogram show?

Apart from the lesion shown in the two films, the rest of the arterial tree was imaged with satisfactory run off into his tibial vessels with no other significant areas of narrowing.

Q7 How are you going to manage this problem?

The patient undergoes a reverse vein femoropopliteal bypass. This is successful in improving his lower limb circulation but is complicated by a cerebrovascular event involving his non-dominant hemisphere for which he requires 3 months of intensive rehabilitation.

Fig 28.1

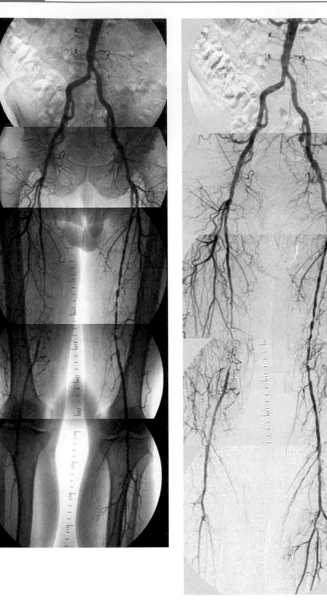

ANSWERS

A1 His history of calf pain on exercise relieved by rest is typical of intermittent claudication. You may also consider spinal cord stenosis in your differential diagnosis, but relief of the pain by rest points to peripheral vascular disease as the cause of the problem. As such, you would like to know if he has risk factors for cardiovascular

disease and any history of other previous or current problems related to his cardiovascular system.

Major risk factors which you must ask about are:

● Hypertension (duration and adequacy of control).

A N S W E R S – cont'd

- Diabetes mellitus (duration, Hb A1C).
- Smoking (pack years).
- Hyperlipidaemia.

Typical cardiovascular co-morbidities are:
- Ischaemic heart disease (especially current but also past symptoms).
- Cerebrovascular accidents or transient ischaemic attacks (TIAs).
- Abdominal aortic aneurysm.

You also want to enquire about any medications that he might be taking such as betablockers, which may exacerbate the symptoms of peripheral vascular disease.

A2 • The cardiovascular system should be examined for hypertension and evidence of cardiac dysfunction. The carotid arteries should be examined for bruits.
- The respiratory system should be examined for evidence of smoking-related chronic airways obstruction.
- His abdomen should be examined carefully for evidence of aortic aneurysm (present in 10–15% of claudicants).
- His peripheral pulses, including the femoral, popliteal, dorsalis pedis and posterior tibial pulses should be examined. Provided a pulse can be felt, the quality of the femoral pulse will be assessed (for strength and dilatation) and bruits listened for.
- The legs should be assessed for evidence of ischaemia. This includes the colour and temperature of the limbs. If ischaemia is advanced, the foot will become pale when the leg is elevated and deeply red when it is then lowered to a dependent position. Reduced blood flow through the capillary bed will result in increased uptake of oxygen from the blood by the tissues and this may cause the limb to take on a cyanotic hue. An ischaemic foot tends to be relatively cool.
- The limb should also be examined for areas of ulceration and necrosis – so-called 'dry gangrene' or mummification. There may also be evidence of muscle atrophy. As the ischaemia worsens, atrophy of the skin progresses and it

appears shiny and scaly. loss of hair and thickening of the nails are unreliable signs of ischaemia because they are widely present in the normal population.
- Objective measurement of foot perfusion with Doppler ultrasound is essential – clinical judgement, including palpation of pedal pulse, is fairly inaccurate.
- You should measure the ankle–brachial index (ABI).

At this stage the patient does not warrant extensive investigation, but the following should be performed:
- Blood sugar.
- Lipid profile.
- Serum biochemistry (looking for any renal impairment).

A3 By comparing the blood pressures in the brachial (which is assumed to be normal) and dorsalis pedis vessels, an estimation can be made of the efficacy of arterial blood flow in the leg. In an individual with normal arteries the ankle–brachial index is expected to be one or greater. A value below 0.5 is often associated with rest pain and when the ratio gets to less than 0.3, viability of the limb may be in jeopardy.

A4 You should advise him in simple language that:
- The pain in his legs is due to arterial occlusive disease, resulting in insufficient blood getting to the muscles, which is most noticeable during exercise
- He should continue to walk. Even when the exercise provokes pain, it will do no harm and this exercise may improve his symptoms due to the development of collateral channels.
- It is absolutely vital that he stops smoking because if he does not the disease will progress and he could develop gangrene or another complication such as a heart attack or stroke.
- He needs to take low-dose aspirin.
- No other drugs will improve his symptoms.
- Apart from Doppler studies, he does not need any other investigations.

ANSWERS – cont'd

- He needs to take care of his feet and avoid local trauma.
- He should reduce his cholesterol intake by following a low-cholesterol diet. If a lipid profile check 3 months later does not show improvement antilipid agents will be started.

A5 He now has rest pain: the blood supply to the limb has deteriorated to such an extent that the leg's viability is threatened. You must take action and:

- Repeat your physical examination.
- Repeat the Doppler studies.
- Reinforce your advice on the need to stop smoking.
- Make the patient aware of the high risk of losing his limb (or part of it).
- Arrange for the patient to be seen by a vascular surgeon, who will:
  - arrange imaging studies
  - suggest some form of intervention to try and improve blood supply to his foot.

A6 Both a non-subtracted and subtracted angiogram are shown to assist with vessel orien-

tation. The angiogram demonstrates normal aortoiliac arteries. The common femoral and pro funda femoris vessels are also widely patent. Both superficial femoral arteries (SFA) (from groin to adductor canal) are extensively diseased, with a 7–8 cm long occlusion of the right SFA being shown. Collateral vessels via the profunda femoris arteries fill the popliteal arteries.

As a result of the more severe occlusive disease on the right side, the contrast filling the popliteal and proximal tibial vessels on this side is reduced, resulting in reduced opacification of the vessels.

A7 As this patient has rest pain, revascularization should be undertaken, assuming his co-morbidities do not preclude intervention.

Approximately 25–30% of patients with disabling claudication or critical limb ischaemia (see Revision points) are suitable for percutaneous intervention (angioplasty, stent, thrombolysis or combinations of these techniques).

The majority of patients require bypass, either due to the length of the stenotic lesion/occlusion or the quality of the vessels above and below the lesion.

REVISION POINTS

Chronic lower limb ischaemia

Incidence
Approximately 5:1000 population/year in developed countries.

Aetiology
- atherosclerosis (>90% of cases)
- thromboangitis obliterans (Buerger's disease)
- vasculitis
- arterial trauma
- rare causes: cystic adventitial disease of the popliteal artery, popliteal artery entrapment.

Differential diagnoses
- spinal canal disease
- sciatica
- peripheral neuropathy.

Note: Presence of pulses, ankle–branchial index (ABI) or exercise ABI should allow differentiation

between claudication and neurological cause of pain.

Risk factors for atherosclerosis
- smoking
- diabetes
- hypertension
- genetic
- hyperlipidaemia.

Classification
See Table 28.1.

Natural history
Claudication
- approximately 5–10% require lower limb intervention within 5 years for disabling claudication or deterioration to critical limb ischaemia
- limb loss in 2% during lifetime: majority of patients managed conservatively

continues overleaf

REVISION POINTS – cont'd

Table 28.1 Classification of lower limb ischaemia

Classification	Doppler ankle–brachial index (ABI) approximate	Fontaine stage
Claudication	0.6–0.9	II
Critical limb ischaemia:		
• rest pain	0.3–0.6	III
• ulceration and/or gangrene	< 0.4	IV

- mortality 30% at 5 years (predominantly MI, CVA).

Critical limb ischaemia
- revascularization attempted in 40–80%
- limb loss in 40% at 1 year
- mortality 20–30 % at 1 year (mainly cardiovascular).

Management

Claudication
- conservative
- aggressive risk factor control

- only consider intervention if symptoms disabling.

Critical limb ischaemia
- angiography with a view to revascularization
- stenting may be possible with durable results obtained in aortoiliac segments
- selected centres rely on duplex ultrasound for planning revascularization
- lower limb bypass using autogenous vein is frequently required for limb salvage.

ISSUES TO CONSIDER

- How successful are conservative measures in the prevention of progression of occlusive vascular disease?
- What is neurogenic claudication and how does it differ from vascular claudication?
- What measures may help this man give up smoking?

FURTHER INFORMATION

www.scvir.org Home page of the American Society of Cardiovascular and Interventional Radiology. Interesting information and links about peripheral vascular diseases and the role of endovascular therapies.

Acute leg pain in a 73-year-old woman

You are sitting in the on call room, enjoying pizza with your fellow interns and about to become immersed in your favourite TV show when you receive a call from the ward.

The nurse would like you to see a 73-year-old woman who is complaining of sudden onset acute severe pain in her left leg. Four days earlier she was admitted to hospital with an anterior myocardial infarction.

Q1 What diagnoses go through your head as you head for the ward?

When you see the patient, you find her distressed with pain. She tells you the pain in her left leg came on abruptly about 40 minutes ago. The leg now feels numb and she cannot move it. She gives no prior history of claudication. Two years previously she underwent a total left knee replacement, which has been trouble free.

Her blood pressure is 130/80 mm Hg and her pulse rate 100 (irregularly irregular). Examination of the chest is unremarkable. There are no abnormalities in her abdomen. Her femoral pulses are of good volume, the pulses in her right leg can all be felt. There are no pulses to be felt below the groin on the left side. The left leg is not swollen, but pale and cool to the touch.

Q2 What do you think has happened? What further information would you like?

You are handed her in-patient notes. She had presented with 7 hours of chest pain. Work-up showed an acute anterior myocardial infarction. As her pain had subsided and she had developed Q waves in the anterior leads, she was not given any thrombolytic therapy.

She was immediately given oral aspirin and betablockers before being transferred for close monitoring in the coronary care unit. She remained there for 2 days before moving to the general ward. Now, 4 days since her admission, she has been slowly mobilizing. She was initially prescribed subcutaneous low molecular weight heparin, but you note on the drug chart that this was not continued on the ward since returning from coronary care.

Her myocardial infarction was complicated by atrial fibrillation, with a rapid ventricular response rate on day 1. She had no ventricular arrhythmias and was treated with digoxin resulting in good rate control. She does not have any other significant past medical history.

Q3 What would you like to do now?

An investigation is performed. One of the results is shown in Figure 29.1.

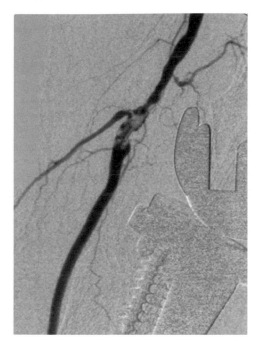

Fig 29.1

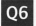 **Q4** What is this investigation? What does it show?

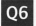 **Q5** What would you like to do now?

The patient underwent thrombolysis of the embolus radiologically using the 'pulse-spray' technique that often results in rapid clot lysis. Standard thrombolytic techniques would take 4–20 hours to achieve clot dissolution, and it was thought this patient's leg was unlikely to be viable if revascularization took this length of time. The 'pulse-spray' technique is much more rapid. After 1 hour of urokinase pulsing, the perfusion of the foot was reassessed and the angiogram repeated (Figures 29.2 and 29.3).

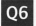 **Q6** What do these new X-rays show?

The patient was anticoagulated with heparin and plans were made to continue anticoagulation on oral warfarin for at least 6 months, or possibly indefinitely depending on her atrial rhythm.

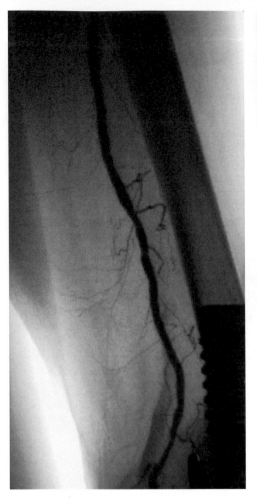

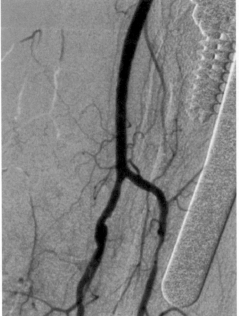

Fig 29.3

Fig 29.2

ANSWERS

A1 There are few possible causes of an acute severely painful leg. The most likely diagnosis is one of arterial embolus to the left leg. Other less likely possibilities include thrombosis of a pre-existing arterial atherosclerotic plaque, an extensive deep thrombosis of the left leg or an aortic dissection extending into the left leg arteries. A muscle haematoma if on thrombolytic or anti-coagulant therapy is also a possibility.

A3 She has a critically ischaemic limb. Her leg is pale, pulseless, painful and perishing with cold.

In addition she may have paraesthesia and paralysis of the affected limb – the classic six Ps.

The presence of a femoral pulse on the left indicates that the occlusion is likely to be in the superficial femoral or popliteal artery.

The sudden onset, lack of previous history and recent myocardial infarction all suggest that this is an embolic phenomenon. She has most probably thrown off an embolus from the heart which has lodged in the femoral artery. Such an embolus would have arisen from a mural thrombus at the site of infarction (in the left

A N S W E R S – cont'd

ventricle) or dislodged from clot in an atrium that is fibrillating. A less likely cause in this instance would be atherosclerosis and femoral or popliteal artery occlusion by acute thrombosis.

After your initial assessment you will want to examine the notes looking for information about her post myocardial infarction course, the timing and duration of arrhythmias and whether or not she has been anticoagulated.

A3 You should contact the vascular surgeons immediately. Emergency arteriography will be required to define the site and extent of obstruction.

Unless angiography can be performed without delay, you should consider anticoagulating the patient with unfractionated intravenous heparin. Baseline coagulation studies (APTT) must be performed before starting the heparin. Heparin is dosed by weight and must be adjusted to maintain the APTT in the therapeutic range. A standard loading dose for an adult would be 5000 units, followed by an infusion of 1000 units/hour. Blood should also be collected for a complete blood picture, electrolytes and type and cross-matching. This patient is not a good candidate for general anaesthesia, but may need it and should be fasted.

A4 This is a digital subtraction angiogram, which demonstrates a filling defect in the popliteal artery at the level of the knee. At the level of the obstruction, there is a large collateral seen filling

the distal popliteal vessel. This is consistent with a popliteal embolus. The proximal vessels (not shown) are normal.

Note that this is a transverse view due to her total knee replacement, which is visible on the right of the scan. The artery would not be able to be seen on an anteroposterior view in this patient.

A5 This patient has a threatened ischaemic leg requiring revascularization within 4 hours (see Revision points at end of chapter).

Management options include:

- Surgical removal of the embolus. However, this would likely require a general or spinal anaesthetic – a high-risk procedure so soon after a myocardial infarct.
- Thrombolytic therapy. Possibilities include a rapid clot thrombolysis technique ('pulse-spray') or suction thrombectomy as a percutaneous radiological procedure. Urokinase and heparin can be 'pulsed' directly into the clot via a catheter traversing the thrombus.

A6 The angiograms performed after 1 hour of thrombolysis demonstrate a good radiological result. Figure 29.2 demonstrates a patent above-knee popliteal artery. The filling defect is no longer seen. Figure 29.3 shows the distal popliteal artery and proximal tibial vessels. These are widely patent. It is important to make sure that no residual thrombus has embolized distally which could cause persistent ischaemia.

R E V I S I O N   P O I N T S

Acute lower limb ischaemia

Incidence
Approximately 2:10 000 population per year.
Aetiology
- Embolus – almost always due to mural thrombus post myocardial infarction or secondary to arrhythmia (occasionally can be from valvular heart disease or proximal aortic disease, e.g. aneurysm).

- Acute thrombosis of diseased artery.
- Bypass graft thrombosis.
- Trauma (e.g. knee dislocation, tibial plateau fracture).

Classification
Table 29.1 outlines classification criteria.
Investigations
- Following examination for pulses and assessment of severity of ischaemia, vascular sur-

continues overleaf

R E V I S I O N   P O I N T S – cont'd

Table 29.1 Classification of severity in limb ischaemia

		Sensation (calf/foot)	Power (foot movement)	Calf tenderness
1	Viable (urgent revascularization not required)	normal	normal	nil
2	Threatened			
	a) needs revascularization (4–8 hours)	slightly reduced	normal	nil
	b) needs *urgent* revascularization (<4 hours)	reduced	decreased	often tender
3	Unsalvageable	numb	decreased/nil	very tender (or paralysed)

geons should be consulted, and ECG, bloods, group and match performed. Doppler pressures (ankle–brachial index) may be performed. Anticoagulation should be commenced unless angiogram can be performed.

- Also search for other sites of embolization (common sites include other leg, arms, brain and gut).
- Angiography will demonstrate the level of occlusion and may clarify the aetiology of acute ischaemia.

Management

Therapy will depend on aetiology, severity of ischaemia and patient co-morbidities.

Options:

- Surgical thrombectomy under local, spinal or general anaesthetic.
- Thrombolysis performed radiologically (using urokinase or ± tissue plasminogen activator: TPA). Advanced catheter techniques such as suction thrombectomy or pulse-spray thrombolysis may be used in highly selected cases

and decrease time taken to reperfuse the lower limb (particularly in cases of profound ischaemia – category IIb).

- Bypass graft thrombectomy, thrombolysis or replacement for occluded (usually prosthetic) grafts.
- Surgical repair of artery ± bone fixation (for trauma).
- Immediate amputation for unsalvageable limb may be required.
- Occasionally palliative care is appropriate in selected cases.

Note: Fasciotomy of lower limb muscle compartments may need to be considered if ischaemia is profound and of lengthy duration prior to revascularization.

Outcomes

- Depend on severity and duration of ischaemia, and co-morbidities.
- Mortality rates are still 15–30%.
- Amputation rates in survivors 20–30%.

- What are the risks of surgery after a myocardial infarction?

- What are the other short- and long-term vascular complications of myocardial infarction? How may this patient's risk have been minimized?

FURTHER INFORMATION

www.freevas.demon.co.uk A superb website from the vascular unit of the Royal Free Hospital, London, with links, an image library and an excellent medical student section.

Ouriel K. **Thrombolytic therapy for acute arterial occlusion**. *Journal of the American College of Surgeons* 2002;194:S32–S39.

A 68-year-old woman with a leg ulcer

A 68-year-old woman attends the outpatient department with an ulcer on her left leg. She tells you it has been present for 2 months. She remembers knocking her leg on the end of her bed. The ulcer on her leg has become fairly painful over the last week. She has had a similar ulcer on her leg in the past which was treated by 'bandaging'.

Q1 What other information would you like from the history to ascertain the cause of the ulcer?

She is not a diabetic, but does take tablets for her blood pressure. She is not sure what these are. She is on no other medications. She has had no other illnesses of note, but has had varicose veins ever since the birth of her children. On further questioning, she reveals that the left leg was very swollen for 2 or 3 months after her third pregnancy but she never had any tests to see why. This has been her 'bad leg' ever since. Her leg ulcer is shown below (Figure 30.1).

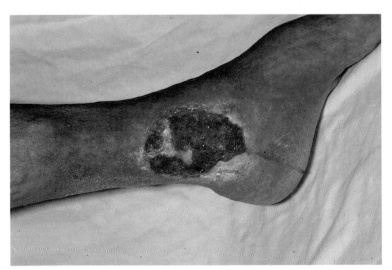

Fig 30.1

Q2 Describe what you see.

In addition to what is shown in the photograph, both legs show evidence of chronic venous insufficiency. There is loss of subcutaneous fat, and this atrophy has caused an 'inverted champagne-bottle appearance'. There is pigmentation above each ankle. There are no ulcers on the feet or toes.

Q3 What else are you going to look for before you complete your examination of her legs?

On general examination she is mildly obese and has a blood pressure of 160/110 mm Hg. The rest of the cardiorespiratory and abdominal examination is unremarkable. Her left leg shows varicosities of the long saphenous vein and at least one incompetent perforating vein in the calf. The right leg is similarly affected with varicosities and changes of chronic venous insufficiency in the lower third of the calf. You note the skin around the ulcer is mildly inflamed and tender and you think the ulcer is infected. The peripheral pulses and neurological exam of the lower limbs are normal.

Q4 What is your diagnosis now? What, if any, investigations should be performed? What is your initial management?

ANSWERS

A1 You would like to know if there is a history of:

- varicose veins or deep venous thrombosis
- previous surgery on this leg
- pain in the lesion
- problems with her legs suggestive of arterial insufficiency, e.g. claudication, rest pain
- diabetes mellitus
- rheumatoid arthritis or other vasculitic process.

You also want to know the patient's general state of health, and occasionally, their place of origin (tropical ulcers). You would also want to know about other medical problems like cardiovascular disease, medications (e.g. steroids) and use of tobacco and alcohol.

A2 There is an extensive ulcerated area over and above the medial malleolus approximately 8 x 5 cm. There is slough on the ulcer but with considerable healthy granulation tissue. The surrounding skin is discoloured, scaly and indurated. There are areas of haemosiderin deposition. This appearance is characteristic of venous ulceration secondary to chronic venous congestion.

A3 On examination you need to ensure that pulses are present in the limbs (i.e. palpable femoral, popliteal and at least one of the dorsalis pedis or posterior tibial pulses). It is also important to exclude neuropathy by performing a screening neurological examination of the lower limbs.

A4 The diagnosis is a venous ulcer. In the presence of cellulitis, take a swab and start antibiotics to cover *Staphylococcus aureus* and Gram-negative bacilli including *E. coli* and *Klebsiella*.

A venous incompetence duplex scan is not essential in this setting but will confirm underlying incompetence of the deep veins (usually secondary to a previous DVT) in approximately 40–50% of cases or of the superficial veins (long or short saphenous ± perforating veins) in a further 40–50% of cases. Some individuals may have incompetence of both deep and superficial venous systems.

Initial management is based on compression therapy. You may delay commencing this for a few days until the cellulitis has settled. Most fre-

ANSWERS – cont'd

quently, a 4-layered compression bandaging system is applied on a weekly basis until the ulcer is healed. Smaller ulcers can be managed with occlusive dressings and class III (20–40 mm Hg) compression stockings. Most clinicians use knee-high rather than full leg stockings because of higher patient compliance levels.

Once healed, compression is maintained using knee-high stockings to reduce recurrence. Patients with isolated venous incompetence of the superficial systems (e.g. long saphenous vein ± perforator incompetence, with normal deep veins) should be considered for surgery to reduce the risk of recurrent ulceration. Skin grafting is infrequently required in venous ulcers.

In this patient healing will take many weeks. Therefore, she will require visits from a nurse who is experienced in wound care and assistance in the activities of daily living.

REVISION POINTS

Assessment of leg and foot ulcers

Table 30.1 describes the assessment of these ulcers.
Note:

- Vasculitic ulcers: exclude above causes, may need biopsy.

- Malignant ulcers: biopsy suspicious ulcers and those not responding as expected.
- Combination of above aetiologies common.

Table 30.1 Assessment of leg and foot ulcers

	Venous	Arterial	Neuropathic
Location	Lower calf area	Pressure areas – toes, 1st–5th MTP joints, heel, malleoli	Pressure areas
Swelling	Yes	Not usually	No
Pain	Usually not (or not severe)	Yes – except if also neuropathic	No
History	Often recurrent DVT/varicose veins likely	May have claudication	'Diabetes', alcohol, spinal pathology
Associated features	Venous skin change/ lipodermatosclerosis		
Presence of pulses	Yes, but may be difficult	No	Yes
Investigations	? Nil initially Venous incomplete duplex scan	Ankle–brachial index (usually <0.7)	Exclude arterial contribution to ulceration
Management	Compression ? Fix isolated superficial incompetence	Revascularize if necessary	Pressure relief/ podiatry/orthotics

ISSUES TO CONSIDER

- What advice can be given to diabetics with neuropathy to avoid lower limb ulceration?

- What is the cause of tropical ulceration?

- What are the features of the various dressings available to specialist teams to manage lower limb ulceration?

- Why do varicose veins form and what are the associated complications?

- Do varicose veins predispose to deep vein thrombosis?

- How can chronic venous insufficiency be treated surgically?

FURTHER INFORMATION

www.bmj.com London N J M and Donnelly R. ABC of arterial and venous disease: ulcerated lower limb. *British Medical Journal* 2000;320: 1589–91. A superb overview of the subject.

www.thediabeticfoot.net An interesting resource about diabetic foot care.

A 38-year-old man involved in a car crash

A 38-year-old man is brought in by ambulance to the emergency department of a district general hospital from the scene of a car crash. The paramedic crew provides a history. The patient was the front seat passenger in a car that was crossing a crossroads when it was struck on the passenger side by a speeding hatchback. The patient was wearing a seatbelt; a headrest was fitted, but the car possessed neither side-impact bars nor passenger airbags although the driver's airbag was deployed. There was significant intrusion into the pas-senger compartment and the patient was trapped for about 30 minutes before extrac-tion, with full cervical spine immobilization, by the emergency services.

During the ambulance journey from the scene of the crash the patient complained of shortness of breath and pain in the left side of his chest. He has been cardiovascularly stable throughout. The patient has been given oxygen by mask, one large-bore intravenous access has been obtained and 500 ml of crystalloid has been infused.

Q1 Describe your initial assessment of this patient? What elements of the history are particularly important?

Your examination reveals the following:

Airway (with cervical spine control): The patient's airway is patent, he is speaking to you and has no evidence of facial trauma or airway foreign body. His cervical spine is immobilized with a hard collar, sand bags and tape.

Breathing: He has a respiratory rate of 30 bpm and his pattern of breathing is shallow. He is not centrally cyanosed. Examination of his chest reveals superficial abrasions and contusion to his left anterior hemithorax and shoulder. There is no evidence of paradoxical chest movement or open wound. He is tender over the anterior aspects of the 6th–10th ribs and crepitus is present. There is a paucity of breath sounds on the left side and the percussion note is increased on that side. His trachea is central. Pulse-oximetry measurement reveals his oxygen saturation is 99% on 15 litres of O_2 by non-rebreather mask.

Circulation: He has a pulse rate of 130/min and a blood pressure of 105/85 mm Hg. His jugular venous pressure is not elevated and he has a slightly delayed peripheral capillary return of 3–4 seconds. He has no obvious external haemorrhage or major long bone fractures. The examination of his abdomen reveals generalized tenderness of both upper quadrants, maximally on the left, with marked guarding.

Disability: A rapid skeletal and neurological survey shows that the patient has no obvious deformity or tenderness of his limbs and has normal sensation. His Glasgow Coma Score (GCS) is 15/15. His pupils are equal and react normally to light.

Q2 Describe your approach to the management of this patient in light of the above findings. What are your priorities? What investigations would you request during the initial management?

A second wide-bore intravenous cannula is inserted into a peripheral vein and 1 litre of a crystalloid solution administered rapidly. Blood samples are collected for cross-matching, complete blood picture and biochemistry. The chest X-ray is shown below (Figure 31.1).

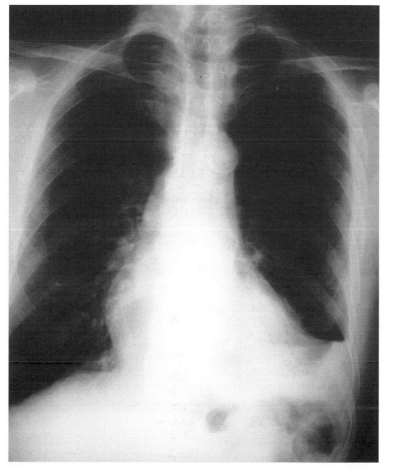

Fig 31.1

Q3 Describe the abnormalities shown in this chest X-ray. In what ways may this condition be complicated?

The lateral cervical spine views are adequate and show no bony injury, the pelvis appears undamaged. The chest X-ray confirms your clinical suspicion of a haemopneumothorax. A chest drain is inserted successfully and connected to an underwater seal. Air and approximately 500 ml blood drain out. The patient confirms that his breathing is much improved.

The initial laboratory results are unremarkable and his haemoglobin is 131 g/l.

One hour after admission and initial resuscitation you reassess the patient and note that although he has received a total of 2 litres intravenous fluid and his pain is adequately controlled with parenteral opiates, his pulse has risen to 145/min and his blood pressure is 90/75 mm Hg. His JVP is not visible. His airway and breathing are stable. Examination of his chest shows reasonable air entry to all areas, but there is still dullness at the left base. There is a further 100 ml fresh blood in the chest drainage bottle. His abdomen is markedly tender in the left upper quadrant.

Q4 What is the probable cause of this change and what needs to be done now?

A further haemoglobin estimation is performed. It is now 102 g/l. He is rapidly transfused 2 units blood and a further 1 litre crystalloid. His urine dipstick is negative for blood and a urinary catheter is inserted. His blood pressure stabilizes at 105/80 mm Hg with a pulse of 120 bpm.

A CT scan of his upper abdomen is performed (Figure 31.2).

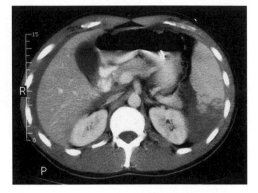

Fig 31.2

Q5 What does the CT image show?

The patient is transfused a further 2 units blood. He remains stable, his tachycardia settles and his injuries are treated conservatively.

He is admitted to an intensive nursing unit where he is monitored closely and has an uneventful course. His chest drain is removed at day 5. His splenic injury is monitored with a further CT, which showed gradual reabsorption of the haematoma. He is discharged home 2 weeks after the accident and advised to avoid strenuous exertion for a month.

ANSWERS

A1 This patient has been involved in a high-speed crash and is likely to be suffering from multiple traumatic injuries. In order to avoid overlooking significant injuries and to treat the most life-threatening conditions first it is wise to take a structured approach. Advanced Trauma Life Support® is such a system (also known as Early Management of Severe Trauma®). This system relies on:

Airway (with cervical spine control).
Breathing and ventilation.
Circulation with haemorrhage control.
Disability (neurological evaluation)
Exposure/environmental control.

The mechanism of injury is especially important. You should establish the speed and type of vehicle and the mode of impact, i.e. direction and

A N S W E R S – cont'd

whether the car hit a mobile or immovable object. Also, the condition of the vehicle after the accident, the provision and use of safety features, the position of the patient and the time taken to release trapped victims are all important features and may give valuable information as to the likely nature and severity of injuries.

A2 As always in any trauma case, your priorities are **A, B, C**.

The assessment of this patient reveals no imminent problems with **A** and the cervical spine is being appropriately managed with 3-way immobilization. Further investigation of the cervical spine with cross table lateral X-ray should be arranged.

The assessment of **B** demonstrates problems that need to be addressed rapidly. The chest wall shows obvious signs of trauma with probable rib fractures of at least four ribs, the underlying lung is probably damaged and the increase in percussion note on the left side suggests a pneumothorax. He does not appear to be deteriorating rapidly, and the pneumothorax does not appear to be under tension. Therefore it is reasonable, in this case, to proceed to imaging of the chest to rule out diaphragmatic rupture and intrathoracic abdominal contents before proceeding to chest drain insertion. Whilst the X-ray is performed you ask for a chest drain set and under-water seal to be prepared and you proceed to assess **C**.

C. This is a relatively young patient who will have a good cardiovascular reserve. This means that even when bleeding and shocked, he can maintain his blood pressure and central perfusion. As he has a marked tachycardia and is diverting his blood from his peripheries (prolonging his capillary return), restoration of his circulating volume should be started immediately. Two large peripheral cannulae should be adequate at this stage. Blood samples should be sent for haematology, biochemistry and urgent 6-unit crossmatch. Two litres of intravenous crystalloid (e.g. Hartmann's solution) should be infused over the first hour.

The history of injury to the left side of the torso must raise the possibility of damage to the rib cage and the abdominal wall, and the contents in the immediate vicinity. Any trauma of suffi-

cient force to break ribs, particularly if associated with shock, may well have produced substantial internal injury.

Disability: A rapid skeletal and neurological survey shows that the patient has no obvious deformity or tenderness of his limbs and has normal sensation. Assessment of **D** may not show any immediate acute problems, but should be repeated later.

Apart from X-rays of chest and cervical spine, a pelvic X-ray should be performed, especially in view of his haemodynamic instability. An ECG should also be performed to look for evidence of cardiac contusion.

A3 The X-ray shows collapse of the upper part of the left lung with air in the pleural space from the mid-zone to the apex. There is blunting and flattening of the left costophrenic angle, suggesting a haemopneumothorax. There are fractures of the 7th–10th ribs.

In this situation the following potential complications must be remembered:

Tension pneumothorax

With a rapidly developing pneumothorax a one-way valve may be created in the lung or chest wall and air enters the pleural cavity with each breath. This is known as a tension pneumothorax. These are dangerous because the accumulating air cannot only collapse the lung, but will push the mediastinum to the opposite side, preventing blood getting to the heart. Features suggestive of a tension pneumothorax include rapidly worsening respiratory function, haemodynamic instability and hypotension, together with engorgement of neck vessels and tracheal deviation. A tension pneumothorax is an emergency and must be dealt with immediately, prior to any imaging. A large-bore cannula should be inserted in the 2nd intercostal space, mid-clavicular line prior to definitive insertion of a chest drain.

Haemothorax

Extensive damage to the intercostal vessels can lead to a rapidly enlarging haemothorax. With this condition the breath sounds on the affected side are diminished, and the percussion note is markedly dull, as is vocal resonance. A chest drain should be inserted and the blood drained.

ANSWERS – cont'd

Flail segment

Multiple ribs fractured in more than one place prevent that section of the chest moving normally. The affected section of the chest moves paradoxically and can limit normal ventilation. It is not this that causes hypoxia, but the associated severe contusion to the underlying lung. Contused pulmonary tissue is very sensitive to both under- and over-perfusion. Very careful fluid balance is needed in these cases. A short period of assisted ventilation may be required to optimize ventilation and perfusion of the affected lung.

A4 Despite your initial resuscitation this patient has become hypotensive and this is likely to be due to hypovolaemia. While other causes of hypotension must be considered, in this setting the cause of the problem is almost certainly blood loss. The patient requires:

- prompt resuscitation (with blood transfusion)
- a careful assessment made for the site of blood loss. This is likely to be either into the left chest, the abdominal cavity or both.

Apart from a further clinical examination, imaging studies must be considered. The two main imaging methods used in these circumstances are the CT scan and ultrasound.

If available, ultrasound examination in the emergency department is useful in the unstable patient, and can be performed in the resuscitation cubicle. It is particularly useful for rapidly detecting free fluid (e.g. haemorrhage) in the abdomen.

A CT scan is the imaging investigation of choice, particularly in the classification of splenic injuries when non-operative management and spleen preservation is the preferred option. If the patient is haemodynamically unstable, moving the patient out of the emergency department or resuscitation area for an imaging investigation may be dangerous.

A5 This is a section through the upper abdomen. Free blood can be seen between the right lobe of the liver and the abdominal wall. There is a large haematoma within the spleen, particularly involving the lower pole. The laceration goes towards the splenic hilum and most of the splenic capsule appears to be intact.

REVISION POINTS

Care of the trauma patient

Multiple and major trauma requires a structured and organized approach. A team approach is essential. Many of the steps discussed will happen simultaneously, but must be coordinated by one individual. Involvement of multiple specialties such as anaesthetists, surgeons and radiologists is frequently essential.

The first hour following major trauma is the most important. Rapid assessment, diagnosis and intervention during this period is essential for favourable outcome.

Many hospitals have dedicated trauma teams and some are designated trauma centres where this approach to trauma care is highly rehearsed and senior staff from all required specialties are on site. Outcomes in these hospitals are significantly better.

The ATLS® approach is pivotal:

- **Airway** (with cervical spine control)
- **Breathing** and ventilation
- **Circulation** with haemorrhage control
- **Disability** (neurological evaluation)
- **Exposure**/environmental control.

Any change in the condition of the patient should make you go back to the beginning and start again.

- How have the implentation of compulsory seatbelt laws and the advent of airbags influenced the severity and nature of road traffic crashes?
- What are the indications for splenectomy in abdominal trauma and what measures need to be taken after an emergency splenectomy has been performed to protect the patient from future infection?
- Discuss the different forms of shock. How is haemorrhagic shock classified?

FURTHER INFORMATION

Advanced Trauma Life Support® student manual. American College of Surgeons, 1997.

Saunders C E, Ho M T. Current emergency diagnosis and treatment. Appleton and Lange, 1992.

www.surgical-tutor.org.uk An excellent website with a good section on trauma as well as a full range of other surgical topics.

Lower limb trauma in a young man

You are on duty in the emergency department. The triage nurse asks you to assess a 24-year-old motorcyclist who has been brought in by ambulance. Witnesses reported that he was travelling at 70–80 kph when he lost control on a bend and crashed. You notice that his jeans are bloodstained and that he has a deformed left leg. He is moaning incoherently.

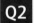 **Q1** What are the principles of early management of this patient?

He is still wearing his full-face motorcycle helmet.

Q2 What do you do?

You perform a primary survey and are reassured that his airway is clear and intact. His breathing is not hampered and his oxygen saturation by pulse oximeter is 98%. His blood pressure is 130/80 mm Hg and his heart rate is 100 bpm and of good volume. His helmet is removed. His initial score on the Glasgow Coma Scale is 12 (E3 V3 M6). A face mask is applied and oxygen delivered at 8 l/min. A wide-bore catheter is inserted into a peripheral vein of his right arm and an infusion of isotonic saline started. His disorientation settles and his only injury appears to be to his left leg. His clothing is removed and his legs are shown in Figure 32.1.

 Fig 32.1

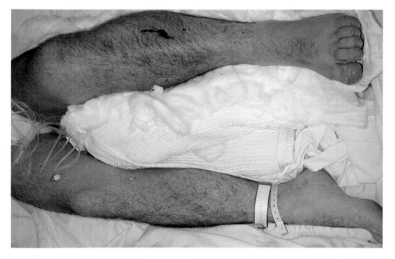

Q3 What do you see? What will you particularly look for on examination?

Motor function, sensation and blood supply to his foot are intact. The radiograph of his left leg is shown in Figure 32.2.

Fig 32.2

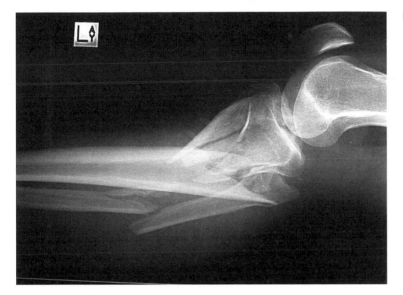

Q4 What does the radiograph show and how should this problem be managed?

The orthopaedic surgeon treats his fracture, and the next evening you come to see him on the ward to check on his progress. He complains bitterly that the pain in his left leg and foot is now worse than it was the night before and he is requesting more morphine. You note from the drug chart that he has been given a total of 50 mg morphine over the last 12 hours. You examine his legs and feet and note what is shown in the photograph (Figure 32.3).

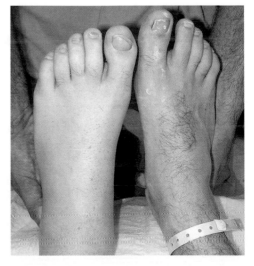

Fig 32.3

Q5 What do you see? What is the explanation for the changes?

The orthopaedic surgeon reviews the patient and agrees that he has sufficient evidence of compartment syndrome to warrant urgent re-exploration of the wound. In the operating room the wound is opened and a fasciotomy is performed. This prompt intervention avoids any serious complications to the wound, and the patient recovers uneventfully. Prior to discharge he shows you the new Kawasaki he has chosen on the internet. You recommend he keep up private health insurance.

ANSWERS

A1 This patient has been involved in a high-speed motorcycle accident and must be assessed using a structured approach (e.g. Advanced Trauma Life Support or ATLS, known as Early Management of Severe Trauma or EMST in Australasia). In a teaching hospital this would involve calling the trauma team. The primary survey is carried out in this order:

- Airway and cervical spine protection. This patient is moaning so his airway is likely to be intact, but may still be compromised by facial, mandibular or tracheal/laryngeal fractures. A cervical spine injury must be assumed and a hard cervical collar must be applied.
- Breathing. The chest must be exposed and examined for injury by inspection, palpation, percussion and auscultation. High flow oxygen must be applied. An oxygen saturation monitor is a useful adjunct to clinical examination. Injuries that can impair ventilation are tension pneumothorax, open pneumothorax, flail chest, haemothorax, pulmonary contusion and fractured ribs.
- Circulation. This can be rapidly assessed on the basis of level of consciousness, skin colour, pulse and blood pressure. Two large-bore intravenous catheters should be inserted and blood taken for baseline haematological studies, type and cross-match. In road trauma there is often a legal requirement to test blood alcohol. Intravenous fluid resuscitation should be commenced immediately. Haemorrhage should be controlled by pressure on obvious external bleeding sites.
- Disability. The level of consciousness should be assessed and recorded sequentially using the Glasgow Coma Scale. Alteration in con-

scious state could be due to hypoxia, hypovolaemia or head injury, and should not be assumed to be due to drugs or alcohol.
- Exposure. The patient should be completely undressed, often by cutting off the garments. A thorough examination is then carried out to look for other injuries. Radiographs must be taken of the chest, pelvis and cervical spine in all patients with major trauma. Further radiographs may be necessary based on the findings of the primary and secondary surveys.

The secondary survey is carried out once the patient is stabilized. This involves a thorough history from the patient and/or witnesses, as well as full reassessment of vital signs and comprehensive head-to-toe examination.

A2 The motorcycle helmet presents a problem. If there is any suspicion of a cervical spine fracture (as there must be in any high-speed road trauma), removal of the helmet is dangerous. On the other hand, the helmet is preventing access to his airway. In the order of ATLS, airway comes first. If you decide to remove his helmet, one possible technique is for someone to slip their hands inside the helmet either side of his temples to steady the head and neck while the helmet is carefully removed. If the patient had obvious facial or head wounds suggestive of impact to the helmet, a cervical spine injury is likely and you may have to call on the anaesthetist or emergency consultant to help with intubation.

A3 The upper part of the left lower leg is swollen, bruised and deformed. There is a 5–6 cm laceration over the anterior aspect of the tibia. The foot and toes are pink. This patient probably

ANSWERS – cont'd

has a compound (open) fracture involving the tibia.

You must look for evidence of any vascular injury.

A4 There is a comminuted fracture of the upper end of the tibia. There is also a fracture through the shaft of the fibula. This is a compound open fracture and is therefore at high risk of infection. The wound should be covered with a sterile dressing. Antibiotics and tetanus prophylaxis should be administered. The patient should proceed to the operating theatre for thorough irrigation and debridement of the soft tissue injury as soon as possible.

The general principles of managing any fracture are to reduce the fracture and to maintain reduction of the fracture until healing. This can be achieved either with closed reduction (without an incision) or open reduction (with an incision). Reduction can be maintained with plaster, internal fixation or external fixation.

This fracture is already open, so reduction will most likely be achieved by open means. The various ways of treating this fracture have different advantages and disadvantages and the decision is complex. Metal fixation devices are foreign bodies that can become infected. A plaster cast will avoid this problem, but will not provide enough stability to allow the soft tissue injury to be examined and to heal. More rigid fixation is required. A plate requires more extensive soft tissue dissection and is a large foreign body at the fracture site. An intramedullary nail would avoid additional soft tissue damage at the fracture site, but is also a large foreign body. An external fixator would avoid both of these problems but has a high risk of infection in the pin sites.

A5 The left foot is white and decidedly pale in comparison with the right foot and the examiner's arms. The foot is ischaemic. This could be due either to compartment syndrome or a primary vascular injury. The latter is less likely as the patient was noted on admission to have palpable pulses distal to the fracture. It is possible that when the fracture was manipulated, reduced and stabilized the adjacent vessels were damaged.

Escalating pain after fracture and surgery demands action. At the very least, the limb and wound must be examined. The potential problem is development of a compartment syndrome. This is a surgical emergency where circulation and function of tissues within a closed space are compromised by increased pressure within that space.

In this case the tight fascial compartments of the leg are not able to expand, and as the injury swells the pressure in the leg compartment rises rapidly. Trauma and hypoxia increase capillary permeability, which increases the amount of fluid contained within the compartment. Bleeding into the compartment from vascular injury and pressure from external dressings exacerbate this. The increased pressure eventually causes venous occlusion, which decreases the arteriovenous pressure difference and exacerbates the hypoxia. The result is a vicious circle of hypoxia, swelling, increased pressure and tissue damage. If unchecked, irreversible muscle necrosis occurs and ischaemic contracture or loss of the limb is the long-term result.

The classic symptoms and signs of compartment syndrome are: pain, pallor, paraesthesia, paralysis, pulselessness and perishing with cold (the six Ps). The earliest and most important symptom is pain. This is described as deep, unremitting, poorly localized and difficult to control, and is exacerbated by passive movement. A high index of suspicion is vital, as the other four signs are those of neurovascular compromise; by the time they develop it may be too late.

The increased pain in this patient – despite large doses of morphine – is of major concern. It is important to look for pain with passive movement of his toes and ankle, and assess the neurovascular status of his foot. Any circumferential dressings should be cut completely. If this does not relieve his symptoms then the orthopaedic surgeon should be contacted. The pressure in his compartments can be measured using a compartment pressure monitor. The normal pressure is zero mm Hg. Any increase is abnormal, but an increase to 30 mm Hg less than current diastolic blood pressure is an absolute indication for urgent surgical release of the compartments.

REVISION POINTS

Emergency management of severe trauma

Primary survey
- airway and cervical spine protection
- breathing
- circulation
- disability
- exposure.

Resuscitation and management of life-threatening injuries as they are identified.

X-rays: chest, pelvis, cervical spine.

Secondary survey
- thorough history
- head-to-toe examination
- X-rays as indicated
- ongoing resuscitation and reassessment of vital signs.

Management of fractures

General principles
- reduce the fracture if displaced, either by open or closed means

- maintain reduction until fracture union, with plaster, internal or external fixation
- specific treatment depends on the fracture.

Open fractures
- high risk of infection
- treat with tetanus immunization, prophylactic antibiotics and early surgical debridement and stabilization of the fracture.

Compartment syndrome

Definition
Circulation and function of tissues within a closed space are compromised by increased pressure within that space.

Presentation
- pain (most important)
- pallor
- paraesthesia
- paralysis
- pulselessness
- raised compartment pressure.

Treatment
Emergency surgical fasciotomy.

ISSUES TO CONSIDER

- What is the cost to the community of motor vehicle crashes, in terms of healthcare and loss of work?
- What other complications can arise in patients suffering major trauma with multiple fractures?
- What different injuries occur with full-face and open motorcycle helmets?

FURTHER INFORMATION

www.rta.nsw.gov.au/roadsafety/index.html Road traffic accident statistics are available online for most countries, states and counties. A particularly good example is from New South Wales.

www.ortho-u.net A privately posted but extremely extensive orthopaedic textbook online with a huge amount of well-written information and lots of links.

A 48-year-old man with chest pain

A 48-year-old man was awoken from his sleep by severe chest pain. The pain was mainly central and crushing in nature but also spread across both sides of his chest and spread into his neck. It was associated with sweating, nausea and mild breathlessness. The pain resolved spontaneously after an hour but the patient was concerned and drove himself to the emergency department of the local hospital.

On arrival the patient is pain free and haemodynamically stable. The physical examination is unremarkable. The ECG shows sinus rhythm at 78 bpm and is normal.

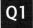 **What further information would you like to aid your diagnosis? What is the most likely diagnosis?**

Over the last few months he reports that he has been suffering from occasional chest pains. They were initially only related to exertion but over the preceding 2 weeks his exercise capacity has reduced considerably and he has noted slight twinges of pain at rest. Yesterday morning he had an episode of quite severe pain that lasted 20 minutes while he was having his breakfast.

The patient has been a heavy cigarette smoker for 30 years. His father died suddenly at the age of 56 but otherwise there is no known family history of ischaemic heart disease. The patient has no previous illnesses, is on no medication and has never had his cholesterol level checked.

 How would you manage this patient initially?

The patient is admitted to a cardiology ward for bed rest, cardiac monitoring and commenced on aspirin, a betablocker and low molecular weight heparin.

Later that afternoon you are called to see him as he is complaining of further ischaemic-type pain. It is of a similar nature although less severe than he experienced earlier. He is not distressed and remains haemodynamically stable.

Figure 33.1 is the patient's ECG during chest pain.

Q3 What does it show and what should be done now?

The patient's pain settled on an infusion of nitrates within 10 minutes. Serial ECGs were unchanged and showed no evidence of Q wave (full thickness) myocardial infarction. Blood tests show a slightly elevated cardiac troponin and serum cholesterol.

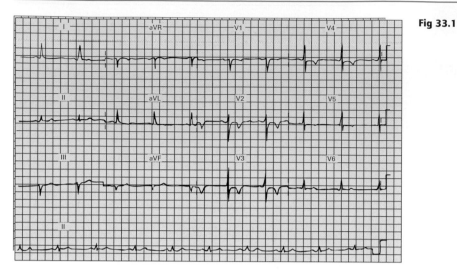

Fig 33.1

 Discuss the further management of this patient.

You telephone the on-call cardiologist, who comes in to perform the following investigation (Figure 33.2).

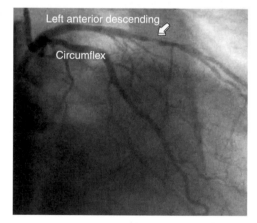

Fig 33.2

 What is the investigation? Describe what it shows. What do you think needs to be done next?

The patient recovers well and has no further chest pain.

 What else should be done once the patient has recovered?

ANSWERS

A1 You must inquire about the following:

- How long did the pain last? Did it wake him from sleep? Was it associated with nausea or vomiting? Was he pale or clammy?
- Cardiac risk factors: smoking, family history, diabetes mellitus, hyperlipidaemia, hypertension.
- Past medical and drug history.
- Any previous episodes of similar chest pain or chest discomfort.
- Previous upper gastrointestinal disorder/heartburn/indigestion.

The most positive predictive test for myocardial ischaemia on first presentation is the history – in other words, if it sounds like texbook classical angina, assume it is, regardless of the ECG findings. Greater difficulties are in patients who present with atypical symptoms, e.g. described as indigestion, jaw pain, pain in the shoulder or left elbow.

The most likely diagnosis in this patient is unstable angina.

A2 This patient is having pain at rest which is likely to be ischaemic in origin, and should be assumed so until proven otherwise. He also has considerable cardiac risk factors. He should be admitted to a cardiac ward with monitoring facilities, such as a chest pain investigation unit. An intravenous cannula is inserted and blood is taken for a complete blood count, total cholesterol, glucose, electrolytes and cardiac enzymes (creatine kinase and cardiac troponin). A chest X-ray should be arranged and must be examined for cardiomegaly and evidence of left ventricular failure. Serial ECGs and measurements of cardiac enzymes should be performed to exclude myocardial infarction not evident on the initial tests.

An immediate oral dose of 300 mg soluble aspirin is given for its antiplatelet effect, and regular daily aspirin commenced. An alternative is to use the antiplatelet agent clopidogrel. Anticoagulation should be commenced with a low molecular weight heparin, and a beta-blocker should be prescribed.

A3 The ECG shows widespread T-wave inversion in keeping with severe myocardial ischaemia. This is an acute coronary syndrome, and you must act to prevent infarction. Intravenous nitrates (such as isosorbide dinitrate) can be started with the dose titrated to the patient's pain and blood pressure. If this does not relieve the pain promptly, an intravenous narcotic should be given, and it would be reasonable to commence a glycoprotein IIb/IIIa antagonist (a potent antiplatelet agent) to try and prevent clot formation in the culprit artery.

A4 This patient has acute coronary ischaemia, positive ECG changes and elevated troponin. He is at high risk of impending myocardial infarction, and should undergo coronary angiography immediately. Angiography will define the anatomy of the coronary arteries and may allow angioplasty and stenting if the lesion is suitable. It will also identify severe coronary disease, for example, stenosis of the left main coronary artery or triple vessel disease, both of which should be dealt with by early coronary bypass surgery. The patient should also be started on a HMG-CoA reductase inhibitor (statin) to reduce his cholesterol.

A5 This is a coronary angiogram. It shows a severe narrowing of the left anterior descending artery.

This is a straight lesion in an accessible artery which is amenable to angioplasty. The patient had a percutaneous dilatation of the narrowed segment with a balloon catheter (coronary angioplasty). Treatment was continued with aspirin, a betablocker and a statin.

A6 This patient still has high risk factors for coronary artery disease and is likely to develop further problems later in life unless aggressive changes are made to his modifiable risk factors. Education is very important in helping the patient understand his risks and that he can effectively reduce them by changing aspects of his lifestyle. The most important of these is his cigarette smoking: it is vital that he be counselled to stop. His lipid profile should be reassessed after several months to ensure that the statin is reducing his cholesterol appropriately, and his blood pressure monitored carefully and treated if even moderately raised.

REVISION POINTS

Acute coronary syndrome

This is a case of acute coronary syndrome leading to unstable angina.

An acute coronary syndrome is caused by rupture or fissuring of atherosclerotic plaque within a coronary artery. Platelets are activated and fresh thrombus is formed over the lesion. This leads to rapid narrowing of the vessel lumen and a reduction in blood flow and the onset of chest pain. An acute coronary syndrome can result in total vessel occlusion and ST elevation on the surface ECG. This usually results in a full thickness, Q-wave myocardial infarction (QMI). It can also cause transient disruption to blood flow resulting in myocardial infarction without ST segment elevation – the non-ST elevation myocardial infarction (NSTEMI) or non-Q-wave myocardial infarction (NQMI) (Figure 33.3).

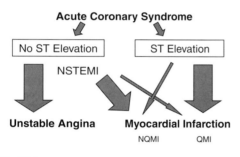

Fig 33.3

- The greatest period of risk of myocardial infarction and death in patients with unstable angina is in the first 6 hours after onset.
- Any person, and especially those with known ischaemic heart disease, must be educated to present immediately to hospital in the event of prolonged chest pain (>15 minutes).
- An attempt should be made to risk stratify patients once medically stabilized. Patients with ongoing chest pain associated with ECG changes or patients with abnormal ECGs and elevated cardiac troponin have been shown to be at high risk of subsequent cardiac events. In those patients, coronary angiography with a view to intervention (angioplasty or coronary artery bypass surgery) should be considered.
- Before discharge from hospital it is important to reinforce the importance of the ABCDE of secondary prevention measures:
  Aspirin and anticoagulants
  Betablockers and blood pressure
  Cholesterol and cigarettes
  Diet and diabetes
  Education and exercise

ISSUES TO CONSIDER

- Should statins be in the water? Find out the latest evidence for the use of cholesterol-lowering medications in patients with and without heart disease.
- How can you help this patient give up smoking?
- What advice are you going to give him about diet and exercise? What rehabilitation programmes exist for cardiac patients in your hospital?

FURTHER INFORMATION

ACC/AHA Guidelines for the management of patients with unstable angina and non-ST-segment elevation myocardial infarction. *Journal of the American College of Cardiologists* 2000;36(3):970–1062.

Clinical outcomes, risk stratification and practice patterns of unstable angina and myocardial infarction without ST elevation: prospective registry of acute ischaemic syndromes in the UK (PRAIS-UK). *European Heart Journal* 2000;21:1450–7.

Invasive compared with non-invasive treatment in unstable coronary-artery disease: FRISC II prospective randomized multicentre study. *Lancet* 1999;354:708–15.

A simple readily available method for risk stratification of patients with unstable angina and non-ST elevation myocardial infarction. *American Journal of Cardiology* 2001;87:1008–10.

Effects of clopidogrel in addition to aspirin in patients with acute coronary syndromes without ST-segment elevation. *New England Journal of Medicine* 2001;345(7):494–502.

www.acc.org The website of the American College of Cardiology. Lots of excellent up-to-date clinical practice guidelines.

Severe epigastric pain in a middle-aged man

It is early on a Monday morning and you have started your shift in the emergency department. Clutching a cup of coffee, you blearily survey the scene in front of you. A 59-year-old man has just been brought in by his wife, and it is obvious that he is in distress. He complains of severe epigastric pain lasting at least 45 minutes. It started during his breakfast and has rapidly increased in severity. It has no radiation but is associated with intense nausea and he has vomited once. He claims that he has never had pain like this before but has occasionally suffered 'indigestion' which was relieved by an antacid. He has had no major medical illnesses in the past and is on no medications. He is an ex-smoker.

On initial examination, you notice the man is clammy and sweaty and is mildly short of breath as he speaks. His pulse is 90 bpm and his blood pressure is 125/80 mm Hg.

Q1 What is your immediate differential diagnosis and what will you do next?

His chest is clear and he has normal heart sounds, blood pressure is equal on both left and right arms. His abdomen is soft and there is no evidence of peritonitis. His femoral pulses are present, equal and of good volume. The distal pulses are also normal. You insert an intravenous line while the nursing staff perform a 12-lead ECG (Figure 34.1).

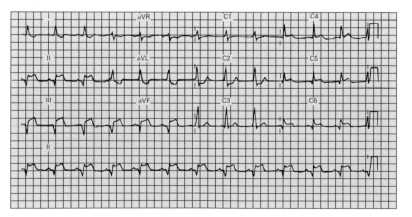

Fig 34.1

What does the ECG show and what is the diagnosis?

The appearances on the ECG startle you into wakefulness and you immediately ask the patient some more questions, as you commence treatment.

Q3 What specific questions should be asked before initiating urgent treatment?

High-flow oxygen is applied by face mask. The man is given morphine 5 mg and metoclopramide 10 mg intravenously, soluble aspirin 300 mg orally and glyceryl trinitrate 600 µg sublingually. He has no contraindications to thrombolytic therapy and gives verbal consent to its use.

You commence an infusion of a thrombolytic drug, and transfer your patient to the coronary care unit. A chest X-ray is performed and shows mild pulmonary oedema with a normal heart size. He continues to have epigastric pain and is given a further 5 mg morphine intravenously.

On examination, his pulse rate has now dropped to 50 bpm and his blood pressure is 95/65 mm Hg. He is sweaty and a little agitated. His jugular venous pressure is elevated 2 cm with the patient at 45°. His apex is not displaced and his heart sounds are normal. He has a few bilateral inspiratory crepitations. Abdominal examination is normal.

Q4 What is the diagnosis and what should be done?

The patient responds well to lying flat with elevation of the legs and 0.6 mg atropine intravenously. After 30 minutes of streptokinase his pulse rate is maintained at sinus rhythm of 72 bpm but his blood pressure remains at 90/60 mm Hg.

Q5 What is the differential diagnosis of the hypotension in the current clinical setting?

Ten minutes later the cardiac monitor alarm sounds and this rhythm is seen on the monitor (Figure 34.2).

The patient is unconscious and has no pulse.

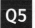

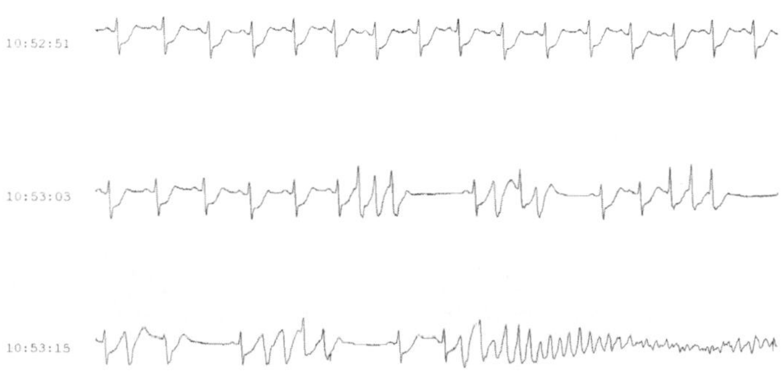

Fig 34.2

Q6 What is the rhythm? What should be done?

The patient returns to sinus rhythm after the second shock at 360 joules. You wipe the sweat off your brow and monitor your patient carefully. He has a few brief runs of ventricular tachycardia (<20 beats) but no sustained arrhythmias. His blood pressure improves after the streptokinase is complete and he remains rhythmically stable and pain free.

He is commenced on metoprolol 50 mg bd after an intravenous dose of 5 mg, a statin to lower his cholesterol, and aspirin 75 mg daily. His serial cardiac enzymes and ECGs confirm a myocardial infarction.

Two days later he starts to mention new chest pain. This is sharp and felt beneath the lower sternum and is different from his original pain. It is aggravated by movement and deep inspiration. He has a fever of 38°C. Examination is normal except for an added harsh murmur heard at the lower left sternal edge during systole.

Q7 What is the diagnosis and what treatment should be instituted?

The patient's pain resolves after 24 hours. On day 3 he is transferred to a general ward and slowly mobilized over the next few days.

Q8 What drug therapy is thought to be 'cardioprotective' in the post-infarct patient?

Q9 What, if any, further investigation should this patient undergo?

The patient has the following study (Figures 34.3 and 34.4).

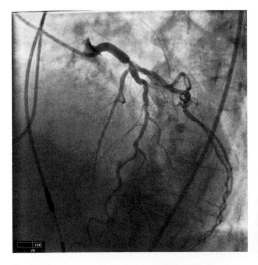 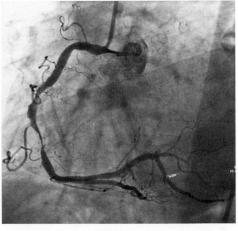

Fig 34.3   **Fig 34.4**

Q10   What do the images show?

The patient underwent triple coronary artery bypass grafting using saphenous vein and internal mammary artery grafts.

Q11   What else should be done for this patient?

The patient remained well after bypass surgery and attended cardiac rehabilitation classes as an outpatient. He was maintained on aspirin 75 mg daily, metoprolol 50 mg bd, pravastatin 40 mg and ramipril 10 mg and had no recurrence of chest pain when reviewed in outpatients 3 months later.

ANSWERS

A1 The important conditions you must consider in this situation include:
- perforated peptic ulcer
- acute pancreatitis
- aortic dissection
- myocardial infarction
- cholecystitis
- biliary colic.

You should rapidly examine him, including palpating his femoral pulses on both sides and compare blood pressures on both upper limbs, and perform an ECG.

A2 The ECG shows sinus rhythm with a rate of 72 bpm and a normal axis. There is an acute inferior myocardial infarction, with ST elevation in the inferior leads (II, III and aVF) caused by occlusion of one of the coronary arteries. There is also slight ST elevation in chest leads 5 and 6 with ST depression in the lateral leads I and aVL. This pattern suggests the involvement of the right coronary artery.

A3 The patient is a candidate for thrombolytic therapy to open up the occluded coronary artery. Any potential contraindications to thrombolytic therapy must be quickly identified. You need to ask about:
- any serious bleeding tendency
- any previous cerebrovascular accident

- uncontrolled hypertension (you would control the blood pressure and if then stabilized, continue thrombolytic treatment)
- any recent major surgical procedure
- any previous exposure to streptokinase (if it is to be used).

Remember – time is of the essence because the sooner the thrombolytic therapy can be given the greater the likely benefits. The diagnosis must be quickly explained to the patient, his consent to thrombolysis obtained and treatment commenced immediately.

A4 The diagnosis is sinus bradycardia, a vagal effect that can complicate inferior myocardial infarction. If the patient does not respond to lowering of the head end of the bed and elevation of the legs, 0.6 to 1 mg atropine can be given intravenously, and a bolus of intravenous colloid can be given. The thrombolytic infusion should be stopped only if the patient does not respond to the above measures.

A5 In this patient with acute inferior myocardial infarction, there are a number of possible explanations for his ongoing hypotension:
- left ventricular failure as a result of extensive myocardial damage
- right heart failure (the infarct is inferior and there may be a component of right ventricular failure). The JVP is elevated

A N S W E R S – cont'd

- drug interaction:
  - intravenous analgesics
  - streptokinase
- intracardiac mechanical complications:
  - papillary muscle rupture
  - ventricular septal defect
  - ruptured free wall of the ventricle.
- bleeding secondary to thrombolysis.

Cardiac ultrasound (echocardiography) is a useful investigation to identify the cause of hypotension after acute infarction. If this patient's hypotension had persisted, an urgent echocardiogram should be performed in the cardiac care ward, to exclude any of the above causes.

A6 The rhythm is ventricular fibrillation triggered by multiple ventricular ectopic beats. When the ectopic beats fall on the T-wave they can lead to the onset of ventricular fibrillation (R on T phenomenon). The patient is unconscious and therefore should immediately be treated with DC electrical cardioversion at 200–360 joules. If he does not revert after the first few electrical shocks then a brief period of cardiopulmonary resuscitation should be performed to improve cardiac oxygenation, adrenaline (epinephrine) administered and the shocks repeated.

A7 The patient has the features of acute pericarditis. The murmur is a pericardial friction rub. Post-infarction pericarditis is treated symptomatically with a non-steroidal anti-inflammatory drug such as ibuprofen.

A8 Aspirin has been shown to reduce non-fatal reinfarction and non-fatal stroke in the post-infarct patient. The antiplatelet agent clopidogrel should be used in those intolerant of aspirin.

Betablockers (e.g. propranolol, metoprolol, atenolol) have been shown to be beneficial both in the acute stages of infarction and in the medium term and should be prescribed to all patients without contraindications (asthma, chronic obstructive pulmonary disease).

Angiotensin converting enzyme (ACE) inhibitors (e.g. ramipril or lisinopril) are beneficial post-infarction to prevent left ventricular dysfunction, particularly in patients with large myocardial infarcts.

Early statin therapy reduces ischaemic events post-infarction and is recommended in most patients.

A9 If the patient has further ischaemic sounding chest pain associated with ECG changes then early coronary angiography should be performed. Younger patients without significant co-morbid illnesses should be considered for an exercise stress test before discharge from hospital. If the test is positive, angiography is performed with a view to performing a revascularization procedure (coronary angioplasty or coronary artery bypass grafting).

A10 Figure 34.3 is an LAO view of a left coronary angiogram. This shows a prominent, tight stenosis in the left main coronary artery prior to its bifurcation. Figure 34.4 is a coronary angiogram of the right coronary artery. This shows a severe stenosis of the artery, and is possibly the lesion responsible for his infarction. This patient has triple vessel disease requiring coronary artery bypass surgery.

A11 The patient's reversible risk factors should be reviewed. He is an ex-smoker and is not hypertensive or diabetic. The main risk factor to concentrate on is his lipid status. Hyperlipidaemia has been shown to encourage development of graft atheroma that will lead to graft occlusion. This lipid status should therefore be reviewed after a few months to ensure that his cholesterol is low. He should be advised to keep to a low-fat diet and take gentle exercise. He should be advised not to drive until he has fully recovered. Cardiac rehabilitation nurses provide outpatient support groups for patients recovering from myocardial infarction and bypass surgery.

REVISION POINTS

Myocardial infarction

Definition

Either one of the following criteria satisfies the diagnosis for an acute, evolving or recent MI:

1 Typical rise and gradual fall (troponin) or more rapid rise and fall (CK–MB) of biochemical markers of myocardial necrosis with at least one of the following:
   - ischaemic symptoms
   - development of pathologic Q waves on the ECG
   - ECG changes indicative of ischaemia (ST segment elevation or depression); or
   - ischaemia requiring coronary artery intervention (e.g., coronary angioplasty).

2 Pathologic findings of an acute MI.

Thrombolysis

- thrombolysis should be administered as urgently as possible to open up the occluded artery and limit the infarct size ('time is muscle')
- it is most effective when it is given 1–2 hours into the acute event but there is still clinical benefit if it is given up to 12 hours
- a number of thrombolytic drugs are available but at the present time there is little difference in clinical outcome between them. Streptokinase is usually the first-line thrombolytic in acute myocardial infarction
- tissue plasminogen activating (TPA) thrombolytics can be used if patients have previously been exposed to streptokinase, or if younger than 75 years with large anterior MI and seen within 4 hours of the onset of symptoms
- TPA appears to be associated with a greater reduction in mortality but a greater risk of cerebral haemorrhage than streptokinase. Alteplase is about 10 times more expensive than streptokinase. The newer drugs reteplase and tenecteplase are given as bolus injections rather than as an infusion
- if patients have absolute contraindications to thrombolysis then many cardiology units are now offering a primary angioplasty service to mechanically open up the artery.

Silent MI

Some myocardial infarcts are painless (particularly in diabetics) and may present as acute pulmonary oedema, a ventricular arrhythmia or hypotension and confusion. Always be alert to the possibility.

Localizing the artery (most common patterns)

- ST elevation in leads II, III, aVF are inferior infarcts (caused by occlusion of the right coronary artery in 80–90% of cases)
- ST elevation in the chest leads (V1–V6) are anterior infarcts (typically caused by occlusion of the left anterior descending artery).

ISSUES TO CONSIDER

- What are the critera for thrombolysis?

- Is immediate angioplasty better than immediate thrombolysis at opening the occluded artery and what difference does that make to long-term outcome?

- How should patients with diabetes be managed during an acute myocardial infarction?

- How do the glycoprotein IIb/IIIa antagonists help during thrombolysis?

FURTHER INFORMATION

Electrocardiographic diagnosis of acute myocardial infarction: current concepts for the clinician. *American Heart Journal* 2001;141:507–17.

Myocardial infarction redefined – a consensus document of the Joint European Society of Cardiology/American College of Cardiology Committee for the Redefinition of Myocardial Infarction. *Journal of the American College of Cardiology* 2000;36(3):959–69.

ACC/AHA guidelines for the management of patients with acute myocardial infarction. *Circulation* 1999;100:1016–30.

GUSTO V Investigators. Reperfusion therapy for acute myocardial infarction with fibrinolytic therapy or combination reduced fibrolytic therapy and platelet glycoprotein IIb/IIIa inhibition: the GUSTO V randomized trial. *Lancet* 2001;357:1905–14.

www.heartcenteronline.com An extremely comprehensive website for patients and professionals alike covering all things cardiological.

Breathlessness in a diabetic woman

A 56-year-old woman was brought into the emergency department by ambulance in the middle of the night. She is acutely breathless and looks extremely unwell. You notice she is wearing a medical alert bracelet with the words 'Diabetes Hypertension Ischaemic Heart Disease' on it.

The woman is severely distressed, unable to speak and is sitting up gasping for breath.

On examination the patient is mildly obese, cold and sweaty. She is peripherally and centrally cyanosed. Her radial pulse is weak, rapid and irregular. Her blood pressure is 160/100 mm Hg. Her jugular venous pressure is elevated to the jaw. Her heart sounds are inaudible and her breath sounds are coarse with an expiratory wheeze and loud inspiratory crepitations to the apices. Her femoral pulses are present and equal. She has mild pitting ankle oedema.

Q1 What should be immediately done for this patient?

While a colleague is searching the woman's hand-bag for a possible list of her medications and a next of kin contact number you start emergency treatment with
- oxygen
- 100 mg intravenous frusemide (furosemide)
- 5 mg morphine intravenously
- 300 mg aspirin
- half a glyceryl trinitrate tablet (600 μg) sublingually.

A 12-lead ECG is obtained which is shown in Figure 35.1.

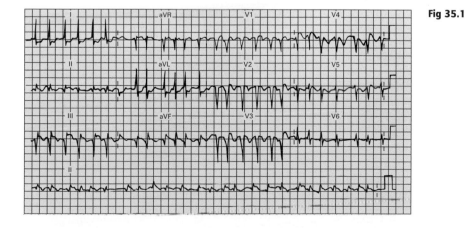

Fig 35.1

Q2   What does the ECG show?

On the monitor her heart rate is now 154 bpm and her blood pressure is 125/90 mm Hg. Blood has been sent for a complete blood picture, electrolytes and cardiac enzymes. A list of her medications is found in her handbag and includes frusemide (furosemide) 40 mg, amiloride 5 mg, aspirin 75 mg, nifedipine (slow release) 20 mg, glibenclamide 10 mg, metformin 500 mg and diclofenac 50 mg. It is unclear how many of each she is taking.

A urinary catheter is inserted and drains 300 ml urine. The woman's casenotes are obtained from records and they reveal the following medical history:

- Type 2 diabetes mellitus for 10 years. Blood glucose difficult to control on oral hypogly-caemics and the patient is not compliant with diabetic diet and reluctant to commence insulin.

- Anterior myocardial infarct 2 years previously. A coronary angiogram revealed inoperable coronary artery disease.
- Hypertension treated with nifedipine. The primary care doctor was monitoring her blood pressure control.
- Diabetic retinopathy requiring laser therapy. Regularly attends diabetic retinal outpatient clinic.
- Ex-smoker until 2 years previously. Until then, had smoked 10–15 cigarettes per day for 35 years.
- Widowed and lives alone. Next of kin is her daughter who lives overseas.
- The casenotes do not document any history of atrial fibrillation.

Q3   She is still acutely short of breath. What further emergency drug therapy should be given to this patient?

The initial blood results show normal values apart from:

- Elevated glucose 18.3 mmol/l.

- Elevated serum creatinine 0.19 mmol/l.

A portable erect anteroposterior chest X-ray is done and shown in Figure 35.2.

Fig 35.2

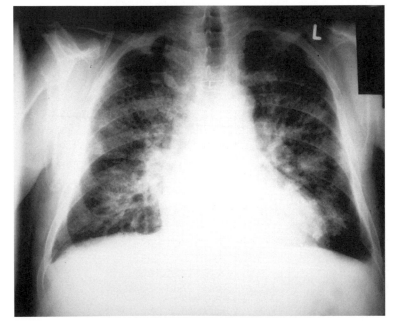

Q4   What does the X-ray show?

An intravenous infusion of isosorbide dinitrate is started and the woman is given 500 μg digoxin and observed. After 40 minutes she has passed a total of 850 ml urine. The patient is now able to talk in brief sentences. She says she has been unwell for 2 days. She had had some mild chest discomfort yesterday and stayed in bed all day. She was planning to see her local doctor the next day but became acutely short of breath and called the ambulance.

Q5   What has precipitated this woman's acute left ventricular failure? What are the likely underlying causes of her cardiac failure?

After 90 minutes of emergency treatment the woman is more comfortable. She has passed a total of 1.8 litres urine. She is admitted to the cardiology ward and has continuous cardiac monitoring. Four hours after the first dose of digoxin a further 250 μg digoxin is given intravenously. She is placed on a sliding scale of short-acting insulin intravenously. All her usual medications are ceased except for the aspirin.

Twenty-four hours later she has improved considerably. Her creatinine kinase peaked at 1486 iu/l and the cardiac troponin is elevated.

These values confirm acute myocardial infarction. You calculate a maintenance dose of digoxin of 62.5 μg per day. Her blood sugar levels are well controlled on the sliding scale of insulin.

An echocardiogram is performed which reveals a moderately dilated left ventricle with severe impairment of function. There is akinesis of anterior and inferior segments and hypokinesis laterally. There is mild mitral regurgitation and the left atrium size is at the upper limit of normal. No thrombus is seen in the left heart. The right heart is relatively normal.

Q6   Briefly describe your further management of this patient in hospital.

Q7   What further cardiovascular drug therapy should be added to this woman's treatment to improve her survival and her quality of life?

The woman spent another 12 days in hospital and made a gradual recovery. Her renal function remained stable. She was discharged on the following therapy: frusemide (furosemide) 80 mg, lisinopril 5 mg, spironolactone 25 mg, aspirin 75 mg; digoxin 125 μg, carvedilol 3.125 mg twice daily, simvastatin 40 mg, warfarin 5 mg and twice daily insulin. The heart failure liaison nurse reviewed her frequently as an outpatient and her medication was gradually increased.

ANSWERS

A1 While a rapid examination is performed the following should be done:
- Apply high-flow oxygen (e.g. 10 litres per minute) by face mask.
- Insert an intravenous line.
- Connect a cardiac monitor to the patient.
- Quickly remove the patient's clothes as necessary to enable free access. This is important in cases of imminent cardiac arrest.

ANSWERS – cont'd

- Take blood for complete blood picture, electrolytes, glucose and cardiac enzymes.
- Obtain any extra information from the patient's belongings and the ambulance driver.

A2 The electrocardiogram shows atrial fibrillation with a ventricular rate of approximately 150 bpm. There is a leftward axis. There is an old anteroseptal myocardial infarct. There is an acute inferior infarct of probably about 12 hours, duration with reciprocal ST segment depression in leads I and aVL.

A3 The patient is still in acute pulmonary oedema. Both frusemide (furosemide) and morphine have immediate effects by venodilatation, but further acute therapy is needed. An infusion of intravenous nitrates should be commenced to offload the heart. The infusion is normally run at a rate of 2–10 mg per hour and titrated such that the highest tolerated dose is used.

Her atrial fibrillation with rapid ventricular rate is also contributing to her pulmonary oedema. Rate control is of paramount importance. Drugs that will control the ventricular rate include digoxin, diltiazem, verapamil, betablockers and amiodarone. In the acute setting they should be used intravenously for more rapid effect. Digoxin is the drug most commonly used, particularly in severe heart failure, and can be given as an oral or intravenous loading dose of 500 μg followed by a further 250–500 μg 4 hours later if required. The maintenance dose for digoxin should take into account her age and renal impairment, based on calculation of her creatinine clearance, e.g. using the Cockroft–Gault equation.

She has had a myocardial infarction, and is in atrial fibrillation. She should therefore be anticoagulated to reduce further infarction and to prevent atrial thrombus formation due to fibrillation. Treatment should start with an unfractionated heparin and only changed to a low molecular weight heparin when it has been established that the patient has normal renal function. The effect of low molecular weight heparin cannot be reversed and it is cleared by the kidneys. As you do not yet know her renal function or her bleeding risks, you should use standard unfractionated heparin intravenously, as this has a short half-life and can be rapidly reversed if necessary. This approach has been shown to improve survival in patients with acute coronary syndromes.

A4 This is a portable anteroposterior view of the patient's chest. The patient has obvious cardiomegaly, even allowing for the anteroposterior projection. The lung fields demonstrate pulmonary oedema and the upper lobe vessels are dilated.

A5 This patient's acute pulmonary oedema has been precipitated by an acute myocardial infarction and atrial fibrillation. Infarction causes loss of myocardial contractility leading to left ventricular failure, and atrial fibrillation causes loss of 'atrial kick' and worsening of cardiac output.

This woman has a history of pre-existing myocardial dysfunction secondary to ischaemic heart disease and previous myocardial infarction, hypertension and diabetes mellitus. She is also on NSAIDs. It is important to note that these can cause fluid retention as well as worsen renal failure, and should be stopped. Her anticoagulation will need to be switched over to warfarin.

A6 The patient has had a myocardial infarct complicated by pulmonary oedema.
- The nitrate infusion can be tailed off gradually once she is out of severe cardiac failure.
- After being monitored for 48–72 hours, provided she is stable, she will need to be mobilized slowly over the following 5–7 days.
- Her diabetes needs to be well controlled. The insulin can be switched over to twice daily injections, and should be reviewed regularly in outpatients.

A7 There are a number of drugs that have been shown to improve symptoms, reduce hospitalization or reduce mortality in heart failure. These include:
- Angiotensin converting enzyme (ACE) inhibitors (such as ramipril or lisinopril).
- Spironolactone.
- Betablockers (such as carvedilol or bisoprolol).
- Digoxin (even when in sinus rhythm).

ANSWERS – cont'd

An attempt should be made to initiate these (particularly the ACE-inhibitors and betablockers) while the patient is still in hospital and then gradually optimize the doses in a careful manner as an outpatient.

Renal function should be closely monitored during the initiation of ACE-inhibitors and during any subsequent dose adjustment. The patient should be anticoagulated to reduce the risk of thromboembolism. The patient should also be maintained on a statin to reduce her cholesterol and reduce the risk of future myocardial infarction.

Her previous angiogram has demonstrated inoperable coronary disease, she has a severely damaged left ventricle and therefore she should be managed medically. Her cardiac failure should be managed with general measures involving a reduced salt diet, rest and drug therapy. Regular outpatient review by specialized nursing and medical staff can prevent hospitalization and improve her symptoms. Cardiac transplantation may be a possibility if she deteriorates further but her age and diabetes make her unlikely to be accepted on to a transplant list.

REVISION POINTS

Cardiac failure

A significant cause of morbidity and mortality resulting in approximately 5% of hospital admissions. In the Framingham study the 5-year mortality was 62% for men and 42% for women.

Aetiology
- coronary heart disease
- hypertension
- valve disease
- cardiomyopathy
- toxins (alcohol and chemotherapy)
- infective (viral myocarditis)
- infiltrative (amyloid, sarcoid, iron)
- incessant tachycardia (tachycardiomyopathy).

Signs
- dyspnoea at rest/tachypnoea
- cool peripheries. Muscle wasting
- low blood pressure and low pulse pressure.
- Tachycardia (sinus or atrial arrhythmia)
- raised JVP
- displaced apex (may be heaving in hypertensive heart disease)
- added 3rd heart sound (S3 gallop)
- hepatomegaly, ascites, oedema (leg and sacral)
- pleural effusions and crepitations.

New York Heart Asssociation (NYHA) classification

Class I   No limitation compared to normal individuals

Class II   Minor limitation of activity by symptoms

Class III   Marked limitation of activity by symptoms

Class IV   Symptoms at rest.

Drug therapy

Drugs that improve symptoms, reduce hospitalization or reduce mortality in heart failure are:
- diuretics
- ACE-inhibitors
- betablockers
- spironolactone
- digoxin
- combination therapy with hydralazine and nitrates.

Drugs that can worsen heart failure:
- non-steroidal anti-inflammatory drugs
- most antiarrhythmic drugs
- most calcium channel blockers.

ISSUES TO CONSIDER

- Diagnostic methods for investigating cardiac failure: echocardiography, nuclear medicine, biochemical markers (natriuretic peptides).

- How can positive pressure ventilation (CPAP, BiPAP) be useful in the treatment of acute heart failure and pulmonary oedema?

- What are the uses, the effectiveness and the hazards of these alternative treatments for severe heart failure?
  - intravenous inotropes
  - biventricular pacing
  - heart assist devices
  - intra-aortic balloon pumping
  - left ventricular reduction surgery
  - artificial heart
  - cardiac transplantation.

FURTHER INFORMATION

ACC/AHA guidelines for the evaluation and management of chronic heart failure in the adult. *Journal of the American College of Cardiology* 2001;38(7):2101–10.

Practical recommendations for the use of ACE inhibitors, beta-blockers and spironolactone in heart failure: putting guidelines into practice. *European Journal of Heart Failure* 2001;3:495–502.

www.bcs.com Comprehensive website from the British Cardiac Society with useful link and cardiology news.

Breathlessness in a 37-year-old woman

A 37-year-old woman presents to the emergency department complaining of breathlessness. Two weeks earlier she had been involved in a car crash and suffered seatbelt trauma to the abdomen, causing a small bowel perforation which required a laparotomy. She also sustained multiple minor lacerations and bruises. She had made an uncomplicated recovery and was discharged home 2 days ago. Yesterday she became short of breath. There were no obvious precipitants and she attributed the problem to being generally unfit and debilitated after the accident. The woman has no fever, cough, or wheeze and has never previously suffered any respiratory complaints. Her health is otherwise good. She has previously had a cholecystectomy and has one healthy child.

Q1 What other history should be sought?

On further questioning, she says the breathlessness is worse on exertion but doesn't change with position or at night. She has no chest pain, chills, sputum, calf pain or ankle swelling. She smokes about 15 cigarettes a day and consumes approximately 80–100 grams of alcohol a week. She has no other past medical history. Her only medication is the oral contraceptive pill.

Q2 What are the possible causes of her breathlessness and what features would you look for on examination?

On examination she is 57 kg, comfortable at rest but tachypnoeic with a respiratory rate of 22 breaths per minute. She is afebrile and neither cyanosed nor clinically anaemic. She is tachycardic with a pulse of 105 bpm. Her blood pressure is 120/74 mm Hg. Otherwise, the examination of her cardiac and respiratory systems is unremarkable, as is examination of her legs. Inspection of her abdomen reveals a healing midline scar but is otherwise unremarkable.

Q3 What investigations are you going to arrange at this stage?

The haematological and biochemical investigations are normal, as is the chest X-ray, and the ECG is normal except for sinus tachycardia. Arterial blood gases on room air are shown in Investigation 36.1.

Investigation 36.1 Arterial blood gas analysis			
pO_2	65 mm Hg	pCO_2	28 mm Hg
pH	7.48	Calculated bicarbonate	29 mmol/l
O_2 saturation (calc.)	90%		

An imaging study is undertaken and two images from the sequence are shown (Figures 36.1 and 36.2).

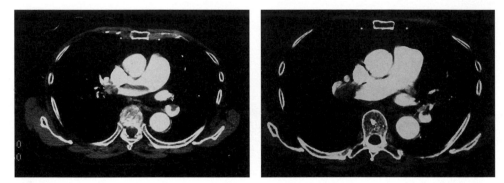

Fig 36.1   **Fig 36.2**

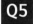 Comment on the blood gases. What is the investigation above and what does it show?

 What action do you take?

The patient is started on unfractionated heparin for 24 hours and then switched to low molecular weight heparin (enoxaparin) at full dose subcutaneously twice daily. She will need a course of warfarin.

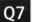 Describe how you would prescribe the warfarin and how you would monitor its effects. How long should this woman stay on warfarin?

After 8 days, her INR has been within the therapeutic range for 3 days; the heparin is stopped. Advice is provided about her condition and taking warfarin tablets. The hospital's outpatient warfarin clinic is going to monitor her INR.

Q7 What advice would you give her before discharge?

The woman's INR is maintained within the therapeutic range. Two months after her hospitalization she presents to the emergency department with an epistaxis. The left nostril has been bleeding for 50 minutes and she has been unable to stop it with simple pressure. She has been unwell with bronchitis and production of yellow sputum

for 4 days and her local doctor prescribed her a course of oral amoxicillin 3 days earlier.

 What do you think has happened?

Her INR is 8.1. The nostril is packed and she is given 3 mg intravenous vitamin K and advised to hold further warfarin.

 What are the potential hazards of intravenous vitamin K? Why can't it be given as an intramuscular injection?

The patient's bleeding is controlled. The next day she returns for removal of packing. The INR returns to 2.2 and the warfarin is restarted with-out the antibiotics. She is instructed to have her warfarin therapy carefully monitored for the remainder of her anticoagulation.

ANSWERS

A1 More specific questions concerning the shortness of breath and associated symptoms may help to support a specific diagnosis. Ask about the following:

- Was shortness of breath sudden (suggesting pulmonary embolus or pneumothorax) or gradual (more suggestive of infective cause)?
- Is there any associated pleuritic chest pain (pulmonary embolus, pneumonia, pneumothorax)?
- Is there any associated haemoptysis (pulmonary embolus or possibly infection)?
- Is there sputum production (suggesting infection)?

A pulmonary embolus (PE) is high on the differential diagnosis list because she has had:

- recent emergency abdominal surgery
- a period of prolonged immobility.

Further questions should therefore look for additional risk factors for DVT/PE:

- Did she receive treatment to prevent clots while an inpatient (sequential compression stockings and/or low molecular weight heparin)?
- Does she smoke?
- Does she use the oral contraceptive pill?
- Any past history of DVT or PE?

- Any history or family history of thrombophilia?
- Additional enquiry should be made about past respiratory disease such as asthma, which may have been exacerbated (e.g. by an intercurrent viral infection).

A2 The most likely diagnosis for this woman's current problem is a pulmonary embolus because she has:

- recently sustained trauma and undergone major abdominal surgery with a period of immobility
- two additional risk factors (cigarette smoking and the oral contraceptive pill).

The next most likely explanation would be pneumonia. Infective respiratory complications are common after abdominal surgery and this diagnosis should be considered except that:

- postoperative pneumonias normally occur in the first 5 days after surgery
- the patient has no cough or sputum production or fever.

A less likely diagnosis would be a pneumothorax. The history of trauma would be in favour of this diagnosis except that:

ANSWERS – cont'd

- it is too long after the event
- the predominant injuries were abdominal rather than thoracic.

An anaemia is a possible cause of the breathlessness and could be related to her injuries. The rapid onset of her symptoms is against this diagnosis.

Asthma is an unlikely cause for the woman's symptoms in the absence of any history.

Your examination would first focus on:

- general appearance
- respiratory rate
- pulse
- blood pressure.

You would examine and auscultate the lungs looking for general and localizing signs, e.g. wheeze, consolidation and hyper-resonance. The signs of pulmonary emboli will generally depend on the size of the embolus. Small emboli may have no signs although multiple recurrent small PE can present with pulmonary hypertension. Haemodynamically significant PE can be associated with:

- tachycardia
- tachypnoea
- atrial fibrillation.

Larger pulmonary emboli can also include all the above and:

- raised JVP
- pleural rub
- cardiovascular collapse
- cyanosis
- sudden cardiac arrest into pulseless electrical activity (PEA).

A3 This woman has had a pulmonary embolus until proven otherwise. It is the most sinister of the possible diagnoses and the one that requires prompt therapy. The following investigations must be undertaken.

- A full blood count looking for anaemia or a leucocytosis, which may suggest infection.
- A chest X-ray. A chest radiograph may show evidence of a pneumothorax or consolidation. The radiograph is normal in most cases of pulmonary embolus unless there has been major pulmonary infarction (wedge-shaped basal pleural infiltrate or a unilateral pleural effusion).

- Electrocardiogram. The ECG is usually normal. The most common abnormality seen is a sinus tachycardia although more extensive emboli may result in new-onset atrial fibrillation. The classically quoted ECG changes of S-wave in lead I with a Q-wave and T-wave inversion in lead III (S1Q3T3) are rarely seen.
- Arterial blood gases on room air.
- Specific imaging. The two standard imaging studies used for the detection and assessment of pulmonary embolus are:

Isotope ventilation–perfusion scan ('V/Q scan'). The ventilation component of the scan is obtained when the patient breathes a radioactive gas (e.g. Xenon 133) and the perfusion scan obtained by injecting the patient with a gamma-emitting radionuclide (e.g. technetium 99m). A pulmonary embolus is detected through the identification of a 'mismatch' between ventilation (normal) and perfusion (reduced). This is the better investigation for detection of small peripheral embolic lesions. There are no concerns about contrast allergies, but it is of limited value in the presence of other forms of lung disease which can include postoperative atelectasis, pneumonia, COPD or pleural effusions.

CT-pulmonary angiography (high-definition spiral CT). This is the better tool if there is co-existent lung disease. These high-resolution scans are capable of detecting small pieces of blood clot in the major pulmonary vessels. Some patients may be allergic to the contrast and there can be concerns about the contrast load in critically ill patients with renal impairment. The use of the spiral CT is also limited by its availability.

A4 The arterial blood gases show the following:

- hypoxia (low oxygen tension)
- hypocapnia (low carbon dioxide tension)
- respiratory alkalosis.

This is the picture seen in type 1 respiratory failure. This suggests that there has been a sudden event, which has caused the patient to become hypoxic and then hyperventilate to compensate. By hyperventilating she has blown off carbon dioxide leading to hypocapnia and an alkalosis.

ANSWERS – cont'd

A similar pattern may be seen in acute asthma, pneumothorax and pulmonary oedema.

The two high-definition images are from a CT-pulmonary angiogram and show clot at the bifurcation of the pulmonary artery into its right and left main branches and a further clot in the first main branch of the right pulmonary artery.

A5 The patient needs immediate anticoagulation. Heparin should be given to achieve rapid anticoagulation followed by warfarin for long-term therapy. You need to make sure you do baseline coagulation studies (INR and APTT). Prolonged APTT is a common presentation of a lupus anticoagulant. This is a very important diagnosis as it may contribute to thrombophilia and will mean the APTT cannot be used to monitor the heparin therapy if unfractionated heparin is to be used.

A choice will need to be made between the use of unfractionated heparin and low molecular weight heparin. Unfractionated heparin has the disadvantage of requiring more frequent monitoring and can be more difficult to dose, which increases the risk of both under-anticoagulation (under-treating the patient) versus over-anticoagulation (increasing the chance of haemorrhage). However, it has the major advantage of being rapidly reversible when given intravenously (by stopping the intravenous infusion and, if necessary, giving protamine). It can also be used in patients with renal impairment. Low molecular weight heparin is more convenient as it is dosed on weight and does not require monitoring in most patients. However, a major disadvantage is that it cannot be reversed which is a serious problem if haemorrhage occurs. Also, use in renal failure is extremely dangerous and is contraindicated. Therefore, it is mandatory to ensure there is no renal impairment before therapy is started.

In view of this patient's recent surgery, it would be prudent to use unfractionated heparin, at least for the first 24 hours or so and watch for any bleeding complications. Because she has had a major pulmonary embolus, it will be very important to ensure rapid therapeutic anticoagulation, but without over-anticoagulation which would increase the chance of a complicating haemorrhage.

If she is stable, she could be switched to low molecular weight heparin, which will facilitate hospital discharge. The patient should be anticoagulated therapeutically with heparin for at least 24 hours before commencing warfarin. Clots of this size are sometimes considered for thrombolytic therapy. This would not be done in this instance, however, in view of the recent major abdominal surgery.

A question also arises as to whether it is necessary to search for an underlying deep venous thrombosis. At this stage it would not change management. It can be useful in cases of bleeding when anticoagulation cannot be used. In this situation, if there is documented clot in the lower limbs or pelvic vessels then an inferior vena cava filter is indicated.

A6 Warfarin can be started once heparin is therapeutic, given at the same time each day, usually in the evening. Some clinicians give a loading dose of 10 mg followed by 5 mg daily for an average-sized adult. Subsequent doses will depend upon the patient's international normalized ratio (INR), which should be measured daily until stable in the therapeutic range. The maximum effect of a dose occurs 48–72 hours later; an INR level will reflect the dose of warfarin given 2–3 days previously. Hospitals have set guidelines as to warfarin loading and monitoring and you need to familiarize yourself with these. The standard therapeutic range is 2–3. It is important to recognize that the patient is not anticoagulated when the INR first reaches 2. Thus, heparin must not be stopped until a minimum of 48 hours (i.e. 2 consecutive days) have elapsed with the INR greater than 2.0. Plans must be made for close monitoring of the INR and warfarin clinics are the best for this. In addition, any doctor involved in the patient's care must be made aware that the patient is anticoagulated with warfarin.

This case is complex because there are some risk factors for thrombosis that are short-lived (i.e. trauma, abdominal surgery and immobility) whereas the patient's risk factors of smoking and use of oral contraceptive pill may be ongoing. Furthermore, we do not know whether there are other factors present that could promote

ANSWERS – cont'd

thrombosis. For example, she may be a carrier of the Factor V Leiden mutation (causes activated Protein C resistance). The first management step is to encourage cessation of smoking. The risks and benefits of discontinuation of the oral contraceptive pill also need to be considered. However, if the pill is stopped, it is mandatory to ensure adequate contraception, as warfarin is teratogenic. It would be reasonable to screen for the Factor V Leiden mutation. If this were present, she will need to stop the OCP.

She should have some basic screens for other thombophilias by checking her complete blood picture (myeloproliferative disorders) and baseline PTT (lupus anticoagulant/antiphospholipid syndrome). A further detailed work-up for inherited thrombophilias would only be necessary if there was a positive family history or prior personal history of thrombosis. Assuming she does not have any major bleeding complications with anticoagulation, 6 months of anticoagulation rather than 3 may be prudent.

A7 The patient should be issued with an information card about warfarin and advised not to commence any new medications without first talking to a doctor. She must understand that warfarin can interact with many drugs and over-anticoagulation can risk life-threatening haemorrhage. The patient should be warned that she may bruise more easily and advised what to do if she has a bleed. This would include coffee-ground vomitus or black melaena bowel actions. Also, contraception while on warfarin is essential. Furthermore, she must stop smoking.

A8 It is likely that the amoxicillin has potentiated the action of the warfarin and now the patient is over-anticoagulated. This complication could have been predicted, had the local doctor and the patient remembered about the warfarin when she sought treatment for her bronchitis.

A9 Severe allergic reactions to intravenous vitamin K are well documented. These can be largely avoided if the drug is given by slow intravenous injection no faster than 1 mg per minute. Intramuscular injections of any drug must be avoided in anticoagulated patients because of the risk of haematoma formation. The management of haemorrhage in anticoagulated patients requires an assessment of how serious the haemorrhage is, to what degree they are anticoagulated and a risk-benefit analysis. Haemorrhage that is life threatening requires immediate reversal and in this instance use of blood products, i.e. fresh frozen plasma, is warranted. However, if the haemorrhage can be controlled with local measures and a reversal is required within 4–8 hours for example, withholding the warfarin and giving vitamin K is perfectly satisfactory and allows the avoidance of the exposure to blood products. If full reversal of anticoagulation is required, then a large dose, e.g. 10 mg vitamin K, can be given. This will, however, make further anticoagulation with warfarin difficult in the immediate future. Therefore, if ongoing anticoagulation with warfarin is required, limited doses of vitamin K (either intravenous or subcutaneous) are appropriate.

REVISION POINTS

Pulmonary embolism

Definition
Clots which, having travelled through the venous system, lodge in the arterial circulation of the lungs. Most arise from thromboses in the deep venous system of the legs and it follows that risk factors for pulmonary emboli are identical to those for deep vein thromboses.

Risk factors
Divided into three groups as first described in Virchow's triad:
- Stasis: e.g. bed rest, immobility.
- Endothelial damage: e.g. surgery, trauma.
- Increased coagulability of blood: e.g. inherited thrombophilia (Factor V Leiden mutation, protein C, protein S deficiency) versus acquired

continues overleaf

REVISION POINTS – cont'd

(malignancy including myeloproliferative disorders, pregnancy, oral contraceptive pill, nephrotic syndrome, heparin-induced thrombocytopaenia, thrombotic thrombocytopaenic purpura).

Clinical presentation

Varies greatly – from mild dyspnoea to sudden cardiovascular collapse and death – depending upon the extent of the embolus. The classic presentation includes sudden onset of shortness of breath, haemoptysis and pleuritic chest pain. In reality only extensive emboli will lead to chest pain and pulmonary infarction as a result of embolism will only be seen in a small number of patients. Pulmonary emboli will have a greater impact on those with poor cardiovascular reserve (e.g. chronic obstructive pulmonary disease, congestive cardiac failure), and a sudden deterioration in breathing of such patients should raise suspicions of an embolus. The investigations of pulmonary embolism are discussed throughout the answer section.

Treatment

Initial therapy is heparin followed by warfarin. Issues involved in the choice of unfractionated versus low molecular weight heparin are outlined in Answer 5. Remember, for the equivalent degree of anticoagulation the bleeding risk for low molecular weight heparin and unfractionated heparin is the same. Low molecular weight heparin should not be used in those with a bleeding risk as it cannot be reversed and must not be used in patients with renal impairment. Patients should continue warfarin for 3–6 months or longer if there are ongoing risk factors for thrombophilia. In massive pulmonary embolism with haemodynamic compromise, intravenous thrombolytic therapy may be indicated or rarely, in critical cases, surgical embolectomy can be performed.

Patients with underlying malignancy have a high risk of developing thromboembolism, and unexplained DVT or pulmonary embolus in a previously well patient may be the first suggestion of occult malignancy. In patients with unexplained DVT/pulmonary embolus, a family history and personal history for previous episodes of clotting is very important in establishing whether they may have an inherited or acquired thrombophilia.

In the near future, oral direct thrombin inhibitors, which are currently undergoing Phase III studies, which have weight-based dosing (making it easier to keep the patient in the target range of anticoagulation), will probably replace the use of warfarin.

ISSUES TO CONSIDER

- What steps can be taken to minimize the risk of post-surgical embolic disease? What protocols exist in your hospital? Which surgical patients are particularly at risk?
- How would your management of this woman's high INR have differed if she had not been bleeding? Again, familiarize yourself with local guidelines.
- What further investigations may be indicated in patients who present with thromboembolic disease in the absence of known risk factors?

FURTHER INFORMATION

Sixth ACCP Consensus Conference on Antithrombotic Therapy. *Chest* 2001;119(1)Supp.

www.umassmed.edu/outcomes/dvt A useful website from the University of Massachusetts with downloadable information on DVT and PE with the emphasis on prevention.

Collapse in a 63-year-old man

A 63-year-old farmer is referred for investigation of recurrent episodes of collapse. He has experienced 5 or 6 attacks over the previous 12 months but had not sought medical advice until the most recent attack, which occurred a few days ago.

What specific questions would you ask to determine the cause of his collapses? Who else would you talk to?

The attacks come on without warning or obvious precipitant. He can be walking or resting and they are not related to a particular posture. The patient thinks he is only 'out' for a short time (seconds to minutes). On two occasions he has fallen and sustained minor head lacerations and bruises. He regains consciousness quickly and is able to continue the day's activities, including driving his tractor. There is no evidence of tongue-biting or incontinence during these episodes.

He has a history of hypertension but rarely has his blood pressure checked because he 'doesn't like doctors'. He has no other significant past medical history and, prior to 12 months ago, had never had any 'faints, fits or funny turns'. He smokes 15–20 cigarettes a day. He consumes 40–50 grams of alcohol a day and more on 'special occasions'. He is on no medications. He denies any symptoms of cardiopulmonary disease such as chest pain or shortness of breath.

His wife is the only person who has been witness to these attacks. In the attack she observed he collapsed to the floor as he crossed the lounge floor. She described him as being pale and suddenly losing consciousness. She says there was no shaking or twitching and that his breathing appeared normal. He always recovered quickly, and he would claim that he had stumbled and fallen over.

On examination, he has a ruddy complexion with sun-damaged skin. His pulse is 85 bpm and regular and his blood pressure is 165/105 mm Hg (lying) with a postural drop of 10 mm Hg. On fundoscopy, he has silver wiring and arteriovenous nipping. His cardiovascular examination is otherwise normal and he does not have an abnormal response to carotid sinus pressure. The remainder of the examination is unremarkable.

The patient has been referred to you for further investigation.

What are the possible causes of syncope in this man?

You explain to the patient that his syncopal episodes are probably related to his heart, and further episodes may be dangerous or even lethal. He begrudgingly agrees to hospital admission for investigation.

Q3 What initial investigations are you going to organize?

Figure 37.1 shows the patient's 12-lead ECG.

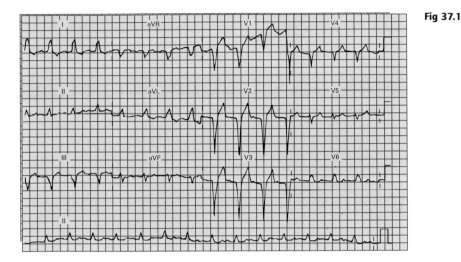

Fig 37.1

Q4 Report the ECG. What abnormalities would you particularly be looking for in this case?

The man's complete blood picture was normal except for a mild macrocytosis thought to be secondary to alcohol use. His biochemistry was normal except for a cholesterol of 7.5 mmol/l and a GGT of 144 U/l; the latter also attributed to his alcohol consumption. A urinalysis was normal.

A chest radiograph revealed a cardiac silhouette at the upper limit of normal and increased lucency of the lung fields and increased airway markings consistent with smoking related chronic airways disease. An echocardiograph revealed mild left ventricular hypertrophy and mild global reduction in contractility. The mitral and aortic valves were thickened but functioned normally and the right heart was normal.

Q5 What other cardiac investigations could help in the diagnosis of this man's syncopal attacks?

A 24-hour period of ambulatory cardiac monitoring was arranged. During this period the patient was asymptomatic and no abnormality of cardiac rhythm was observed.

By this time the patient is fed up with being in hospital and agitating to go home. You have one more investigation up your sleeve: an implantable loop recorder (ILR) is implanted under local anaesthesia, and the patient returns home. Five weeks after the procedure the patient suffers another syncopal attack, and the following rhythm is retrieved from the recorder (Figure 37.2).

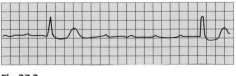

Fig 37.2

Q6   What does the rhythm strip show and what is the appropriate management?

The ILR was removed and replaced with a dual-chamber pacemaker. This was associated with a resolution of his syncopal episodes. The man declined further study of his hypercholestero-laemia or advice concerning his tobacco and alcohol abuse. He was also uninterested in monitoring or treatment of his hypertension and promptly returned to work on his farm.

ANSWERS

A1 The history is a vital part of the evaluation of a patient with syncope and will often indicate what type of syncope the patient is suffering. It is important to establish the frequency, precipitating factors and symptoms associated with each attack. The presence of warning symptoms and the speed of recovery are also important. In addition, a full past medical and drug history must be sought.

- Lightheadedness, pallor, sweating and nausea associated with a particular environmental stimulus (e.g. prolonged standing, pain) are characteristic of vasovagal syncope.
- Syncope due to cardiac obstructive causes or severe myocardial ischaemia may be associated with exertion.
- Symptoms of brainstem ischaemia (e.g. diplopia, vertigo, dysarthria, bilateral limb weakness or paraesthesia) usually indicate that the cause of the syncope is a vertebrobasilar transient ischaemic attack (TIA).
- An epileptic aetiology may be associated with a premonitory aura, evidence of tongue biting or incontinence and prolonged post-ictal confusion. In addition, there may be an eyewitness account of seizure activity.
- 'Drop attacks' are characterized by a sudden abrupt collapse with little or no warning. Recovery is usually rapid. These attacks are typically due to cardiac dysrythmias
- Witnesses to any form of collapse are the source of invaluable information. You should talk to this man's wife and enquire about any collapses she may have seen, especially asking about any seizure activity and other symptoms.

A2 The causes of syncope include:
- Cardiac dysrythmias

- bradycardia: sinus node dysfunction, intermittent complete atrioventricular block (Stoke–Adams attacks), sustained complete AV block
- tachycardia: ventricular, supraventricular
- Obstructive cardiac conditions:
  - severe aortic stenosis, hypertrophic cardiomyopathy, cardiac tumours, pulmonary embolism.
- Autonomic reflex:
  - vasovagal and orthostatic syncope (tilt table testing can be useful in diagnosis)
  - carotid sinus hypersensitivity.
- Neurological:
  - seizure disorders
  - vertebrobasilar transient ischaemic attacks. NB Carotid territory TIAs do not cause syncope
- Metabolic, e.g. hypoglycaemia.
- Psychiatric or functional.
- Unknown aetiology: up to 50%.

The history is of sudden syncope in an older man who is a smoker and without premonitory aura, associated symptoms or obvious precipitants. On occasions the syncope has resulted in significant trauma. He makes a relatively rapid recovery. No incontinence is reported. These features are suggestive of a cardiac arrhythmia.

A3 Due to the severity and frequency of his syncopal episodes, this patient should be admitted for cardiac monitoring.
- 12-lead ECG can provide valuable information but rarely reveals the diagnosis.
- A complete blood picture and biochemistry should be performed.
- In view of his hypertension, a urinalysis and microscopy should be done, as should lipid

ANSWERS – cont'd

studies as part of a global risk assessment for cardiovascular disease.

- Echocardiography should be performed to detect any structural abnormality as well as assessing left ventricular size, wall thickness and systolic function. Regional wall motion abnormality on the echocardiogram may reveal undiagnosed asymptomatic ischaemic heart disease and infarction. Rarely, problems such as cardiac tumours, right ventricular dysplasia or unsuspected valvular disease are detected on echocardiography.
- A significant proportion of syncope and left ventricular dysfunction will be caused by ventricular arrhythmias (e.g. intermittent VT). Prompt diagnosis of this particular cause of syncope is important as it is associated with a high mortality if not appropriately treated.

A4 On reviewing an ECG from a patient with syncope you should look for evidence of:

- Myocardial ischaemia and previous myocardial infarction.
- Ventricular hypertrophy.
- Obvious rhythm and/or conduction abnormalities, e.g. bifascicular block, intermittent or permanent atrioventricular block, sinus bradycardia/sinus arrest.
- Pre-excitation delta waves in Wolff–Parkinson–White syndrome which predispose to tachyarrhythmias such as paroxysmal SVT.
- The long Q-T syndrome and the Brugada changes predisposing to paroxysmal wide complex tachycardias such as *torsades de pointes* VT.

This is an abnormal ECG, which shows a regular sinus rhythm of 90 bpm with a normal axis. There is a prolonged PR interval. The QRS complexes are wide and have the configuration of left bundle branch block.

A5 In patients with a suspected cardiac cause of syncope, a recording of the heart rhythm during an episode of syncope or pre-syncope is the most valuable piece of information. There are a number of ways to achieve this,

depending on how often the patient experiences symptoms.

In-patient cardiac monitoring may capture the rhythm in patients with very frequent attacks.

External ambulatory cardiac monitoring can be used in patients experiencing symptoms every few days. These devices use a number of surface electrodes with a battery-powered unit worn by the patient. They are activated by the patient during a symptomatic event and keep a rhythm strip of cardiac activity prior to and subsequent to the episode. They are most useful in patients with brief events from which they have a rapid recovery. The diagnostic yield from this form of patient-activated ambulatory recording is substantially greater than that achieved utilizing continuous 24/48-hour ECG monitoring ('Holter' monitoring).

In this case the events occur too infrequently for an ambulatory event recorder to capture an attack. Two further options are available.

An electrophysiology study (EPS) could be performed in hospital using an electrical probe which is guided into the heart from a peripheral artery. The probe is used to detect sinus or atrioventricular nodal disease or to provoke inducible ventricular tachycardia. The yield from an electrophysiology study is low and it is sometimes difficult to be certain that any abnormal findings at EPS are related to the clinical presentation.

More recently, implantable loop recorders (ILR – shown in Figure 37.3) have provided an additional tool for evaluation of patients with recurrent syncope.

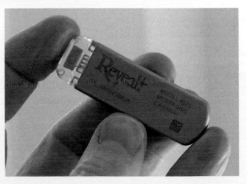

Fig 37.3

A N S W E R S – cont'd

This device is a miniaturized electrogram recorder, which is implanted subcutaneously in the infraclavicular fossa. It continuously monitors the patient's cardiac rhythm and stores the rhythm when the device automatically detects an arrhythmia or if the patient activates the device during a symptomatic event. In this patient an ILR would be useful following the failure of the initial investigations to yield a definitive diagnosis. Many patients with syncope of unknown cause may have potentially lethal arrhythmias

which are as yet undiagnosed. ILR is particularly useful in this group in whom the one-year mortality approaches 30%.

A6 This trace demonstrates complete atrioventricular dissociation (3rd-degree heart block). There is a very slow ventricular escape rhythm at a rate of 18 bpm on this strip. The likely cause of this man's syncope is therefore intermittent complete heart block.

R E V I S I O N   P O I N T S

Complete heart block

- A common cause of syncope.
- Atria and ventricles contract independently.

Aetiology

- Degenerative diseases of the conducting system (Lev's and Lenègré's disease).
- Myocardial infarction or ischaemic heart disease.
- Drug toxicity (e.g. digoxin, calcium channel blockers, betablockers).
- Mitral and aortic valve disorders.

Diagnosis

- On ECG during an event.

- During continuous monitoring as an in-patient.
- Implantable loop recorders (ILRs).

Treatment

Permanent pacing with a pacemaker.

Note: Syncope in patients with chronic bundle branch or bifascicular block may be due to intermittent complete heart block, or due to intermittent ventricular tachycardia. This difference is important because insertion of a pacemaker will *not* help syncope due to ventricular tachycardia.

ISSUES TO CONSIDER

- What other cardiac disorders may benefit from pacemaker insertion?
- What are the different types of pacemaker? How do they differ in function?
- What other forms of implantable cardiac devices are available? In whom are they indicated?

FURTHER INFORMATION

www.medtronic.com Useful commercial site from the makers of an ILR with lots of information on ILRs and links to related articles.

Krahn A P et al. **Randomised assessment of syncope trial: conventional diagnostic testing versus a prolonged monitoring strategy.** *Circulation* 2001;104(1):7–8.

A 62-year-old man with breathlessness and yellow sputum

You are working in the emergency department one winter evening. A 62-year-old man is brought in by ambulance acutely short of breath. The history is obtained mainly from the patient's wife. She claims he has had difficulty with his breathing for about 4 years and can now only walk at a slow pace for 50 metres and then has to stop due to breathlessness. He has had a smoker's cough for as long as she can remember and has produced phlegm on most days for many years. He has had a number of chest infections this winter despite repeated courses of antibiotics and as a result the local doctor placed him on theophylline tablets.

On this occasion the man has been unwell for 1 week. During this time he has been producing thick yellow-green sputum which he has found difficult to cough up. He has been sitting up at night in a chair and has been unable to do anything due to his breathlessness and extreme fatigue. He has become nauseated and is eating very little. He has not had a temperature or shivers or chest pain. He has not noticed any blood in his sputum and he has not had ankle swelling. The patient has been on antibiotic tablets for 5 days but there has been no improvement.

The man suffered a myocardial infarction at the age of 60 and underwent a right femoropopliteal bypass 4 years ago. He has not had angina since his heart attack and is not on any cardiac medication. He does not have hypertension or diabetes mellitus. He had experienced pain in the left calf on walking up until the last 6 months when he has been more troubled by breathlessness.

He is on a salbutamol puffer, 2 puffs 4 hourly, theophylline slow-release tablets 300 mg bd and amoxicillin 250 mg 3 times a day. He currently smokes 5 cigarettes a day but until 3 months ago smoked 30–60 a day and had done so since the age of 17. He claims he finds benefit from the smoking as it seems to aid the clearing of his sputum.

Q1 What is the likely diagnosis? What factors may have precipitated his recent deterioration?

In this case, it appears that a respiratory tract infection may be contributing to his present state of ill-health.

Q2 Describe the key components of the examination.

The man is agitated and looks exhausted and cyanosed. He sits up on the examination couch clutching the sides in obvious respiratory distress. He is tachypnoeic with a respiratory rate of 30 breaths/minute. He has prolonged expiration with a loud wheeze. He is coughing frequently, producing thick yellow-green sputum. He has a ruddy complexion, and appears moderately dehydrated.

His temperature is 38°C, his pulse 140 bpm, regular and bounding and his blood pressure is 150/100 mm Hg with a paradox of 25 mm Hg. The patient has marked overinflation and a tracheal tug with use of his sternocleidomastoid muscles and intercostal recession. There is no finger clubbing or flap.

His jugular venous pulse is raised 4 cm. His apex is not palpable and his heart sounds are inaudible. His chest is hyper-resonant with globally reduced breath sounds, a prolonged expiratory phase and a loud wheeze. There is no cervical lymphadenopathy and the abdomen is not examined formally due to the patient's distress. There is mild ankle oedema. He is unable to use the peak expiratory flow meter due to the severity of his breathlessness.

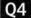 **Q3**   What investigations would you like at this stage?

The following result is obtained:

Investigation 38.1 Arterial blood gas analysis on air	
pO_2	41 mm Hg
pCO_2	75 mm Hg
pH	7.25
HCO_3	32 mmol/l

Q4   What does this investigation show?

The patient is placed on 3 l/min oxygen via nasal cannulae. The arterial blood gas estimation is then repeated after 30 minutes. Other blood tests, an ECG and a chest X-ray are obtained.

Investigation 38.2 Arterial blood gas analysis on 3 l/min O_2	
pO_2	58 mm Hg
pCO_2	89 mm Hg
pH	7.21
HCO_3	32 mmol/l

Investigation 38.3 Complete blood picture			
Haemoglobin	181 g/l	White cell count	14.3×10^9/l
Platelets	259×10^9/l	Neutrophils 86%	12.3×10^9/l

The electrolytes are normal other than bicarbonate. The serum theophylline concentration is 48 µmol/l (therapeutic range 55–110).

The chest X-ray is shown in Figure 38.1.

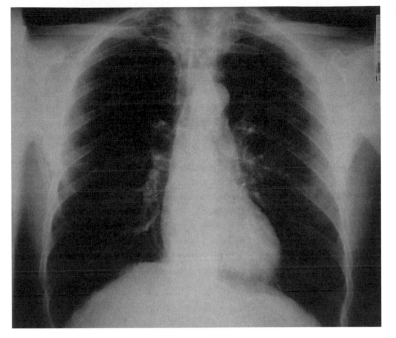

Fig 38.1

An ECG shows a sinus tachycardia with a right axis deviation and a prominent R wave in lead V1.

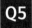 What do these results indicate?

 How are you going to manage this patient?

The patient is managed in an intensive care unit. His blood gases are maintained within a satisfactory range using nasal cannulae at 1 l/min oxygen. Salbutamol nebulizers are given hourly.

The intensive care resident commences an aminophylline infusion of 1000 mg in 1 litre 5% dextrose running over 24 hours. After blood cultures have been taken, he is started on intravenous amoxicillin and clarithromycin. A trial of oral steroids is given starting at 30 mg prednisolone. Hourly chest physiotherapy and endotracheal suction is performed to clear purulent sputum.

 If his respiratory failure had continued to worsen, what options would have been open to you?

Twenty-four hours later you are called to see the patient because he has begun vomiting bile-stained vomitus. He has suffered extreme nausea for 3 hours. His respiratory distress is much improved and he has no abdominal pain. He has an obvious tremor and a temperature of 37.6°C. His pulse is 146 bpm and his blood pressure is 140/90 mm Hg.

Q8 What are the possible explanations for his deterioration? What should you do?

His chest findings are unchanged and abdominal examination is unremarkable. A repeat chest X-ray shows no change and an ECG shows a sinus tachycardia with a rate of 146 bpm.

A theophylline estimation is performed and it is 155 μmol/l. His aminophylline infusion is ceased.

The patient slowly improves with cessation of the aminophylline and switch of the antibiotic therapy. His nebulized salbutamol is decreased to 4 hourly. He slowly improves and 12 hours later he is recommenced on slow-release theophylline tablets 300 mg bd. He admitted that before coming into hospital he had missed taking some of his theophylline tablets. The pred-nisolone dose is decreased and then ceased over 5 days. An ipratropium bromide puffer is instituted on discharge to act as a bronchodilator. His peak expiratory flow rates are performed regularly on the ward before and after nebulized salbutamol. They improve slowly but plateau at about 180 to 200 l/min. He has a small improvement with salbutamol.

Seven days after admission he has improved to the extent where he can walk slowly around the ward. Formal pulmonary function tests are done prior to discharge. The results are as follows.

The patient is told firmly that he must stop smoking immediately.

Investigation 38.4 Forced expiratory volumes			
	pre-bronchodilator	post-bronchodilator	predicted
FEV$_1$	0.81 (28%)	1.37 (48%)	(2.89)
FVC	2.84 (78%)	3.71 (102%)	(3.62)
FEV$_1$/FVC	29%	37%	(80%)
Single breath diffusing capacity			
DLCO corrected for haemoglobin		observed	predicted
(ml/min/mm Hg)		10.2 (42%)	24.5

Investigation 38.5 Arterial blood gases on air	
pO$_2$	50 mm Hg
pCO$_2$	61 mm Hg
pH	7.40
HCO$_3$	34 mmol/l

Q9 What do these results tell you? How will you manage the patient before discharge and in the future?

The patient ignores your advice on smoking. He is placed on home oxygen 4 months later. He survived another 18 months, dying of another episode of acute on chronic respiratory failure.

ANSWERS

A1 He has at least an 80-pack/year history of smoking and chronic obstructive pulmonary disease secondary to cigarette smoking is the most likely diagnosis. This includes chronic bronchitis and emphysema and there may also be an element of reversible airways obstruction, i.e. asthma. Infection of the tracheobronchial tree causing an increase in airway inflammation and volume and viscosity of sputum (known as mucus plugging) is the most common precipitant of deterioration in these patients.

Other factors contributing to deterioration may include increased tobacco use, non-compliance with medication, use of sedative drugs, intercurrent pneumonia, left ventricular failure, pneumothorax, thromboembolism and development of a bronchogenic carcinoma or development of anaemia.

The differential diagnosis includes adult-onset asthma and bronchiectasis, but these are less likely.

Occupational history is important as the man may have pneumoconiosis in addition to his smoking-related disease. This must always be asked about, even with an obvious smoking history. A history of childhood respiratory problems including exposure to pulmonary tuberculosis may also be relevant.

A2 During the examination of this patient, focus on:
- Disturbance of the mental state, e.g. agitation or drowsiness suggesting underlying hypoxia or hypercapnia.
- Cyanosis and polycythaemia.
- Clubbing (which may suggest an underlying carcinoma).
- Metabolic flap (hypercapnia).
- Fever (suggests sepsis).
- Tachycardia and arrhythmia (e.g. sudden onset atrial fibrillation could contribute to decompensation).
- Blood pressure including pulsus paradox.
- Degree of over-inflation.
- Pursed lips respiration.
- Use of accessory muscles and intercostal recession.
- Chest signs of over-inflation (increased resonance, reduced breath sounds) and airways

obstruction (wheeze). Also evidence of pneumothorax (reduced breath sounds) or consolidation (bronchial breath sounds).
- Evidence of right heart failure (cor pulmonale).
- Evidence of primary and metastatic malignancy (e.g. cachexia, pleural effusion, supraclavicular lymphadenopathy, hepatomegaly).
- Sputum.
- Peak expiratory flow rate.

A3 Initial investigations should include:
- Arterial blood gas analysis (an objective measure of the degree of derangement of lung function and to detect respiratory failure).
- Chest X-ray (evidence of emphysema, consolidation, airways thickening, pneumothorax, cor pulmonale and primary lung malignancy).
- ECG (arrhythmia, right ventricular hypertrophy or hypoxia-induced ischaemia/infarction).
- Complete blood picture (anaemia or polycythaemia, leucocytosis).
- Biochemistry (baseline electrolytes).
- Sputum culture and cytology (bacterial pathogens by Gram stain and culture, malignant cells).
- Blood serology (raised titres of antibodies against bacteria, e.g. *Legionella*).
- Theophylline level (compliance, toxicity and guide to further theophylline therapy).
- Blood cultures (septicaemia).

A4 The initial blood gas indicates acute on chronic respiratory failure. The bicarbonate is halfway between what is expected in acute respiratory acidosis (lower bicarbonate) and chronic respiratory acidosis (higher bicarbonate). This suggests renal (metabolic) compensation for chronic hypercapnia and acidosis by bicarbonate retention. This would normalize the pH in the chronic state. With an acute deterioration this compensation cannot occur, resulting in a moderate acidosis.

A5 With the application of 3 l/min of oxygen there has been improvement in oxygenation but also further CO_2 retention and exacerbation of the acidosis.

ANSWERS – cont'd

The patient has a raised haemoglobin, which is likely to reflect a secondary polycythaemia induced by chronic hypoxia. He has a neutrophilic leucocytosis, which indicates infection.

The chest X-ray reveals a cardiac size within normal limits and prominent pulmonary arteries. The lung fields are grossly inflated and there is some scarring at the lung apices. There is no evidence of consolidation. This suggests chronic obstructive pulmonary disease (COPD) with pulmonary hypertension. This diagnosis is supported by the ECG changes of right ventricular strain (right axis deviation and a prominent R wave in V1).

Overall, the clinical picture indicates that the patient has COPD with probable cor pulmonale. There has been an acute deterioration precipitated by infection but there is no evidence of pneumonia.

The serum theophylline concentration is just below the therapeutic range. It will be important to make enquiries about compliance, particularly in the last few days.

A6 Oxygenation is the key. Patients need oxygen if they are hypoxic, but excessive supplemental oxygen can result in dangerous hypercapnia with mental stupor or coma and respiratory arrest. A compromise is needed. Improvement of the pO_2 towards 50–60 mm Hg should be attempted using the smallest amount of oxygen possible. At this level pulmonary vasodilatation is achieved. This is when Venturi masks are useful: low-dose oxygen via 24% Venturi mask improves oxygen without causing dangerous respiratory depression. If these cannot be tolerated, nasal cannulae can be substituted at 1 l/min. A modest rise in pCO_2 is acceptable provided that the patient remains alert. If a 24% Venturi mask is tolerated, particularly if the patient improves, a 28% mask (or nasal cannulae at 1.5–2 l/min) may be tried. The blood gases will need to be checked to exclude deterioration in ventilation.

In addition to oxygen, the treatment of any reversible airways obstruction by removing secretions and treating infection will help. If this cannot be done by conservative means the issue of mechanical ventilation will have to be considered, including continuous positive airways pressure (CPAP) or intubation.

The patient may only have a small component of reversible airways obstruction but attempted bronchodilatation by frequent salbutamol nebulizers is accepted practice. Salbutamol intravenous infusion is also a possibility.

This patient has a theophylline level just below the therapeutic range and therefore should *not* be loaded with aminophylline. The role of theophylline in the management of chronic airways disease is markedly diminishing because of the high risk of complications related to toxicity and the availability of effective and safer long-acting inhaled bronchodilators.

Steroids are used in acute exacerbations of chronic airways obstruction, although they are less important than with exacerbations of asthma, and their effectiveness in the management of the former condition is not uniform. A similar dose is often used during the acute phase of the illness, but unless there is a significant component of bronchospasm in the obstruction, the chronic use of steroids is not recommended.

Clearance of airway secretions in this patient is important. In the acute stage he would not tolerate routine chest physiotherapy, but regular encouragement of coughing and possibly nasotracheal suction should be performed.

Although the patient has no consolidation he has a fever and a severe deterioration associated with purulent sputum; intravenous antibiotics such as amoxicillin (or amoxicillin/clavulanic acid), doxycycline or roxithromycin should be added. It must be remembered that the macrolide antibiotics (erythromycin, roxithromycin, clarithromycin) interact with many medications including theophylline, warfarin, anticonvulsants, oral contraceptives and any drugs metabolized by hepatic cytochrome P450. Intravenous erythromycin is now avoided wherever possible, as it can be associated with a highly irritant superficial thrombophlebitis.

This patient is critically ill with respiratory failure, and should be admitted to an intensive care ward. If repeated gas measurements are necessary, an arterial line can be considered.

A7 He would need some form of respiratory support. This would probably be non-invasive in the form of CPAP or NIPPV in the first instance.

ANSWERS – cont'd

Both these forms of ventilatory support are supplied via well-fitting face or nasal masks. If his respiratory failure worsened further or his conscious level decreased then he would need endotracheal intubation.

A8 The most likely explanation for this is theophylline toxicity. The dose of aminophylline has been prescribed without taking into account the reduced clearance of theophylline induced by clarithromycin. In addition, he may have cor pulmonale which causes decreased theophylline clearance. Hypoxaemia may also result in delayed hepatic clearance of theophylline.

Severe theophylline toxicity may require charcoal haemoperfusion or continuous veno–veno haemodialysis. Theophylline is now much less commonly used in the management of chronic obstructive airways disease. It is best to avoid theophylline/aminophylline in most cases of acute exacerbations of this condition.

Other possibilities for his deterioration include a cardiac arrhythmia secondary to his lung disease and hypoxia.

You should arrange an ECG, a chest X-ray and an urgent measurement of his theophylline levels.

A9 His lung function tests show a very marked obstructive pattern but with significant reversibility to salbutamol. The reduced DLCO demonstrates markedly impaired gas exchange.

His gases show a return to his chronic state. He is no longer acidotic and his bicarbonate has risen back to its chronically elevated level.

In the short term he should finish his course of antibiotics and tail off his steroids over the following week. Theophylline levels must be measured regularly, and attention paid to any drugs which change the clearance of theophylline, of which there are many. It should be noted that on stopping his clarithromycin, his levels may drop again and his dose may need to be increased.

He should have education about use of his inhalers and his technique should be checked. He should be discharged with inhalers of corticosteroids and salbutamol, possibly in conjunction with ipratropium bromide. He should be considered for a home nebulizer.

He must stop smoking. Tobacco smoke inhibits mucociliary function and hence clearance of airway secretions. Smoking also stimulates increased airway mucus production so cessation of smoking will decrease sputum production and bronchospasm. In addition home oxygen cannot be prescribed if the patient continues to smoke, because of the fire hazard.

This patient should have the pneumococcal vaccine and an annual influenza vaccine. Compliance with salbutamol, ipratropium and theophylline should be ensured and puffer technique should be checked regularly. Infective exacerbations should be treated early with oral antibiotics, and intensive chest physiotherapy. If manifestations of cor pulmonale (such as ankle swelling) worsen, they may have to be treated with diuretics.

Referral to a respiratory rehabilitation programme is helpful, and provision of home improvements may improve the ability of the chronically breathless person to cope. This patient would fit the criteria for home oxygen provided he can become an established non-smoker and that there is reversal of hypoxaemia with domiciliary oxygen without progressive hypercapnia.

REVISION POINTS

Chronic obstructive pulmonary disease

Cigarette smoking is by far the most important aetiological factor in this disease. Cessation slows the progression of the disease and there may be improvement in airway obstruction.

Chronic bronchitis is a clinical diagnosis, i.e. the condition of excessive production of mucus by the respiratory tract such that the patient has a sputum-producing cough for at least 3 months of the year for more than 2 consecutive years.

continues overleaf

REVISION POINTS – cont'd

Patients with predominant bronchitis are the 'blue bloaters'. They have a decreased respiratory drive and are therefore less dyspnoeic, but at the expense of severely deranged gases.

Emphysema is a pathological diagnosis and is defined as distension of air spaces distal to the terminal bronchioles resulting from destruction of alveolar septa. High-resolution CT scanning nowadays can provide accurate morphological imaging of the lung parenchyma and therefore allow the premortem diagnosis of emphysema. 'Pink puffers' have predominant emphysema and maintain reasonable blood gases at the expense of increased ventilatory drive and severe dyspnoea.

Significant obstruction is always present in both disorders, which may improve with bronchodilators and will worsen with respiratory infection.

Diagnosis

- Spirometry shows slowing of forced expiratory flow rate (FEV_1).
- More complex pulmonary function tests include measurement of the gas diffusion coefficient (DLCO), static lung volumes and lung elastic recoil or compliance.

Infective exacerbations

- Respiratory infections are the commonest precipitants of acute-on-chronic respiratory failure in these patients.
- Cor pulmonale is a bad prognostic indicator.
- Likelihood of acute respiratory failure increases when the FEV_1 is below 25% of the predicted normal values.
- In-hospital mortality rate averages 30% for a single episode and 5-year mortality rate after the initial episode of respiratory failure averages 15–20%.
- Patients with predominant emphysema have a poorer prognosis after the onset of respiratory failure than those with predominant bronchitis.
- In both cases long-term oxygen therapy prolongs survival as well as improving their quality of life.
- Blood gas analysis in the acute setting must be interpreted in the light of the patient's chronic status. The renal bicarbonate compensation for chronic hypercapnia will usually cause the pH to be within the normal range. This means that a patient with acidosis has usually had a major decompensation.

Treatment

- Extent of reversible airways obstruction must be determined in the lung function laboratory. Any reversibility (asthmatic component) should be treated.
- Bronchodilator drugs such as the beta agonists (e.g. salbutamol, and long-acting agonists such as efermoterol). Small changes in the degree of obstruction can make a significant improvement.
- Ipratropium bromide, an anticholinergic (antimuscarinic) agent available as a metered inhaler, is an effective bronchodilator and decreases mucus production in chronic bronchitis.
- Steroids are indicated in acute airflow obstruction exacerbations. They have a much less useful action in long-term treatment of chronic bronchitis and are of no benefit in emphysema.
- Theophylline has a narrow therapeutic window and can have significant toxicity. Viral febrile illnesses, hepatic and cardiac impairment and use of cimetidine, erythromycin and allopurinol will all decrease theophylline clearance.
- Vaccination against pneumococcus and influenza virus is advisable and early treatment of chest infections is important.

ISSUES TO CONSIDER

- How do you clinically measure pulsus paradox?
- What disorders, other than smoking, can cause chronic respiratory failure?
- How are patients assessed to qualify for home oxygen therapy?

FURTHER INFORMATION

www.lungusa.org Directed at patients, but with lots of interesting information on COPD, smoking and other lung diseases.

www.emedicine.com/emerg/topic99.htm Another thorough review, this time on emphysema.

Persistent cough in a young woman

A 37-year-old woman of Caucasian origin presents with an irritating cough of 3 months' duration and recent episodes of small amounts of bloodstained sputum. She is a non-smoker. She has consulted her family doctor twice during this period and has had only a modest response to successive courses of antibiotics.

She has also noticed some lethargy and more recently occasional night sweats.

On examination she appears mildly unwell, has evidence of recent weight loss and a temperature of 38.2°C. No other abnormal findings were elicited.

Q1 What further history should be obtained?

You question the patient further. Five years ago she spent 2 years as a volunteer teacher in Malawi. When she returned she underwent TB screening and had a 'positive' tuberculin skin test and a normal chest X-ray. The clinic placed her on a 6-month course of isoniazid, which she completed.

You arrange a chest X-ray. The PA and lateral views are shown in Figures 39.1 and 39.2.

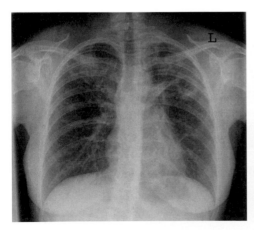

Fig 39.1

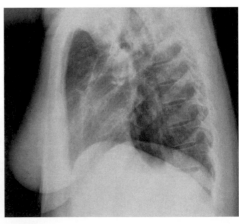

Fig 39.2

Q2 What does the chest X-ray show? What might the findings suggest? Would any other imaging be of help?

Your suspicions have been aroused, and you admit her to an isolation ward for investigation and treatment.

 Q3 What simple investigation would you request urgently? Are there any other investigations that may assist in making the diagnosis?

Your lunch is interrupted by a call from the microbiology laboratory advising that the smear from her sputum is heavily positive for AFBs.

 Q4 Why does this result necessitate an urgent call? What should you do now? What additional investigations are indicated?

 Q5 What treatment would you recommend initially and why? What are the main treatment concerns?

 Q6 Are there any other issues that you need to address promptly?

Your patient is surprised and concerned that she is so sick, and wants to know if this could have been prevented.

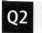 **Q7** Could this illness have been prevented?

ANSWERS

A1 A careful history in a patient with persistent cough and haemoptysis may provide clues about a possible diagnosis before any definitive investigations are undertaken.

Causes include:
- Chronic bronchitis.
- Lung abscess/pneumonia.
- Bronchiectasis.
- Active tuberculosis (TB).
- Mycetoma in an air space caused by inactive TB.
- Carcinoma.
- No cause is found in up to 30% of cases.

This patient's fever and night sweats strongly imply an infective cause. Her history does not imply lung abscess nor carcinoma. Tuberculosis must be excluded. You need to specifically enquire about any TB risk factors:

ANSWERS – cont'd

- Known close contact with a TB case (especially family).
- Past residence or visits to a high-risk country for an extended period, including India, Asia, Africa and Aboriginal settlements in rural Australia.
- History of previous treatment for TB disease or 'preventive' treatment for latent TB infection.
- Other causes of immunocompromise such as HIV infection, immunosuppressive medications and steroids, etc.
- Disease caused by a non-tuberculous *Mycobacterium* can present a similar clinical picture to TB but in this instance is unlikely to be the causative agent.

A2 The chest X-ray shows a cavitating lesion in the left upper lobe, with some air space opacity in slightly contracted upper lobes.

These chest X-ray findings are highly suspicious of post-primary TB disease, especially in this clinical context. However, no pattern is absolutely diagnostic. Pneumonic shadowing of a segmental or lobar distribution in the upper zones due to a bacterial or viral illness could be confused with TB but are usually more acute in nature. In the older person carcinoma of the bronchus needs to be considered and may co-exist. Disease that follows primary infection can produce lower zone infiltrates, hilar or mediastinal lymph node enlargement or pleural effusions. More varied and less specific features can be seen in up to a third of cases, particularly the elderly and immunosuppressed. This can include those of primary disease, a miliary pattern, solitary or multiple nodules or even 'normal' chest films. Remember TB is the 'great mimicker'.

The radiological changes seen so far are virtually pathognomonic of pulmonary tuberculosis and a CT scan is unlikely to provide any more definitive information. The CT scan is more sensitive than the standard chest X-ray in the examination of the lung parenchyma, mediastinum and pleura. It may be useful in those patients with less obvious or atypical features.

A3 An urgent sputum sample is required to screen for acid-fast bacilli (AFBs). Collection of

the specimen should be in a well-ventilated area. A further two specimens on consecutive days must also be requested. One specimen alone will fail to detect about 25% of smear positive cases and about 50% of culture positive cases. For the patient unable to produce sputum, inhalation of nebulized hypertonic saline may help. Otherwise bronchoscopy and lavage has a good yield and would also be indicated in the smear negative case with these symptoms and chest X-ray findings.

- An elevated ESR, normocytic anaemia and depressed sodium are non-specific findings which may be present.
- The tuberculin test is not indicated. It cannot distinguish latent TB infection from active disease and false negative results occur in as many as 20% of active cases.
- Presently there are no validated serological tests for TB.
- Nucleic acid amplification tests have been recently developed, making it possible to detect *M. tuberculosis* directly from a smear positive specimen within 24 hours (~95% sensitivity). Due to the urgent treatment and public health implications, nucleic acid amplification could be requested if your clinical suspicion of TB is high but other results are less certain.

A4 TB is the likely diagnosis requiring the following measures:

- Isolation, in a room with negative pressure ventilation if available, and treatment.
- Strict infection control measures need to be followed, as TB is highly infectious, especially in its 'open' pulmonary form as in this case.
- Sputum culture will provide a definitive answer and importantly allow for drug sensitivity testing.
- Urine should be tested for AFBs as a positive urine culture is not an uncommon finding in pulmonary TB cases. Screening for HIV infection is also indicated given the history of residence in an endemic area. The possibility of undiagnosed diabetes also should not be overlooked. Checking for evidence of impaired renal or hepatic function and a baseline ophthalmology review is important with respect to treatment choices.

ANSWERS – cont'd

A5 Standard four-drug treatment (isoniazid, rifampicin, pyrazinamide, ethambutol) initially is indicated to cover for suspected drug resistance (isoniazid resistance is most likely). Pyridoxine is often recommended as a supplement to isoniazid to prevent peripheral neuropathy.

Important treatment principles need to be followed to prevent disease relapse and acquired drug resistance:

- Always use at least two drugs to which the organism is fully sensitive.

- Treatment adherence is essential and direct observation should be considered in all patients especially in the initial 2-month intensive phase.
- Never add one drug alone to a failing regimen.
- Duration needs to be for a minimum of 6 months (dependent on drug sensitivity, tolerance and extent/site of disease).

Correct application of these rules results in a failure rate of less than 5%.

Adverse drug reactions are common (Table 39.1).

Table 39.1 Important side effects and drug interactions

Drug	Side effect	Interaction
Isoniazid	Peripheral neuropathy, hepatitis, rash	Anticonvulsants (increased level)
Rifampicin	Hepatitis, rash, 'flu-like syndrome, thrombocytopenia	Warfarin, oral contraceptives, oral hypoglycaemics, anticonvulsants (reduced level)
Pyrazinamide	Hepatitis, rash, arthralgia, gout	
*Ethambutol	Optic neuritis	

* Modify dose or avoid in those with renal impairment. Do not use in children whose visual acuity cannot be assessed

Discharge of this patient can occur when there is evidence of good clinical improvement, cough reduction or absence, the quantity of AFBs on smear is substantially reduced and treatment is assured. Regular follow-up is required to monitor disease response, check for side-effects and assess compliance.

A6 Prompt notification to the relevant public health authority is required for surveillance purposes and to facilitate contact investigation. The infectious risk of this person is potentially high, based on her sputum smear result. It is important to promptly identify close contacts, particularly children and the immunosuppressed; the risk of progression to disease if infected is greatest in these latter groups.

Contact tracing for notifiable diseases should be performed by a specialized service as there is a delicate balance between preservation of patient confidentiality and protecting public health.

A7 You suspect that this woman became infected during her 2-year stay in Africa. The doctor correctly assumed the tuberculin result reflected TB exposure (no evidence of disease) and advised isoniazid 'preventive' treatment. Isoniazid for 6 months (minimum) is generally recommended, but at least 9 months is preferred for children and the HIV-infected. If resistance to isoniazid is strongly suspected or known then rifampicin and pyrazinamide for 2 months or rifampicin alone for 4 months are the recommended options. Failure to prevent disease may have reflected poor compliance or an isoniazid resistant strain.

This case also highlights the need to be watchful for TB, as its worldwide incidence is on the rise once again, particularly in high-risk populations such as individuals with HIV.

REVISION POINTS

Pulmonary tuberculosis

Causative organism
Mycobacterium tuberculosis.

Mode of transmission
Inhalation of airborne droplet nuclei.

Incidence
- Uncommon in industrialized countries: rates >5–10:100 000.
- 90% of cases occur in resource-poor countries: rates >50–100:100 000.

Risk groups
- People from endemic areas.
- Recent close contacts of infectious cases.
- The socially disadvantaged.
- The elderly, particularly those with medical co-morbidities or who are on immunosuppression.
- HIV co-infected patients.

Pathology
- Primary TB infection is usually asymptomatic.
- Risk of progression is about 5% within the first 2 years; lifetime disease risk of 10–15%.
- If HIV co-infected the risk of developing active TB is 8–10% per year.
- Most disease is pulmonary from reactivation of latent infection (post primary or secondary).
- Extrapulmonary disease occurs in 15–20% but is more frequent with increasing immune suppression. The more common sites include lymph nodes, pleura, bone and kidney.
- The classic histological feature is necrotizing epithelioid granuloma.

Immunopathology
Immune responses in TB are complex and mediated mainly by T cells. They cause either a necrotic hypersensitivity or immune protective reaction but the factors responsible for these responses are not well understood.

Clinical
Classic presentation of pulmonary disease not always the case. Atypical presentations are frequent in the elderly and immunosuppressed, and TB should always be in the back of the mind as a differential diagnosis. Patients who become immunosuppressed, or have been started on immunosuppressant medication should be watched for symptoms suggestive of TB. Symptoms are often non-specific and insidious and the diagnosis often not considered. Extrapulmonary symptoms will be site dependent.

Diagnosis
- Chest X-ray abnormalities can be consistent with active pulmonary TB but are not diagnostic. Atypical features will be present in up to 30% of cases and CT scan may assist.
- The tuberculin test cannot distinguish active TB from latent infection. Serological tests are unreliable with poor sensitivity and specificity.
- Sputum smear microscopy is rapid but insensitive for detection of AFBs, i.e. may miss mycobacteria if there are only a few per high-powered field.
- Culture remains the gold standard but confirmation takes 10–14 days in smear positive specimens and 3–6 weeks in smear negative specimens. Drug susceptibility testing requires a further 10–15 days.
- The development of nucleic acid amplification tests makes diagnosis from some specimens possible in 24 hours but is not an alternative to conventional methods.

Treatment
Principles and drugs have changed little in 30 years. Directly observed treatment should be considered in all cases. Intermittent 2–3 times weekly treatment (directly observed) is as effective as daily treatment. Surgery is rarely indicated and mainly used if complications arise.

Public health
Notification is usually a legislative requirement and allows for contact investigation.

Prevention
Treatment of those recently infected/exposed (no active disease) is ~90% effective.

BCG vaccination has protective benefit in neonates and young children but its value to adults remains unclear. Patients who become immunosuppressed and who also have a clear history of prior exposure to TB should be considered for anti-TB medication as a secondary preventative measure.

ISSUES TO CONSIDER

- What is the role of screening programmes in the detection of tuberculosis?
- What would you do if a patient refused to give information for tracing contacts who may be at risk of contracting TB (or any other infectious disease)?
- Why is tuberculosis on the increase in developed nations?

FURTHER INFORMATION

www.nlm.nih.gov/medlineplus/tuberculosis.html A National Library of Medicine website. Comprehensive coverage of tuberculosis with links to a wide variety of sites dealing with many aspects of this disease.

www.who.int/gtb A superb web resource from the World Health Organization dealing with the global fight against tuberculosis infection.

Fever, cough and breathlessness in a middle-aged man

A 55-year-old market gardener is brought into the emergency department by his family. He has been unwell for 3 days. The illness started with general weakness and aches and pains all over his body and he thought he was in for a bout of the 'flu. He has suffered a persistent generalized headache, which has not responded to paracetamol. He then developed an irritating dry cough and bouts of diarrhoea.

In the last 24 hours he has become very unwell. He has developed a high fever and sweats and has vomited a number of times. He is breathless, the cough has worsened and he is now producing scant amounts of clear sputum. He has no pleuritic pain but has a dull generalized ache in his abdomen. He has no significant past medical history. He smokes about 20 cigarettes a day and consumes 30–50 grams of alcohol daily. He does not take any medications and has no known allergies.

On examination he looks ill. He is flushed, orientated but agitated and easily distracted. He has a temperature of 39.5°C. The patient is not cyanosed, clubbed, jaundiced or anaemic. He has dry mucous membranes and a coated tongue. His pulse rate is 105 bpm and regular, his blood pressure is 120/75 mm Hg and his oxygen–haemoglobin saturation is 90%. His cardiovascular system is otherwise normal. His respiratory rate is 30 breaths per minute and he has a hacking cough productive of small amounts of mucoid sputum. His chest is resonant and the breath sounds vesicular. There are scattered inspiratory crepitations throughout the right lung only. His abdomen is soft and non-tender. There is no neck stiffness and no focal neurological signs.

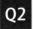 **Q1** What is the likely diagnosis?

The patient is placed on oxygen via nasal cannula at 4 l/min. An intravenous line is inserted and 1 litre isotonic saline is set up running over 2 hours to rehydrate the patient.

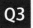 **Q2** What investigations would you perform?

The results in Investigation 40.1 are available.

Q3 Interpret the results. Do they help you with your diagnosis?

A chest X-ray is performed and is shown (Figure 40.1).

Investigation 40.1 Summary of results

Haemoglobin	161 g/l	White cell count		12.2 x 10^9/l
RBC	4.39 x 10^{12}/l	Neutrophils	50%	6.1 x 10^9/l
PCV	0.53	Lymphocytes	38%	4.6 x 10^9/l
MCV	86.9 fl	Monocytes	7%	0.9 x 10^9/l
MCH	29.5 pg	Eosinophils	2%	0.2 x 10^9/l
MCHC	340 g/l	Basophils	3%	0.4 x 10^9/l
Platelets	278 x 10^9/l			
Sodium	128 mmol/l	Calcium		2.16 mmol/l
Potassium	3.1 mmol/l	Phosphate		1.15 mmol/l
Chloride	106 mmol/l	Total protein		66 g/l
Bicarbonate	25 mmol/l	Albumin		39 g/l
Urea	10.1 mmol/l	Globulins		27 g/l
Creatinine	0.19 mmol/l	Bilirubin		16 μmol/l
Uric acid	0.24 mmol/l	ALT		62 U/l
Glucose	4.9 mmol/l	AST		75 U/l
Cholesterol	3.5 mmol/l	GGT		80 U/l
LDH	212 U/l	ALP		131 U/l
INR	1.0	APTT		35 secs

Arterial blood gases on room air

pO$_2$	61 mm Hg	pCO$_2$	32 mm Hg
pH	7.50	Calculated bicarbonate	25 mmol/l

Urinalysis: 1+ (0.3 g/l) protein, 1+ (5–10 red cells/μl) blood – no active sediment

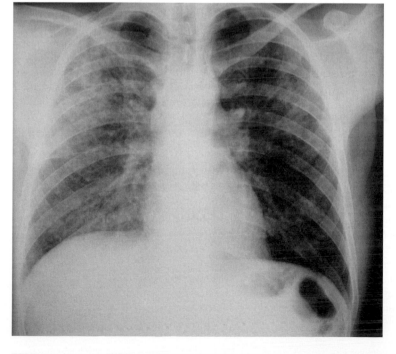

Fig 40.1

Q4 Describe the abnormalities on the chest X-ray.

The radiological features are consistent with pneumonia.

Q5 What organisms are likely to have caused this man's illness? How would you expect the clinical signs to differ with different pathogens?

Blood is taken for cultures and respiratory serology. You specifically request testing for antibodies against influenza A and B, respiratory syncytial virus, adenovirus, Q fever, psittacosis, mycoplasma and legionella. Nasopharyngeal swabs are taken for rapid antigen testing for respiratory viruses. Sputum is taken for Gram stain and culture; fluorescent antibody staining and culture for a particular organism is requested.

Your patient has a radiologically proven community acquired pneumonia.

Q6 How are you going to manage this patient at this stage?

The patient was commenced on erythromycin 1 g 6-hourly and ceftriaxone 1 g intravenously. He was rehydrated using isotonic saline so as not to exacerbate the hyponatraemia. The hypokalaemia was corrected.

His sputum showed polymorphs and oral flora. Sputum culture on special medium was positive for *Legionella pneumophila* after 3 days. Urine was positive for legionella antigen (specific for *Legionella pneumophila 1*). Blood cultures were negative. His respiratory status was closely monitored with the assistance of oximetry and serial blood gases.

He improved after 72 hours and made a slow recovery over the following 10 days. Initial serology for *Legionella* species by indirect fluorescent antibody was <1:4. At 16 days the *Legionella pneumophila* titre was 1:1024. Intravenous erythromycin was continued for 7 days and an oral dose of clarithromycin 500 mg 12-hourly was given for a further 2 weeks. The disease was notified to the Department of Health and *L. pneumophila* was subsequently isolated from a sprinkler system in the patient's greenhouses. The water system was decontaminated. The patient was told that his cigarette smoking and alcohol intake had put him at increased risk of contracting this illness. He was advised to stop smoking and was given options to assist with this process.

ANSWERS

A1 He has a febrile illness with cough and dyspnoea and abnormal respiratory signs but no hard clinical signs of consolidation. He had a prodrome of marked constitutional upset and does not have purulent sputum. Community acquired pneumonia is suggested by this presentation. His respiratory rate is markedly increased, which is an important sign of respiratory compromise.

Possible causes include:
- mycoplasma
- pneumococcus
- psittacosis
- legionella
- viral
- tuberculosis or an opportunistic pneumonia like pneumocystis with underlying AIDS less likely.

ANSWERS – Cont'd

A2 This patient requires the following investigations:

- complete blood picture and coagulation studies
- serum biochemistry
- chest X-ray
- blood cultures
- arterial blood gas analysis on air to ascertain the degree of respiratory impairment that is present, and oximetry performed for ongoing assessment
- nasopharyngeal swabs for the respiratory viruses (influenza, parainfluenza, respiratory syncytial virus, adenovirus)
- serology for respiratory pathogens including:
  - viral
  - *Mycoplasma pneumoniae*
  - *Chlamydia pneumoniae*
  - *Legionella* spp.
- sputum collection for Gram and acid-fast stains and for culture (including for *Legionella*, mycobacteria)
- urine assay for legionella antigen detection.

A3 There is only a mild leucocytosis (much lower than would be expected for pneumococcal pneumonia).

The patient has hyponatraemia, which is not uncommon with some pneumonias. It may be the result of pulmonary production of ADH-like substances. A hyponatraemia of less than 130 mmol/l can be associated with legionella pneumonia, but is not diagnostic. There is mild renal impairment, which may be due to dehydration or the underlying illness. There is a hypokalaemia which needs correction.

- The liver enzymes are abnormal. This is often feature in pneumonias caused by 'atypical' organisms such as *Legionella* and *Mycoplasma* but is non-specific and may occur in any septic patient.
- The urinalysis is abnormal, highlighting the systemic illness, which is not just limited to the lung.
- The coagulation studies are normal and this excludes disseminated intravascular coagulation.
- The arterial blood gas shows moderate hypoxaemia with hyperventilation and respiratory alkalosis.

These findings are in keeping with a severe pneumonia with systemic sepsis. They would be consistent with legionellosis but could still represent a severe pneumococcal infection.

A4 The chest X-ray shows an infiltrate within the right lung, particularly the upper lobe. There is a mixture of small segment consolidation and atelectasis. The appearances suggest bronchopneumonic change without major lobar volume loss. There is also more subtle patchy infiltrate in the left mid and lower zones, suggesting more extensive involvement of the pneumonic process. The heart size is normal.

A5 Community acquired pneumonia in the immunocompetent host can be caused by a broad range of pathogens (see Answer 1), which differ from those seen in hospital acquired pneumonias and pneumonias in immunocompromised hosts.

In the immunocompetent host, community acquired pneumonia is usually bacterial, most commonly due to *Streptococcus pneumoniae*. It may be of abrupt onset and marked by rapid progression with evidence of toxaemia, i.e. prostration, fever and rigors with respiratory symptoms (cough, dyspnoea) from the outset. The sputum is usually purulent, but cough may not be productive in the early phase. The patient may experience pleuritic chest pain and on examination there is likely to be evidence of consolidation, e.g. dullness to percussion and bronchial breathing, if lobar pneumonia is present. There will be marked neutrophilic leucocytosis and the organism may be cultured from the sputum and/or the blood. The chest X-ray will show evidence of consolidation.

In the past, the distinction has been made between 'typical' and 'atypical' pneumonia. This is not truly valid as there are no highly specific clinical symptoms or signs nor radiological findings which clearly discriminate on the basis of causative pathogen. Sometimes, the patterns on chest X-ray may assist in suggesting a particular pathogen, such as tuberculosis or *Pneumocystis carinii*, and helps to direct investigations in addition to those done to look for more common causes.

ANSWERS – Cont'd

A6 You should assess this patient in terms of his risk of complications and the severity of the pneumonia (Box 40.1).

The patient is a high-risk patient who has a severe, multilobar pneumonia with a range of possible causes. Although there are several features suggestive of a non-pneumococcal cause such as a prodromal period, gastrointestinal symptoms and deranged renal function and liver enzymes, accurate differentiation can only be made from specific microbiologic investigations.

Empirical antibiotic therapy should be introduced to cover both pneumococcus and other less common organisms such as *Legionella*, *Mycoplasma* and *Chlamydia* pneumonias. The presence of hypoxaemia and tachypnoea are both indications of severe pneumonia, and parenteral antibiotic therapy is necessary.

An intravenous penicillin in association with a macrolide antibiotic (erythromycin, clarithromycin) to cover the less common organisms mentioned above would be a reasonable initial antibiotic protocol. You must check with the patient and his family to ensure he is not allergic to penicillin. An alternative to penicillin would be an intravenous cephalosporin. In less severe pneumonia, oral therapy with amoxicillin and clarithromycin could be used. It is essential to familiarize yourself with local guidelines for the management of community acquired pneumonia and to adjust therapy according to culture results and advice from microbiologists.

Supplemental oxygen and intravenous fluids should be given. The patient's clinical status should be closely observed to watch for deterioration in respiratory, renal or cerebral status.

Response to treatment should be assessed through observation of the symptoms (particularly fever and respiratory compromise), white cell count and temperature. If there is no improvement the diagnosis should be questioned and alternatives considered. A CT scan would then be appropriate, as would consultation with respiratory and infectious diseases specialists.

Box 40.1 Risk analysis in severe pneumonia

Risk analysis	Severe pneumonia
Low risk	Clinically
• younger i.e. <65 years	• temp >40
• previously well, no co-morbidities	• respiratory rate >30
	• hypotensive BP <90 systolic
High risk	• confusion
• >65 years	• mechanical ventilation required
• nursing home resident	Bloods
• aspiration pneumonia	• PaO_2 <60 mm Hg on air
• Co-morbidities:	• $PaCO_2$ >50 mm Hg
– all smokers and chronic lung disease	• WCC <4 or >30
– liver disease	• metabolic acidosis
– renal disease	• abnormal creatinine
– cardiac failure	• abnormal LFTs
– diabetes	X-ray
– splenectomy	• bilateral involvement
– malignancy	• multilobar involvement
– alcohol abuse and malnutrition	• pleural effusion

Table adapted from Royal Adelaide Hospital Community Acquired Pneumonia management protocol (with permission)

REVISION POINTS

Community acquired pneumonia

Aims of management at presentation:

Assess severity
- respiratory rate
- mental state
- blood pressure and heart rate
- blood gases
- extent of infiltrate or pleural effusion on chest X-ray.

Identify aetiologic agent
- sputum microscopy and culture
- blood culture
- baseline serology
- nasopharyngeal aspirate or sputum for viruses
- urine for *Legionella pneumophilia* 1.

Remember underlying illnesses that impair the patient's immune system will extend the spectrum of possible infecting agents (so-called opportunistic infection).

Exclude other diagnoses
- thromboembolic disease
- malignancy
- hypersensitivity lung disease
- connective tissue disorders.

Initiate treatment appropriately
- high-flow oxygen
- intravenous rehydration and monitoring of fluid balance and renal function
- antibiotic therapy as guided by local policy and microbiology results
- early admission to an intensive care unit for ventilatory support in severe cases.

Remember to consider the patient's fitness. For the elderly, those with serious co-morbid conditions such as diabetes, COPD or cardiac failure or those with immune compromise, pneumonia may be rapidly life-threatening and may require specialized management.

Legionella

Legionella species
- Gram-negative aerobic bacilli

- intracellular bacterium in humans
- responsible for community acquired and nosocomial pneumonias.

Legionellae abound in aquatic environments and infection occurs via inhalation of contaminated aerosols. For examples, sources such as air-conditioning units, cooling towers and humidifiers have been identified in outbreaks of *Legionella* pneumonia. Contaminated water systems can be disinfected, although often with difficulty.

Legionella pneumonia
- most caused by *Legionella pneumophila*
- can be severe and fatal
- most common in adult males
- a notifiable disease
- person-to-person transmission does *not* occur: transmitted environmentally.

Risk factors
- advanced age
- chronic illness
- immunosuppression
- alcohol abuse
- cigarette smoking.

Diagnosis
- culture the organism
- identify the antigen (immunofluorescent antibody testing in sputum or material obtained at bronchoscopy) or by:
- rise in antibody titre in acute and convalescent sera (a fourfold rise).

Management
- erythromycin
- additional antibiotics if the pneumonia progresses
- ciprofloxacin and the newer quinolones (moxifloxacin, gatifloxacin) are very active against *legionella*.

Note: Respiratory failure requiring ventilation can occur. If the pneumonia progresses while the patient is on erythromycin, additional antibiotics may be necessary.

ISSUES TO CONSIDER

- How would you treat a hospital acquired pneumonia?
- What are the implications of the widespread use of parenteral cephalosporins in the management of community acquired pneumonia?
- What other respiratory disorders can be transmitted from environmental exposure?

FURTHER INFORMATION

www.brit-thoracic.org.uk The website of the British Thoracic Society, with access to the excellent guidelines for the management of community acquired pneumonia.

www.legionella.org Public access website from the US with plenty of information on this organism and the public health issues surrounding it.

www.nlm.nih.gov/medlineplus/ency/article/000616.htm National Library of Medicine website for *Legionella*.

Breathlessness and weight loss in a 58-year-old man

A 58-year-old accountant presents with 3 months of progressive breathlessness on exertion. He has no associated chest pain or wheeze but has had a smoker's cough for years. He has lost 5 kg over the last 3 months but says that his appetite is normal. He complains of a 'frog in his throat' for the last 6 weeks, which he has put down to his smoking. His breathlessness has progressed to such an extent that he has been unable to work for the last few days and was only able to walk up the one flight of stairs to your clinic with difficulty. Apart from feeling generally lethargic, he reports no other symptoms.

He has a history of hypertension for which he takes an ACE inhibitor. He smokes 20–30 cigarettes a day; his alcohol consumption is regular and has never exceeded an average of 20 gm a day. He is in his second marriage and has two young children aged 9 and 14.

Q1 What other information would you like from the history? What will you look for on examination?

On examination he is slightly plethoric and has signs of recent weight loss. He has a hoarse voice. His pulse is 80 bpm, his blood pressure is 155/95 mm Hg and he is afebrile. He is tachypnoeic with a respiratory rate of 25 breaths per minute and appears to be centrally cyanosed. Cardiovascular examination is normal.

His trachea is in the midline and the chest is not obviously over-inflated. The percussion note is dull in the lower half of the right chest. The breath sounds are reduced in this area and there is an associated increased vocal resonance. There is a widespread polyphonic wheeze throughout both lung fields. There are no other clinical signs on full examination.

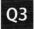

Q2 What are the possible diagnoses?

The man looks ill and dyspnoeic and you decide to admit him to hospital for further management.

Q3 What investigations will you order?

You receive the results shown in Investigation 41.1.

Investigation 41.1 Summary of results

Haemoglobin	175 g/l	White cell count		18.5 x 10^9/l
Platelets	500 x 10^9/l	Neutrophils	80%	14.8 x 10^9/l
Sodium	123 mmol/l	Calcium		2.85 mmol/l
Potassium	4.2 mmol/l	Phosphate		0.65 mmol/l
Chloride	106 mmol/l	Total protein		59 g/l
Bicarbonate	27 mmol/l	Albumin		32 g/l
Urea	5.1 mmol/l	Globulins		27 g/l
Creatinine	0.076 mmol/l	Bilirubin		12 µmol/l
Uric acid	0.24 mmol/l	ALT		22 U/l
Glucose	4.4 mmol/l	AST		32 U/l
Cholesterol	3.5 mmol/l	GGT		17 U/l
LDH	212 U/l	ALP		230 U/l

Arterial blood gases on room air

pO_2	52 mm Hg	pCO_2	50 mm Hg
pH	7.38	Base excess	−2.5

Q4   What do these results tell you?

A chest X-ray is shown (Figure 41.1).

Fig 41.1

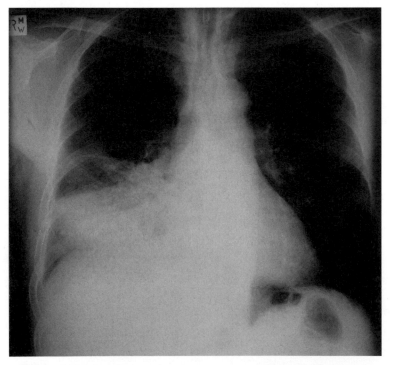

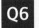 What does the chest X-ray show? How are you going to manage this patient?

 What further investigations should now be considered?

A further radiological investigation is performed. Two representative films are shown (Figures 41.2 and 41.3).

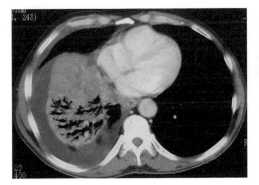 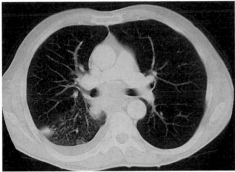

Fig 41.2   **Fig 41.3**

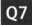 What do these CT scans show?

A bronchoscopy is performed and a tumour is found, obstructing the right middle and lower main lower bronchi. Biopsy of this tumour reveals a poorly differentiated adenocarcinoma.

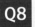 What treatment options are open to you at this stage? What will you tell the patient?

Five days after admission you are called to see him on the ward. He has become confused over the past 24 hours. A decision has been made not to proceed with chemotherapy or radiotherapy. The nurses report that he has not opened his bowels for 4 days.

On examination he is mildly confused with a GCS of 13. Despite his humidified oxygen he has dry mucous membranes and has decreased skin turgor. He is afebrile. The examination is otherwise unchanged since admission.

Q9 What are the possible causes for his confusion? What would you like to do?

Some serum biochemistry had been performed earlier that day. The results are shown in Investigation 41.2.

Investigation 41.2 Summary of results			
Sodium	130 mmol/l	Calcium	3.8 mmol/l
Potassium	4.4 mmol/l	Phosphate	0.16 mmol/l
Chloride	102 mmol/l	Total protein	57 g/l
Bicarbonate	27 mmol/l	Albumin	30 g/l
Urea	15.6 mmol/l	Globulins	27 g/l
Creatinine	0.28 mmol/l	Bilirubin	16 μmol/l
Uric acid	0.24 mmol/l	ALT	28 U/l
Glucose	4.4 mmol/l	AST	40 U/l
Cholesterol	3.5 mmol/l	GGT	17 U/l
LDH	212 U/l	ALP	354 U/l

Q10 What is the problem and what would you like to do now?

He received rehydration and a single dose of pamidronate. This was associated with clearing of his confusion and after discussion with his wife he elected to be transferred to inpatient hospice care. His hypercalcaemia rapidly recurred and he died peacefully surrounded by his family 3 weeks after his initial presentation.

ANSWERS

A1 Find out the following:

- The nature and severity of his shortness of breath. After how much exertion does he get short of breath? Does it occur at rest, during the night or when he lies flat? How many pillows does he sleep with?
- The nature of his cough. Has it changed? Is it productive and if so is it purulent? Has he coughed up any blood?
- Has he had any other symptoms to explain his weight loss? Has he had fevers or night sweats?
- Enquire further about his smoking history. How long has he smoked? Express the smoking history in 'pack-years' where 20 cigarettes a day for 1 year is 1 pack year. Thus a comparative figure can be derived for overall consumption of tobacco measured in terms of the total number of pack-years.
- Are there any other risk factors for lung disease such as industrial exposure to asbestos in the past? Does he keep birds? Has he had any recent foreign travel? Is there a family history of pulmonary disease?

On examination you should look for signs or evidence of the following:

- Respiratory distress, e.g. tachypnoea, cyanosis and the use of accessory respiratory muscles.
- Chronic lung disease, e.g. clubbing, wheeze and hyperinflated lungs.
- Pneumonia, e.g. fever and lobar consolidation.
- Malignant lung disease, e.g. pleural effusions, lymphadenopathy, hepatomegaly and ascites.
- Anaemia.
- Cardiac disease, e.g. cardiomegaly, raised jugular venous pressure, atrial fibrillation or peripheral oedema.

In addition you should measure oxygen saturation via pulse oximetry and perform a peak flow measurement.

A2 His smoking history makes it likely that he is suffering from a degree of chronic obstructive pulmonary disease (COPD). Patients with severe end-stage COPD often suffer from weight loss and become cachectic but this is usually in the context of a reduced intake due to severe dyspnoea at rest.

He may be suffering from an infective process but the length of the history makes it unlikely that this is bacterial in nature. The presence of weight loss raises the possibility of tuberculosis and you should ask about risk factors.

Other intrinsic lung diseases such as fibrosing alveolitis are possibilities but the presence of weight loss, the problems with his voice and his smoking history all make this a less likely diagnosis.

Cardiac failure leading to weight loss (cardiac cachexia) is unlikely in the absence of paroxysmal nocturnal dyspnoea or orthopnoea.

Anaemia may explain both his shortness of breath, lethargy and, depending on the cause, his weight loss.

By far the most likely diagnosis in this man who is a heavy smoker, has experienced recent weight loss and shortness of breath and has localizing pulmonary signs is lung cancer. The hoarseness of his voice is an extremely sinister symptom and may be due to malignant infiltration of the right recurrent laryngeal nerve by a hilar tumour causing a vocal cord paralysis.

A3 Perform these investigations:
- Complete blood picture: look for evidence of anaemia or infection (leucocytosis).
- Urea, electrolytes, creatinine, calcium, liver function tests.
- Chest X-ray.
- Arterial blood gases, looking for evidence of respiratory failure.
- Sputum collection for microscopy, culture, AFB and cytology.

A4 He is likely to have polycythaemia secondary to his long history of smoking (you would like to see his haematocrit). He has a neutrophilia which raises the possibility of an underlying infective process but may be a non-specific finding in any inflammatory condition. His mild thrombocytosis also supports an inflammatory process.

He has a moderately severe hyponatraemia in the context of otherwise normal renal function and in the absence of any culpable drugs. This

may well be the syndrome of inappropriate ADH (SIADH) seen in many pulmonary conditions and particularly in bronchogenic adenocarcinoma. Paired serum and urine osmolalities would help to confirm this. If SIADH is present you would expect to see inappropriately concentrated urine in the presence of dilute or normal serum.

He has a raised alkaline phosphatase which may be due to liver infiltration with metastatic carcinoma (expect to see a raised GGT in addition) or due to bony involvement. The mild hypoalbuminaemia is likely to be due to his chronic illness or, if there is liver involvement, synthetic liver dysfunction. It is highly unlikely to be due to nutritional deficiency despite his recent weight loss.

He has a mild hypercalcaemia. This may be due to production of a parathormone-like peptide by a lung adenocarcinoma. Alternatively, in conjunction with the raised ALP, bony involvement is a distinct possibility.

His blood gases show that he has severe established type 2 respiratory failure with both hypoxia and hypercapnoea. The normal pH implies that this is a relatively well compensated and, therefore, a chronic process.

A5 The chest X-ray is reported as follows:
There is partial collapse and consolidation in the right middle lobe. There is also an abnormal convexity to the posterior aspect of the right hilum and the appearances are suspicious of a right hilar mass resulting in the collapse and consolidation of the right middle lobe. There is some increased opacity in the subcarinal region and lymphadenopathy in this region is suspected. The left lung and pleural reflection appear clear.

He is in respiratory failure. You should administer oxygen by Venturi mask to correct his hypoxia. Repeat his blood gas analysis in 30 minutes to ensure he does not decompensate due to carbon dioxide retention.

In view of the X-ray appearances and the leucocytosis, the administration of antibiotics would be appropriate. An intravenous penicillin and oral macrolide would be suitable until the results of microbiological culture are known.

Remember that although the history and investigations so far point towards an advanced

ANSWERS – cont'd

lung cancer, this has not yet been proven. He should be managed in a high dependency unit and intensive care support requested should he deteriorate.

If he is suffering from SIADH then fluid restriction may be appropriate. However, in the presence of hypercalcaemia, fluid restriction may lead to profound dehydration. It would be wise not to restrict his fluid intake and, if he is unable to drink, to provide the patient with maintenance intravenous fluids using isotonic saline. Daily checks on his electrolytes and calcium will help you adapt his fluid and electrolyte regimens accordingly.

A6 Once he is stabilized he will need:
- A CT scan of his chest to further define the hilar and mediastinal abnormalities.
- A fibreoptic bronchoscopy to look for a bronchial tumour and to obtain histological samples for diagnosis.
- If the bronchoscopy is normal, a CT guided biopsy or mediastinoscopy may be necessary.

A7 The CT scans are reported as follows:

There is a large soft tissue mass in the subcarinal region of the mediastinum consistent with lymphadenopathy. This is associated with soft tissue enlargement with surrounding of the right pulmonary artery by the soft tissue mass lesion. The appearances are consistent with bronchogenic carcinoma with involvement of the mediastinum. There is distal consolidation and partial collapse of the lung within the right middle and lower lobes. The left lung shows no evidence of any sinister parenchymal lesion. There is a right pleural effusion. The appearances are consistent with a bronchogenic carcinoma involving the right hilum.

A8 This man clearly has advanced lung cancer with respiratory failure, hypercalcaemia, SIADH and probable liver and/or bone involvement. Any treatments that you offer him at this stage are palliative.

The presence of mediastinal involvement, respiratory failure and probable metastatic disease rule out the possibility of surgery. Surgery remains the only real option for cure in non-small cell lung carcinoma but is only effective if the lesions are small, usually peripheral and the patient has good respiratory reserve. Surgery is now being performed in some centres for more advanced disease often in conjunction with either chemotherapy or radiotherapy.

Radiotherapy has resulted in 'cure' in a small number of reported cases but is largely used for palliation.

Chemotherapy for non-small cell tumours has also produced disappointing results. Aggressive regimens involving the taxanes and platinum-based drugs have been shown to be useful as palliation in selected patients. This man's respiratory failure and metabolic upset make him poorly suited for any such treatment.

His outlook is poor. When breaking bad news it is important to be in possession of all the facts and prepared for questions. If possible, the most senior member of your team should be present when bad news is broken. It is important that you speak to him in a quiet, private environment in the presence, if he wishes, of friends and family. Allow good time, as he is likely to have many questions. Be honest and frank but avoid medical jargon and don't remove all hope. It is important to avoid phrases such as 'there is nothing we can do' as, although there is no chance of a cure, there are many interventions which can relieve symptoms and improve his quality of life in his final days. The main fear of many patients told they have a terminal disease is that they will die in pain or without dignity. With modern palliative care, this need not be the case. He has a young family and the effects of his diagnosis on them must not be forgotten. The involvement of palliative care professionals at an early stage is important.

A9 There are several possible causes for confusion in this man:
- Hyponatraemia: his sodium was low on presentation, this may have worsened.
- Hypercalcaemia: he may have worsening hypercalcaemia.
- Respiratory failure: he may have become more hypoxic or have increasing hypercapnia.

ANSWERS – cont'd

- Sepsis: keep in mind common causes of confusion. Is there any sign of sepsis?
- Cerebral metastases: he has widespread disease. The presence of cerebral metastases with attendant cerebral oedema needs to be considered.
- Alcohol withdrawal: the patient stated when first seen that he 'drinks regularly', and you must remember that most patients will underestimate their alcohol consumption.
- You should check his electrolytes, calcium and blood gases. If it looks likely that there is no metabolic causes for his symptoms then you could consider a CT scan to identify metastases.

It is important to identify easily treatable causes of his deterioration if such treatment will result in improved symptomatology and quality of life. However, in the setting of palliative care, investigations and interventions should only be carried out if they are likely to lead to such improvements. If not then treatments should aim for symptom control and comfort. Always involve his relatives

particularly his next of kin. Palliative care professionals can also be very helpful.

A10 He has hypercalcaemia with associated dehydration and renal failure. Fluid restriction for his hyponatraemia may have exacerbated this situation.

Hypercalcaemia of malignancy often occurs in the presence of bone metastases but may also be mediated by the production of a parathormone-like peptide from malignant cells; a so-called paraneoplastic syndrome. It often produces a dramatic clinical picture and should be treated in all but the most terminal of cases.

Treatment involves initial rehydration with isotonic saline. This man is likely to need 3–4 litres over the next 24 hours. Bear in mind that this may exacerbate his hyponatraemia.

A biphosphonate such as pamidronate can be added to palliate the hypercalcaemia if this were thought appropriate. These drugs work by inhibiting the mobilization of calcium from the skeleton.

REVISION POINTS

Lung cancer

Epidemiology
- The most common form of cancer in men and now, in most developed countries, in women.
- Causes more deaths in the USA than breast, prostate and bowel cancer combined.
- On the increase, especially in women due to a dramatic rise in female smoking. Also increasing in developing societies.
- Almost all forms of lung cancer are a direct result of tobacco smoking, making it the West's biggest preventable health problem.

Presentation
- Always suspect in smokers with unexplained deterioration in health and/or weight loss.
- May have no pulmonary symptoms. The presence of shortness of breath, pain and haemoptysis often imply advanced disease. Hoarseness of voice if recurrent laryngeal nerve involvement.

- Sometimes picked up incidentally in medical assessments.

Types
Two major groups:
1 Small cell lung cancer
  - accounts for 10-15% of total number of cases
  - tumours tend to be rapidly progressive
  - responds to high dose chemotherapy regimens +/− radiotherapy but have a very high recurrence rate following treatment. Metastatic disease is common.
2 Non-small cell lung cancer (NSCLC).
  Three subtypes:
  - **Adenocarcinoma**
    40–50% of total
    Most common lung cancer in women
  - **Squamous cell carcinoma**
    30–40% of total

continues overleaf

REVISION POINTS – cont'd

More common in men and with advanced age

- **Large cell carcinoma**
  10–15%
  Declining incidence.

Treatment

Treatment depends on stage.

Surgical resection +/− adjuvant therapy are options for early stage tumours (1A–2B).

For later stage tumours, treatment is largely palliative. New high-dose chemotherapeutic regimens may improve quality and prolong length of life.

Current research involves a variety of approaches, e.g. novel chemotherapy agents, photodynamic therapy and vaccine therapy.

Palliative care measures and psychological support especially important in patients with advanced disease.

Prognosis

Prognosis of NSCLC depends on stage at presentation. 1A (small volume local disease with no nodes or metastases) has a 5-year survival of up to 70%. Only 1% of patients with stage 5 disease (the presence of metastases) will be alive at 5 years.

Overall, prevention by not smoking is the most important approach for this disease. Advising patients and their relatives not to smoke should be the responsibility of all healthcare professionals.

ISSUES TO CONSIDER

- What are the factors that influence the incidence of smoking in various countries? Are there any effective measures that might be used to reduce the incidence of cigarette smoking?

- What other paraneoplastic phenomena occur in advanced lung cancer? How can they best be treated?

- What palliative care options exist for the treatment of respiratory distress in this situation?

FURTHER INFORMATION

www.lungcancer.org Excellent website with links and information for patients and healthcare professionals alike.

www.cancerresearchuk.org Website of the Cancer Research Campaign in the UK with lots of information and links for lung and other tumours.

A 63-year-old woman presents to her local doctor's surgery complaining of breathlessness on exertion. She is divorced and lives alone. On reflection, she has noticed this problem for the last 2 months but it has become particularly severe in the last 2 weeks. She now finds it an effort to perform any of her daily activities and recently has spent much of her time resting. She is not short of breath at rest or during the night. She is able to sleep flat and uses only one small pillow. She has no cough, wheeze or phlegm. The patient has not noticed any chest pain or discomfort or any pain on inspiration. She notices palpitations on exertion and feels lightheaded on standing. She has noticed some swelling of her ankles. She admits to feeling weak and despondent. The remainder of the systems inquiry is unremarkable. Her weight is stable. The patient has a past history of a myocardial infarction 2 years ago, which was managed medically. She has no other medical illnesses and has never smoked. She consumes alcohol only rarely. She eats a balanced and varied diet.

Q1 Are there any features from the history that suggest an underlying cause for her dyspnoea?

On examination, her respiratory rate is 14 breaths per minute at rest. She is not jaundiced or clubbed or cyanosed, but her skin folds and conjunctival mucosa are noticeably pale. She has a resting tachycardia of 100 bpm with a blood pressure of 135/70 mm Hg. Her jugular venous pressure is not elevated. Her apex beat is not displaced but she has a hyperdynamic cardiac impulse. Auscultation of the chest reveals a soft ejection systolic murmur, loudest at the apex. No radiation of the murmur is detected. She has minor pitting oedema of the ankles. Respiratory and abdominal examinations were unremarkable. Rectal examination was normal with normal coloured stool. This stool tests positive for blood.

Q2 What initial tests should be performed?

The blood test results are shown in Investigation 42.1.

A chest X-ray is normal and the ECG shows sinus tachycardia with Q waves in the inferior leads suggestive of an old myocardial infarction.

Investigation 42.1 Summary of results

Haemoglobin	68 g/l	White cell count	6.3 x 10^9/l
MCV	69 fl		
MCH	28 pg		
MCHC	300 g/l		
Platelets	332 x 10^9/l		
Sodium	132 mmol/l	Calcium	2.41 mmol/l
Potassium	4.3 mmol/l	Phosphate	0.98 mmol/l
Chloride	106 mmol/l	Total protein	60 g/l
Bicarbonate	27 mmol/l	Albumin	35 g/l
Urea	4.2 mmol/l	Globulins	25 g/l
Creatinine	0.10 mmol/l	Bilirubin	22 µmol/l
Uric acid	0.24 mmol/l	ALT	40 U/l
Glucose	4.4 mmol/l	AST	26 U/l
Cholesterol	3.5 mmol/l	GGT	45 U/l
LDH	212 U/l	ALP	119 U/l
Ferritin	4 µg/l		
Vitamin B$_{12}$	519 µg/l	Red cell folate	4.9 µg/l

Q3 What is the differential diagnosis of the full blood count? What do the haematinics (iron studies) tell you?

Q4 Would you alter your management of this patient if the stools are negative for occult blood?

Q5 What treatment and investigations would you organize now?

Based on the patient's symptoms of increasing breathlessness, a decision is made to transfuse her. Two units of matched blood are slowly transfused, with a clinical review after each unit.

A colonoscopy is performed. Figure 42.1 shows a view from the right colon.

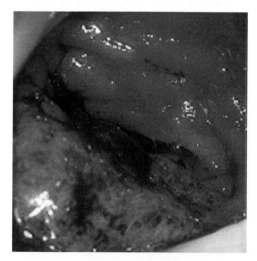

Fig 42.1

Q6 What does the photograph show?

The patient underwent a right hemicolectomy. The pathology of the specimen revealed a Duke's C adenocarcinoma with 3 of 6 resected lymph nodes involved with tumour.

ANSWERS

A1 There are many causes of dyspnoea. They can be divided into categories as follows:

- Lung disease: this includes airway disorders, parenchymal disease or diseases of the respiratory neuromuscular apparatus.
- Cardiac disease, e.g. left ventricular failure, valvular disease.
- Others: anaemia, psychogenic, metabolic disturbances.

The history is the key to the diagnosis:

- It is unlikely that she has chronic obstructive pulmonary disease as she is a life-long non-smoker, and does not have the cough, wheeze and nocturnal symptoms of asthma or the sputum production of bronchiectasis.
- It is possible she has a restrictive lung disease, such as some type of interstitial pneumonitis or fibrosis. Pulmonary vascular disease such as multiple pulmonary emboli is also possible.
- She has a past history of myocardial infarction and mild ankle oedema, but such a degree of dyspnoea is likely to cause orthopnoea if it was due to cardiac failure.
- Anxiety is a potential cause, but functional dyspnoea is often marked at rest whereas this patient's dyspnoea is always precipitated by exertion which is characteristic of an organic disorder.

Overall, there are features to suggest that anaemia is the likely cause: weakness, lethargy, dyspnoea on exertion, palpitations and lightheadedness on standing. However, other conditions such as those listed above are possible diagnoses, and further investigation is required.

A2 As anaemia is suspected, a full blood count is required. If anaemia is confirmed, then haema-tinics and a blood film should be requested. A group and save sample is taken in case cross-matching for transfusion is required. Underlying cardiorespiratory conditions may be exacerbated by anaemia, and therefore a chest X-ray and ECG should be performed.

A3 The blood picture shows a marked anaemia with microcytic red blood cells. The most likely cause of this would be an iron deficiency anaemia. Haematinics show a low serum ferritin confirming an iron deficiency picture. Measurement of serum iron and total iron binding capacity may be of value if there is doubt over the validity of the ferritin result (ferritin may occasionally be spuriously raised – it is an acute phase protein, and so it should be interpreted with caution in the presence of inflammatory conditions). Serum B_{12} and red cell folate are within normal limits, and therefore are not contributing to the anaemia.

A4 Even in the presence of negative faecal occult blood testing, it is important to investigate the gastrointestinal tract. In post-menopausal women and adult men with no obvious source of blood loss, the gastrointestinal tract is the most common source of occult blood loss.

A5 The patient is symptomatic, has a history of coronary artery disease and has signs of a hyper dynamic circulation. An important consideration is whether she requires transfusion. This is a clinical decision. Ideally, transfusion could be avoided provided she does not have any sign of cardiac compromise such as angina or orthopnoea and provided she does not develop any evidence of acute bleeding. It would be appropriate to commence aggressive oral iron replacement, e.g.

ANSWERS – cont'd

ferrous sulfate 200 mg 3 to 4 times daily. If she is intolerant of oral iron, intravenous iron is an alternative, although it has the potential risk of adverse reactions. She should show evidence of a reticulocyte response within seven days and she will need to be monitored closely. If she develops any evidence of cardiac compromise she will need to be transfused. In this case 2–3 units of packed red blood cells should be given slowly with a small dose of frusemide (furosemide) to prevent volume overload.

She must be investigated for the cause of her iron deficiency. As she has no upper gastrointestinal symptoms, her colon should be investigated first, preferably by colonoscopy. If this does not show the cause of the anaemia, she should have a gastroscopy with duodenal biopsies in order to exclude coeliac disease.

Small bowel contrast studies or enteroscopy, labelled red blood cell scans, and mesenteric angiography can also be used to find the source of occult gastrointestinal blood loss.

Virtual colonoscopy is a new technique which uses sophisticated software in tandem with CT scanning to recreate a 3-D image of the colon, which can demonstrate tumours and polyps. Plain CT colography can also be useful especially in elderly frail patients who would not tolerate a barium enema.

Patients may have several digestive tract diseases, and finding a duodenal ulcer does not exclude a co-existent colon cancer.

A6 Occupying the bottom half of the photograph and 50% of the circumference of the bowel wall there is a fleshy tumour. There is fresh blood on its surface. This is the characteristic appearance of an exfoliative neoplasm.

REVISION POINTS

Investigation of anaemia

Definition

Reduction in red cell mass, may be acute or chronic. Not a diagnosis in itself. A cause should be sought in all cases.

Symptoms

Dyspnoea, fatigue, palpitations, dizziness, syncope and headache.

The degree and type of symptoms will depend on the severity and speed of onset of the anaemia, the age of the patient and the presence of underlying medical conditions, e.g. ischaemic heart disease.

Signs

- pallor
- tachycardia
- tachypnoea.

Causes

- blood loss
- decreased red cell production (dietary deficiencies, renal failure, diseases of the bone marrow)
- increased red cell destruction (haemolysis).

Investigations

Mean cell volume (MCV) helps to establish cause:

1 Microcytic: Iron deficiency (commonest cause), thalassaemia, sideroblastic anaemia. Iron deficiency can be caused by:
   - blood loss: menstruation, GI blood loss, haematuria
   - dietary deficiency
   - malabsorption: coeliac disease,* postgastrectomy.

   Investigate with gastroscopy and distal duodenal biopsy, and colonoscopy. Reserve barium enema for patients unable to tolerate colonoscopy.

   Obtain dietary history, urinalysis. Further gastrointestinal investigations may be required, e.g. small bowel radiology, enteroscopy.

2 Normocytic: Anaemia of chronic disease, haemolysis and marrow failure.

   Investigate with reticulocyte count, serum bilirubin and haptoglobin. Bone marrow biopsy if bone marrow failure suspected (indicated if other lineages affected).

continues overleaf

REVISION POINTS — cont'd

3 Macrocytic: B_{12} or folate deficiency (mega-loblastic), alcohol, liver disease, drugs, myelodys-plasia, hypothyroidism, and pregnancy (non-megaloblastic). Haemolysis may cause a macrocytosis and is recognized by polychro-masia, an increased reticulocyte count, increased unconjugated bilirubin, decreased haptoglobin and abnormalities on the blood smear such as spherocytes.

Investigate with serum B_{12}, red cell folate, Schilling test, small bowel barium follow-through, haemolysis screens, bone marrow biopsy.

*Combined folate and iron deficiency is the classical anaemia seen in coeliac disease but may manifest as an apparent normocytic anaemia (due to two populations of red cells – one microcytic, the other macrocytic).

ISSUES TO CONSIDER

● What simple laboratory test may suggest that there are two populations of red cells (one macrocytic, one microcytic) in an apparently normocytic blood count?

● What role does screening play in the early detection of colonic carcinomas? Which populations should be offered screening? How should it be performed?

● What dietary advice should be given to a vegan with recurrent iron deficiency anaemia with no other known cause?

FURTHER INFORMATION

www.bsg.org.uk/clinical_prac/guidelines/iron_def.htm A useful website from the British Society of Gastroenterology with up-to-date guidelines for the management of iron deficiency anaemia.

www.gastro.org Website of the American Gastroenterological Association. Follow the links to practice guidelines on colonic cancer screening and many other issues.

Acute breathlessness in a 21-year-old woman

A 21-year-old female student is brought into the emergency department by ambulance. She is acutely breathless, and cannot speak full sentences. Her mother provides the background history, explaining that her daughter has been asthmatic for 3 years. The girl has recently had a sore throat and runny nose and her asthma has flared up. Over the last 4 days the mother has heard her daughter wake in the early hours of the morning coughing. The patient has become increasingly breathless and wheezy over the last 12 hours. She regularly uses a salbutamol puffer but has used it repeatedly over the last 2 days without much effect.

Q1 What should be done immediately? What information should be sought from the history promptly?

The mother states that her daughter's breathing has been abnormal for some weeks and on reflection it has been getting progressively worse for 4 or 5 days. Her daughter is not a smoker and has never had a hospital admission for asthma. She had an asthma attack last winter for which the local doctor prescribed tablets, the name of which the mother cannot recall. The general practitioner continued them for 2 weeks before tailing off. The daughter had also previously had tablets that had made her feel sick but she had not taken tablets of any kind for many months. The girl indicates that she has produced small amounts of clear sputum but no yellow phlegm.

Q2 What specific features will you look for on examination?

On examination the patient is sitting up grasping the sides of the examination trolley. She is anxious and tears are running from her eyes. She is not cyanosed. She is tachypnoeic at a rate of 30 breaths/minute and has a loud wheeze. She will not speak spontaneously but can briefly answer questions if pressed. Her pulse rate is 130 bpm and her blood pressure is 150/80 mm Hg with a paradox of 20 mm Hg. She is afebrile. Her chest is hyper-resonant and the breath sounds have markedly prolonged expiration with a loud wheeze. There is no evidence of consolidation. She is unable to perform a peak flow measurement.

Q3 What is your assessment of the patient so far and what would you do next?

The patient is given continuous nebulized salbutamol for 30 minutes and then it is reduced to 2.5 mg nebulized every 15 minutes. 200 mg intravenous hydrocortisone is given, followed by 100 mg every 6 hours.

Thirty minutes after admission, she remains tachypnoeic, tachycardic and distressed. She is still unable to speak in long sentences. The following blood gas analysis is performed on high-flow inspired oxygen.

Investigation 43.1 Blood gas analysis	
pH	7.52
pO$_2$	139 mm Hg
pCO$_2$	18 mm Hg
HCO$_3$	24.1
Base excess	4.3

Q4 What do these blood gas results tell you and what will you do now?

After 2 hours, with further management the patient has significantly improved. A chest X-ray is performed which shows bilateral hyperinflation but no evidence of segmental or lobar collapse (from plugging with mucus) or pneumothorax or pneumomediastinum. A complete blood picture and electrolytes are normal.

The patient is transferred to a high dependency unit and closely observed. The nebulized salbutamol is reduced to hourly administration and after 12 hours changed to a 4-hourly dose. After 12 hours the patient is able to use a peak flow meter and her peak flow rates are charted pre- and post-nebulized salbutamol for the remainder of her admission. After 24 hours the young woman has improved sufficiently to be transferred to a general medical ward.

The hydrocortisone is changed to prednisolone 50 mg daily and the dose is tapered off over the next 10 days. Her peak flow rates slowly improve but plateau at approximately 400 l/min and continue to show an improvement of about 30% post bronchodilator.

The patient states that her asthma has been worse over the last 6 months. She has been a regular smoker but ceased 3 months ago because it aggravated her asthma. She says the main precipitants for her asthma are colds, exercise and cold air but that it can also occur without any obvious cause. She has seen a local doctor about her asthma and salbutamol was prescribed. She stopped seeing him 3 months ago when her family moved house and she has yet to register with another GP.

Q5 Describe the further management of this patient.

ANSWERS

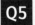 **A1** This girl is having an acute asthma attack. She is unable to speak sentences so the attack is likely to be severe. You should administer high-flow oxygen immediately. She should be moved to a high dependency area and nebulized salbutamol should be administered.

Information should be sought on the following:

• The length of the attack (often underestimated by the patient and observers).

• When the patient's breathing was last normal. This will give an idea of the severity of the overall attack. The time taken for improvement is often proportional to the duration of the attack. This question may also give an idea of whether the patient has chronic asthma or recurrent episodes with normal functional status in between.

• Is there sputum production during coughing: if so, clear or purulent? Discoloured sputum in

ANSWERS – cont'd

asthmatics is often present because of non-infective inflammation and this alone does not indicate infection or a need for antibiotics. Some clinicians will empirically use antibiotics if the patient is also a smoker. Antibiotics would be necessary if there was other clinical evidence of bronchitis or pneumonia, e.g. fever or leucocytosis.

- Any other medications being used for her asthma (e.g. preventative medication or in older patients, enquire about concomitant use of betablockers).
- Any hospitalization over the last 12 months for her asthma. If the answer is yes, then this is a risk factor for severe disease.
- Any previous use of oral steroids for her asthma – if yes, when was the last time steroids were taken? Previous use of systemic steroids indicates severe asthma. If steroids were recently ceased then steroid withdrawal may be a significant factor in exacerbation of her asthma.
- Has she ever been in intensive care or intubated due to her asthma? If so, this indicates very high risk and you should be alert for rapid deterioration.
- Smoking habits. If the girl is a smoker the issue of stopping will need to be addressed at a later time.

A2 You should look for indicators of severity of the asthma attack, including:

- The inability to speak full sentences.
- Tachycardia >110 bpm.
- Tachypnoea >25.
- Pulsus paradoxus >20 mm Hg.
- Peak flow rate <50% predicted.

Subsequent bradycardia, the silent chest and reduced conscious level are all indicators that the attack is life-threatening and anaesthetic assistance should be summoned.

Your initial assessment should also include the exclusion of a pneumothorax, particularly if the onset of the attack is very sudden and severe. Look for chest asymmetry, reduced air entry, tracheal deviation and the circulatory disturbances associated with tension pneumothorax.

A3 The patient has severe acute asthma. The attack has been present for days and has culminated in a medical emergency. There is no obvious evidence of a bacterial chest infection and the likely trigger is an upper respiratory tract viral infection. It is probable that the tablets given last winter and tapered off were oral steroids, and this is confirmatory evidence for severe asthma.

Treatment must begin immediately. This should consist of:

- Continuous high-flow oxygen (which you have started).
- Initial therapy with a continuous nebulized bronchodilator (e.g. salbutamol.) In severe cases this may be combined with intermittent ipratropium bromide nebulizers.
- Intravenous glucocorticosteroids (benefit may not be obtained for 6–8 hrs). The correct dose is controversial. Some clinicians give 200 mg hydrocortisone intravenously followed by 100 mg 6-hourly. Others give higher doses so that failure of treatment will not be ascribed to insufficient steroid therapy.
- Constant monitoring of the patient. The respiratory rate, pulse rate, pulsus paradoxus and peak flow must be measured frequently to provide objective measurement of the severity of the asthma and assessment of response to therapy.
- Arterial blood gas analysis is only necessary if there is no response to therapy or there is deterioration. Transfer to an intensive care unit and assisted ventilation may be required if the patient goes into respiratory failure.
- A chest X-ray is only performed once the patient has shown substantial improvement. However, if a pneumothorax is suspected, an urgent radiograph should be performed.
- Intravenous fluids to prevent dehydration.

A4 The gases show a type 1 pattern secondary to hyperventilation. She is blowing off her CO_2, which has lead to a respiratory alkalosis. Although not hypoxic, her pO_2 is less than you would expect in a healthy individual receiving high-flow oxygen.

A rising CO_2 in the context of hyperventilation, even into the normal range, is an indicator

ANSWERS – cont'd

of deterioration and should alert you to the need for assistance from intensive care staff.

The next step in treatment would either be intravenous salbutamol or aminophylline. There have been concerns about the use of aminophylline in certain circumstances, especially in patients who are taking the drug orally (an intravenous bolus should never be given in these circumstances) and in those who are taking drugs which may potentiate its effect. However, if used carefully it can be an extremely useful drug in the acute setting and is still widely prescribed in the UK and USA.

One of the keys to successful management of severe asthma is being able to recognize that the patient is likely to require intubation and ventilatory support early on and summoning the required help.

A5 There are four components to the further management of this patient:

1 Patient education. Once she has recovered from the acute episode the first important action is to take the time to educate the patient about her illness. She needs to understand that:
   - asthma involves inflammation and narrowing of the airways
   - it is a chronic condition and there is no known cure
   - the disease can be life-threatening, but there is effective treatment available
   - treatment is directed at modifying the inflammation of the airways
   - bronchodilators (e.g. salbutamol). Inhalers act only to relieve the symptoms of asthma and do nothing to alter the underlying problem of airways inflammation. This usually means more treatment than just salbutamol inhalation is necessary.

2 Define the aims of treatment. These are to obtain and maintain normal lung function by preventing airways obstruction and thus maintain a normal lifestyle, and to prevent death from asthma. In addition to symptomatic relief with bronchodilators (inhaled beta-agonists), this patient will need disease-modifying agents that will reduce airways inflammation

and hyper-responsiveness. An inhaled steroid (e.g. beclometasone, budesonide or fluticasone) at a dose of 250–500 µg twice daily given 10–15 minutes after the salbutamol inhaler would be appropriate. If she develops problems with oral candida or a hoarse voice these can be avoided by using a spacing device and mouth washes. Chloride channel blockers such as sodium chromoglycate or nedocromil may also be used as a disease modifier. Oral steroids may be required for rescue from acute exacerbations of the disease.

3 Monitoring and a plan of management. The patient will need to monitor her own disease regularly with a home peak flow meter. Intensive therapy will be needed after this attack to optimize her lung function. Her best peak flow can then be used as a reference level to guide subsequent therapeutic targets.

An 'Acute Asthma Management Plan' should be drawn up which the patient and her family understand. It must be emphasized that this is the best way to avoid having another episode of life-threatening asthma. The plan relies on peak flow measurements, e.g.:
   - If peak flows after salbutamol inhalation drop below 80% of normal for more than 12 hours, then the frequency of inhaled salbutamol should be increased and her inhaled steroid therapy should be doubled.
   - If the flow rate is below 60%, a course of oral steroids should be given by her local doctor.
   - If below 40–50% the patient should present immediately to hospital.
   - She should also wear a medical alert bracelet.

4 Identification of trigger factors. The patient should be questioned about any relationship of her asthma to certain foods which may have chemical additives, and common aeroallergens such as animal danders or house dust. If triggers can be identified then avoiding contact or exposure to these may lead to better disease control in an atopic asthmatic. Some people can have acute asthma triggered by

A N S W E R S – cont'd

taking aspirin and if there is a history of this then aspirin and other non-steroidal anti-inflammatory drugs must be avoided. It should be remembered that many foods contain salicylates so aspirin-sensitive individuals may need to see a dietician to seek advice regarding an elimination diet. This is particularly important in patients who have a history of nasal polyps, allergic rhinitis or peripheral blood eosinophilia.

R E V I S I O N   P O I N T S

Asthma

Aetiology
- Airway inflammation and greatly increased reactivity and irritability of the bronchial tree.
- Contraction of bronchial smooth muscle, mucosal inflammation and increased secretions lead to airway obstruction.
- The disease affects at least 10% of children and 5% of adults in Australia and can be a fatal disease. Asthma deaths are higher in Australia and New Zealand than in the UK or USA and the reasons for this are unclear.

Stimuli/triggers
- In some patients distinct allergens can be identified (extrinsic asthma), while others are not prone to allergy and have so-called intrinsic asthma.
- Upper respiratory tract viral infections are potent causes of airway hyper-irritability and this may last for weeks after the infection.
- Drugs can induce prominent bronchospasm. About 10% of asthmatics will have acute bronchospasm precipitated by aspirin or other NSAIDs. Food colouring agents (e.g. benzoites) and preservatives (e.g. metabisulfite) have been implicated.
- Betablockers are obvious asthma inducers and should be avoided.
- Exposure to substances in the work place can also be important.
- Exercise is a common precipitant of bronchospasm.
- Gastro-oesophageal reflux may exacerbate asthma.

Acute asthma
- Acute asthma is a common medical emergency.
- The use of accessory muscles, tachycardia, tachypnoea and a paradox of greater than 10 mm Hg are all markers of significant obstruction.
- Any patient with a peak flow rate of 150 l/min or less pre-bronchodilator must be considered for admission.
- Blood gas analysis in acute asthma is best used as a guide to whether the patient should be transferred to an intensive care unit for intensive therapy and possible ventilation. The pCO_2 will indicate the state of ventilation, i.e. a normal pCO_2 may indicate impending respiratory failure, as it should be below the normal range due to hyperventilation, and a raised pCO_2 reflects established respiratory failure.

Treatment
- Inhaled steroids are the most effective disease-modifying agents: they are the 'preventers'.
- Bronchodilators are important in symptomatic management and acute exacerbations: they are the 'relievers'.
- Long-acting bronchodilators and combined steroid-bronchodilator inhalers have simplified the maintenance treatment of asthma, but these should be introduced after effective treatment has been titrated up with short-acting agents.

Many patients underestimate the severity of their disease and this may delay seeking medical attention. High-risk patients must understand the importance of monitoring their own peak expiratory flow rates regularly. Therapy must be altered according to an individually tailored acute asthma management plan, as already explained. The patient must be reviewed regularly to ensure good control is maintained.

ISSUES TO CONSIDER

- What are the consequences of long-term untreated asthma?

- How does asthma present in older patients? What are the differences in adult-onset asthma?

- What are the possible explanations for the increasing incidence of childhood asthma in developing countries?

FURTHER INFORMATION

www.aaaai.org Website of the American Academy of Allergy, Asthma and Immunology with links, case scenarios and patient information.

www.asthmalearninglab.com Superb website directed at sufferers but with a wealth of information including inhaler technique.

Haematemesis in a 40-year-old man

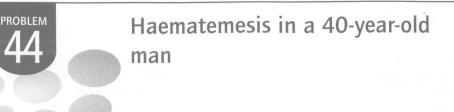

A 40-year-old journalist is brought to the emergency department by ambulance. His work colleagues say he vomited a very large amount of blood at work. He is confused and unable to give a history, and looks very ill. On examination he is listless, pale and obviously jaundiced. He is cool and clammy and you note that he has a flapping tremor when his hands are outstretched. His pulse is 120 bpm and weak. His blood pressure is 80/50 mm Hg, lying. He is thin, has palmar erythema and a number of bruises. He has spider naevi on his upper chest. Cardiopulmonary examination is otherwise unremarkable. His abdomen is distended with shifting dullness but no palpable organomegaly. The patient has shrunken testicles and rectal examination reveals no melaena. His Glasgow Coma Score (GCS) is 13/15. There are no focal neurological signs. He is afebrile.

 Q1 What should you do immediately?

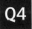 **Q2** What do you think is the likely diagnosis? What leads you to this conclusion?

One hour later, he has improved following 2 litres isotonic saline. His blood pressure is now 120/60 mm Hg with a pulse of 95 bpm. His colour has improved, but he still has orthostatic hypotension. Also, he has not improved neurologically. His work colleagues say that he was mentally sharp until this morning when the vomiting began. They have noticed that he has been jaundiced for several weeks.

Q3 What do you think is the reason for his sudden neurological deterioration this morning?

Some investigations are performed (see Investigation 44.1).

 Q4 Interpret these blood results.

Q5 What do you do now?

Investigation 44.1 Summary of results			
Haemoglobin	95 g/l	White cell count	7.8 x 10⁹/l
MCV	105 fl	INR	2.1
MCH	29.5 pg		
MCHC	340 g/l		
Platelets	60 x 10⁹/l		
Sodium	128 mmol/l	Calcium	2.26 mmol/l
Potassium	3.8 mmol/l	Phosphate	0.91 mmol/l
Chloride	106 mmol/l	Total protein	48 g/l
Bicarbonate	27 mmol/l	Albumin	21 g/l
Urea	12.3 mmol/l	Globulins	27 g/l
Creatinine	0.11 mmol/l	Bilirubin	35 µmol/l
Uric acid	0.24 mmol/l	ALT	75 U/l
Glucose	4.8 mmol/l	AST	185 U/l
Cholesterol	4.2 mmol/l	GGT	165 U/l
LDH	212 U/l	ALP	141 U/l

You continue with the resuscitation, arrange for an intensive care bed and contact the on-call gastroenterological team. You arrange an endoscopy. There is copious fresh and altered blood in the stomach but no active bleeding. However, this is what the endoscopist sees at the lower end of the oesophagus (Figure 44.1).

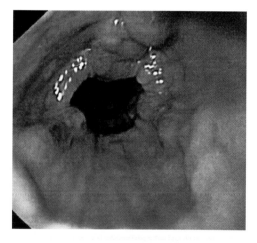

Fig 44.1

 Q6 What does this endoscopic picture show? What can the endoscopist do now?

The patient starts bleeding during the procedure. Despite all efforts, the endoscopist is unable to stop the bleeding.

Q7 What options are now available to control the haemorrhage and to reduce his portal hypertension?

Following a long stay on the intensive care unit, the haemorrhage is controlled and the patient's neurological status returns to normal. He gives a history of 20 years of heavy alcohol use, most recently up to a bottle and a half of wine a day.

Q8 What measures can be taken to reduce the risk of further bleeding in the future? What further investigations would you like to arrange before discharge?

ANSWERS

A1 This man is bleeding profusely from his upper gastrointestinal tract. His hypotension, tachycardia and clinical anaemia all suggest a significant blood loss. In addition, he has obvious clinical signs of chronic liver disease which suggest this may be a variceal haemorrhage. The initial management of acute gastrointestinal bleeding is the same regardless of whether the bleeding is variceal or non-variceal:

1 Airway   Especially important in confused/ encephalopathic patients who are vomiting. Secure the airway, intubate if necessary.
2 Breathing Apply high-flow oxygen.
3 Circulation Two large-bore peripheral cannulae.

- Send blood for full blood count, coagulation studies including fibrinogen, and biochemistry
- Cross-match 6 units packed cells urgently
- Restore circulating volume with colloid initially and then blood. May require group specific or O-negative blood initially
- Prevent hypothermia
- Involve intensive/critical care teams early
- Central venous monitoring useful for fluid balance, but insertion should not delay resuscitation as above.

Move the patient into a high dependency area, remove his clothes and set up suction. Do not leave the patient alone.

A2 You have noticed jaundice with probable ascites plus spider naevi, bruising, palmar erythema and hypogonadism. The most likely diagnosis is variceal haemorrhage in the context of decompensated chronic liver disease. Patients with chronic liver disease often have bleeding from non-variceal causes. Until an endoscopic diagnosis is made, nothing should be assumed.

A3 This is likely to be encephalopathy. The bleeding into his gut is a huge protein load, which is broken down by intestinal bacteria, pro-

ducing a large quantity of ammonia and other toxic materials. The damaged liver is unable to metabolize these materials and encephalopathy ensues. Shock and hypoxia are also likely to be contributory to his confusion. His neurological status has not improved following resuscitation, and this suggests acute encephalopathy is the major cause of confusion in this man.

A4 He is already anaemic prior to resuscitation. Most importantly, his haemoglobin will drop further once he has been resuscitated with fluids, due to haemodilution. He has therefore suffered massive blood loss.

His low platelet count is likely to be secondary to his chronic liver disease. Increased splenic blood flow and subsequent hypersplenism in patients with portal hypertension leads to increased platelet consumption. Alcohol can also have a direct toxic effect on the bone marrow. Massive blood loss and subsequent consumption of platelets and clotting factors can also lead to thrombocytopenia and coagulopathy.

His raised INR is likely to be the result of liver synthetic dysfunction. The liver is unable to make sufficient clotting factors. Other markers of synthetic dysfunction are his low albumin (inadequate synthesis) and high bilirubin (inadequate processing).

His macrocytosis points towards alcohol as a possible aetiological factor.

His hyponatraemia is consistent with chronic liver disease and associated water and salt retention. This is in effect dilutional hyponatraemia, i.e. his total body sodium is normal or raised. The uraemia is due to the high blood load in his upper gastrointestinal tract.

The derangement of liver function tests is consistent with, but not diagnostic of, alcohol-related chronic liver disease. He has modestly elevated transaminases with the AST > ALT, which favours alcohol as a cause. This is because alcohol causes mitochondrial damage and AST is a mitochondrial enzyme. The raised GGT implies a

A N S W E R S – cont'd

degree of cholestasis and is often raised in alcohol-related liver disease.

A5 He needs an urgent blood transfusion. Four units of packed cells should be given initially. The blood bank should be warned to stay at least 4 units ahead. In addition, his coagulopathy should be treated with 6 units of fresh frozen plasma. His fibrinogen should be measured and if low can be replaced with cryoprecipitate (start with 6 units). Platelets should be considered. Stores of vitamin K are often depleted in malnourished alcoholics and this patient should be give 10 mg of vitamin K by slow intravenous infusion.

This man needs an urgent upper gastrointestinal endoscopy. Because he is encephalopathic this should be performed with an endotracheal tube in situ. This is because the risk of aspiration in this group of patients is very high and endoscopic procedures may be long and difficult. He will need an intensive care bed following the procedure.

He needs high-dose parenteral vitamins, especially thiamine. Patients with presumed alcohol-related liver disease are likely to be thiamine deficient and are at risk of Wernicke's encephalopathy.

Following endoscopy, his encephalopathy can be treated with laxatives. High-dose lactulose, a synthetic osmotic laxative, is the drug of choice in these situations as it produces low intestinal pH, inhibiting bacterial production of ammonia. There is no benefit in the use of antibiotics such as neomycin.

A6 There are three large variceal cords running up the oesophagus from the oesophagogastric junction at 12, 5 and 7 o'clock. The endoscopist should look for stigmata of recent haemorrhage which, in the case of suspected variceal bleeding, would be platelet clots or 'cherry red spots'.

The endoscopist has several options. Ideally, if experienced, the endoscopist should attempt to ligate the variceal cords using band ligation. This technique involves placing a tight elastic band over the varix via the endoscope, thereby cutting off the blood supply to the vessel and collapsing the varix. Other options include injection of a

sclerosiant, but this method is inferior to banding and can produce severe ulceration. Some specialized units use tissue glue (histoacryl) although the efficacy and safety of this technique is not fully established.

A7 Further endoscopic therapy is unlikely to be of use. The immediate priority is to control the bleeding. The endoscopist should insert a balloon tamponade tube (Sengstaken–Blakemore, Minnesota or Linton) to occlude blood flow in the varices. A Minnesota tube is shown in Figure 44.2. It consists of a rubber or plastic tube that is inserted into the stomach, preferably under endoscopic guidance. The large gastric balloon is then inflated with a combination of water and radiographic contrast (approximately 150–300 ml). Gentle traction is then applied to pull the balloon up into the gastric cardia, pulling the oesophagogastric junction up and stopping inflow of blood into the varices. Traction is normally maintained for 12–24 hours and if bleeding has stopped when traction is released, then the balloon can be deflated and the tube removed. Some tubes also have an oesophageal balloon. This is very rarely used owing to the risk of oesophageal necrosis and perforation. Variceal tamponade tubes are specialized pieces of equipment and should only be used by personnel experienced in the procedure. They should never be inserted in cases of gastrointestinal bleeding before an endoscopic diagnosis of varices has been made.

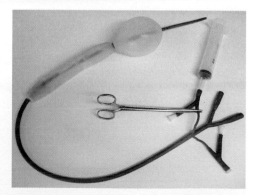

Fig 44.2

ANSWERS – cont'd

Patients with these tubes in situ are best managed in an intensive care unit.

There are several non-endoscopic therapies available to help control variceal haemorrhage.

1 Terlipressin is a vasopressin analogue. It causes vasoconstriction within the splanchnic bed, reducing portasystemic blood flow. It has been shown to be highly effective in the control of acute variceal bleeding. Unlike vasopressin, terlipressin is relatively selective for the splanchnic bed, reducing the problems of coronary vasoconstriction associated with the former drug. It is not, however, without vascular side-effects.

2 Intravenous nitrates can be useful adjuncts in reducing portal pressure although as with non-selective betablockers, their use in this setting is often contraindicated due to acute hypotension from blood loss.

3 Transjugular intrahepatic portasystemic shunt (TIPSS). This radiological procedure involves the insertion of a metal stent from a hepatic vein to the portal vein across the liver parenchyma. By allowing portal blood flow to 'bypass' the liver, there is a significant risk of worsening hepatic encephalopathy, relevant with this patient.

4 Surgical procedures are rarely indicated. Oesophageal transection has now been virtually abandoned. Surgery is usually aimed at portasystemic decompression and this may be achieved by either a portacaval H-graft or a splenorenal shunt.

A8 As alcohol is the suspected cause of this man's liver disease, he should be strongly advised to abstain indefinitely and given the support to enable him to achieve this. Abstention alone can produce enough improvement in portal pressure to prevent further bleeding in some cases.

His portal pressure should be chronically lowered with non-selective betablockers such as propranolol. His response to these drugs should be ideally monitored with portasystemic gradient measurement on treatment. However, this is rarely practical or available in most cases and a reduction in his resting pulse of 25% is usually a reasonable guide to successful treatment. Oral nitrate preparations can be added if tolerated or if he is unable to tolerate betablocker therapy.

Most endoscopists would advocate regular endoscopy and band ligation following a variceal bleed, with the aim of 'eradicating' the variceal cords. This remains controversial and there is little evidence for its superiority over medical therapy alone. Endoscopic therapy is relatively ineffective in cases of gastric or duodenal varices, which can occur alone or in conjunction with oesophageal varices.

The role of TIPSS in the long-term management of varices is controversial. There is evidence that this procedure reduces rebleeding rates when compared to medical therapy but it does not appear to confer a survival benefit and the complication rate is significantly higher.

Despite his alcohol history, chronic liver disease should never be assumed to be alcohol-related until other causes have been excluded. He should, therefore, be screened for viral hepatitis (HCV, HBV), metabolic disorders such as haemochromatosis and autoimmune disease. He should have an ultrasound and Doppler examination of the hepatic vasculature. His alpha-fetoprotein should be checked to screen for hepatoma. Liver biopsy may be helpful but some clinicians would only perform this test if he stopped drinking alcohol or if a diagnostic dilemma remained.

REVISION POINTS

Portal hypertension

Definition

Reduced blood flow through the portal venous circulation with diversion of flow (up to 90%) into the systemic circulation through collaterals. High blood flow through these portasystemic collaterals results in varices.

Causes

Prehepatic

- obstruction of portal vein by thrombus, external compression or developmental anomaly
- thrombosis of splenic vein.

Intrahepatic

1 Presinusoidal
- idiopathic
- congenital hepatic fibrosis
- primary biliary cirrhosis
- sarcoidosis
- schistosomiasis
- drugs and toxins, e.g. methotrexate, azathioprine
2 Sinusoidal
- cirrhosis of any cause

- nodular regenerative hyperplasia
- alcoholic hepatitis (common)
3 Post-sinusoidal
- veno-occlusive disease.

Posthepatic

- Budd–Chiari
- IVC obstruction
- constrictive pericarditis.

Consequences of portal hypertension

- varices and gastrointestinal haemorrhage
- ascites (causes actually multifactorial).

Investigations

- screen for underlying liver disease
- ultrasound and Doppler studies of vasculature +/– CT/MRI
- endoscopy
- hepatic venography.

Treatment

- depends on underlying cause
- lower portal pressure as discussed
- TIPSS, surgical shunting
- liver transplantation.

ISSUES TO CONSIDER

- How would the initial management differ if the haemorrhage was non-variceal?

- How does portal hypertension produce ascites?

- Do you think this man should be considered for a liver transplant? What are the criteria for transplantation in alcohol-related liver disease?

FURTHER INFORMATION

Garcia N, Sanyal A. **Portal hypertension**. *Clinics in Liver Disease* 2001;5(2):509–40.

Lake J R, Howdle P D. **Gastrointestinal hemorrhage and portal hypertension**. In O'Grady J, Lake J, Howdle P (eds) *Comprehensive Clinical Hepatology*. London: Mosby, 2000.

www.emedicine.com/med/topic745.htm
A detailed account of the pathophysiology and management of bleeding oesophageal varices.

A young woman with jaundice

A 19-year-old woman presents with a 2-week history of feeling generally unwell. Her symptoms began with a sore throat and fever. She then developed nausea and infrequent diarrhoea. She has vomited bile-stained fluid on several occasions in the last week and has been eating little. Yesterday a friend noticed that her eyes had turned yellow. On direct questioning she admits that her urine has turned dark brown but she has not noticed what colour her bowel motions are.

On examination she is thin, looks generally unwell and is jaundiced. She is afebrile. She has several tattoos. She also has puncture marks in her antecubital fossae and tracks along the lines of her veins in her forearms. She has no lymphadenopathy. Cardiovascular and respiratory examinations are normal. Her abdomen is soft and there is no ascites. Her liver is palpable 4 cm below the costal margin and is smooth and tender. The spleen is not palpable. There are no stigmata of chronic liver disease. She is not encephalopathic. Her urine is positive for ketones and bilirubin and she has no proteinuria or haematuria.

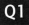 **Q1** What extra information would you like to obtain from the history? What is the most likely diagnosis?

You arrange some blood tests, the results of which are shown below.

Investigation 45.1 Summary of results			
Haemoglobin	125 g/l	White cell count	6.2 x 10⁹/l
Platelets	475 x 10⁹/l	Lymphocytes 50%	3.1 x 10⁹/l
Blood film: occasional atypical lymphocyte			
INR	1.2		
Sodium	145 mmol/l	Calcium	2.16 mmol/l
Potassium	4.4 mmol/l	Phosphate	1.15 mmol/l
Chloride	106 mmol/l	Total protein	67 g/l
Bicarbonate	27 mmol/l	Albumin	40 g/l
Urea	5.9 mmol/l	Globulins	27 g/l
Creatinine	0.12 mmol/l	Bilirubin	171 μmol/l
Uric acid	0.24 mmol/l	ALT	1563 U/l
Glucose	4.4 mmol/l	AST	1284 U/l
Cholesterol	3.5 mmol/l	GGT	75 U/l

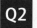

Q2 How do these results help you? What further investigations would you now like to arrange?

The following investigations are now available.

Investigation 45.2 Summary of results	
Anti-hepatitis A IgM:	negative
Hepatitis B surface antigen:	positive
Anti-hepatitis B core IgM:	positive
Anti-hepatitis C IgG:	negative

She is admitted to the ward. When questioned, she admits that she has used intravenous drugs intermittently for 2 years. She said that she has only ever shared needles with her current boyfriend of 4 months.

Q3 What is the diagnosis? Would any other serology be useful?

Q4 How would you further manage this woman?

The patient's HIV serology is negative. A few days after admission the patient's boyfriend visits her in hospital and is accompanied by a 4-year-old boy. It is revealed that the boy is the patient's son by another man. They agree for blood to be taken from the man and the child. The following results are obtained.

Investigation 45.3 Boyfriend's test results			
Albumin	34 g/l	Bilirubin	20 μmol/l
ALP	150 U/l	GGT	85 U/l
ALT	102 U/l	AST	99 U/l

Hepatitis B surface antigen:	positive
Anti-hepatitis B surface IgG:	negative
Hepatitis B 'e' antigen:	positive
Anti-hepatitis B 'e' antibody:	negative
Anti-hepatitis B core IgG	positive
Delta antibody:	positive
Anti-hepatitis C IgG:	negative

Investigation 45.4 Son's test results	
Liver function tests:	normal
Hepatitis B surface antigen:	negative
Anti-hepatitis B surface IgG:	negative
Anti-hepatitis B core IgG:	negative
Anti-hepatitis C IgG:	negative

Q5 How would you interpret these results? What further follow-up should be arranged for these three patients?

ANSWERS

A1 In the assessment of any patient with liver disease the history is extremely important. Small points that could easily be missed may be essential in making the final diagnosis.

This woman has all the hallmarks of a viral hepatitis.

You have noticed a major risk factor on your examination; probable needle tracks from intravenous drug use. Tattoos are less of a risk factor

these days but still can be a risk if they have been done by an amateur.

It is important, therefore, to ask her sensitively about recreational drug use. How much? Which drugs? For how long? With whom has she shared needles?

Other important points in the assessment of an acutely jaundiced patient are summarized in Table 45.1.

Table 45.1 Risk factors for hepatitis in the acutely jaundiced patient

Diagnosis	Important points in history
Hepatitis A	Contacts, foreign travel, recent diarrhoeal illness, dietary risk factors, e.g. shellfish ingestion, recreational risk factors, e.g. swimming and surfing, especially on urban beaches
Hepatitis B	Close contacts, sexual history, blood transfusion, intravenous drug use, foreign travel, tattoos and body piercing
Hepatitis E	As for hepatitis A. Travel to endemic areas important. Rare in US, Australia, New Zealand and Europe
Other viruses e.g. EBV	Contacts, sore throat, age
Drug-induced hepatitis	Recent prescription and non-prescription medications, especially antibiotics. Complementary therapies, Chinese medicines, Ecstasy use
Alcohol-related hepatitis	Alcohol history
Autoimmune hepatitis	Age, female sex, history of other autoimmune disease e.g. thyroid

A2 These blood tests suggest a hepatitic cause for her jaundice with a predominant elevation of her transaminases (ALT and AST). The normal albumin and INR imply that the synthetic function of the liver is relatively well preserved. She has a thrombocytosis which is likely to represent an acute phase reaction. Her lymphocytosis and the presence of atypical lymphocytes raise the possibility of a viral infection.

With this patient's history, a diagnosis of viral hepatitis is likely. Serology should be taken for hepatitis A and hepatitis B. Hepatitis C is extremely unlikely to present acutely in this way as it rarely

causes a severe acute hepatitis. However, in view of her history and risk factors evidence of hepatitis C infection should be looked for. Serology for hepatitis E could be sent if the patient is thought to be at risk. This RNA virus, transmitted by the faecal–oral route, is endemic in India, the Middle East, South East Asia and parts of Latin America and Africa.

Of course, this may not be acute viral hepatitis. The possibility of autoimmune liver disease means that an autoantibody screen and immunoglobulins should also be checked (a raised IgG fraction is in favour of autoimmune

ANSWERS – cont'd

disease). An ultrasound of the liver will also be useful to exclude biliary obstruction as a cause and to look for evidence of chronic liver disease.

A3 The diagnosis is acute hepatitis B infection. This is shown by her presentation with the presence of both Hepatitis B surface antigen and core antibody.

She is at increased risk of other parenterally transmitted viruses. Hepatitis D (delta agent) serology should be checked. This 'defective' RNA virus requires co-infection with hepatitis B to replicate successfully. Superinfection with the delta agent in a patient with pre-existing chronic hepatitis B may cause an acute hepatitis with the above features. She should also be tested for hepatitis C virus infection. Although this will be unlikely to cause an acute hepatitis, the incidence of this infection is very high in intravenous drug users (greater than 90% in some series) and superinfection may reactivate chronic hepatitis B. She is also at risk of HIV infection and consent should be sought to test for HIV 1 and 2.

A4 Management is generally supportive with good hydration and nutrition especially important. The majority of patients will clear the virus completely and develop lifelong immunity (>95% in adults). Most will improve enough to be discharged home relatively early on. A very small proportion of patients (0.1–0.5%) may develop acute liver failure. For this reason close monitoring is important with regular blood testing.

Worrying features would include the development of hepatic encephalopathy, worsening coagulopathy and hypoglycaemia. If any of these occurred then she would need to be transferred to a specialist liver unit.

Contact tracing is extremely important and is discussed in the next answer. Support for her drug addiction should be offered.

A5 Her boyfriend is positive for hepatitis B surface antigen and is therefore a hepatitis B carrier. The presence of the e-antigen and absence of anti-e antibodies indicates persistent viral replication and a high level of infectivity. In addition he is co-infected with the delta agent. These findings, in conjunction with his abnormal liver function tests, suggest chronic hepatitis B although further tests such as Hepatitis B DNA and liver biopsy will be required to quantify this.

The immediate priority is to prevent him infecting others. Involvement of local public health services will be required to identify contacts at risk and to offer them immunization. Hepatitis B can be transmitted to intimate non-sexual contacts such as close family. The woman's son, who is currently negative for hepatitis B, should therefore be immunized as should other close contacts. The woman will need follow-up in approximately 6 months to check that she has cleared the virus. A negative hepatitis B surface antigen at this stage will confirm that this is the case. She will also need repeat testing for the delta agent.

REVISION POINTS

Hepatitis B virus

Epidemiology
- In excess of 300 million HBV carriers worldwide.
- Prevalence of chronic HBV between 0.1–2% in the developing world to 20% in sub-Saharan Africa.

Clinical features
The incubation period is from 1–6 months from exposure.

Acute hepatitis with jaundice presents similarly to the above case. Prodromal symptoms are common. However, 70% of patients will develop subclinical disease without jaundice.

Serology
- HBsAg: The hallmark of hepatitis B infection. Appears in the serum soon after exposure and up to 6 weeks prior to the onset of symptoms. In acute hepatitis B, it may take up to 6 months to disappear from the serum in patients who

continues overleaf

REVISION POINTS – cont'd

clear the virus. Persistence of HBsAg implies chronic infection.

- HBsAb: Surface antibody confers immunity and appears soon after the disappearance of surface antigen.
- HBcAb(IgM): Core antibody, the first antibody to appear, is a marker of acute or recent HBV infection. May also be seen in exacerbations of chronic HBV.
- HBeAg: A marker of viral replication and therefore infectivity.
- HbeAb: This antibody may take years to appear in chronically infected patients. Implies

remission but not clearance of the virus. Usually coincides with the disappearance of detectable HBV DNA from the serum.

Treatment and course

A proportion of patients with chronic infection will develop cirrhosis. There is an increased risk of hepatocellular carcinoma.

Treatment is evolving but may include antiviral drugs, e.g. lamivudine. In some cases liver transplantation may be required.

Prevention

Vaccination of all those at risk, e.g. health workers.

ISSUES TO CONSIDER

- The A to G of viral hepatitis.
- What's the risk of hepatitis B transmission in healthcare workers? How is this reduced?
- What other health problems do you foresee for intravenous drug users?

FURTHER INFORMATION

www.cdc.gov/ncidod/diseases/hepatitis/ index.htm An excellent resource from the CDC in the USA with links to clinical guidelines, related sites and patient support groups.

www.british-liver-trust.org.uk Website of the British Liver Trust. Primarily directed at patients but with lots of information and links to related sites including to its American counterpart.

www.liverfoundation.org

A 34-year-old man with abdominal discomfort

A 34-year-old married dockworker comes to see you with a 2-month history of vague intermittent abdominal discomfort and malaise. The abdominal discomfort is focused in the right upper quadrant, does not radiate and does not seem to have any specific exacerbating or relieving factors. He has not lost any weight and apart from feeling 'under the weather' complains of no other symptoms.

He has never been unwell and takes no medications. He smokes 20 cigarettes a day and states he drinks 'a couple of beers a day'.

His general practitioner has organized an abdominal ultrasound which has shown a hyperechoic mass in the right lobe of the liver. The rest of the liver appears nodular and consistent with cirrhosis.

Q1 What further information would you like from the history? What will you look for on examination?

Q2 What are the possible causes of the mass seen on ultrasound?

You ask him about risk factors for chronic liver disease, and in particular his alcohol consumption. While he used to have the occasional binge drink as a teenager, he states his alcohol has otherwise always been about 20 gm per day.

On examination he appears fit and well. He has several tattoos on his torso, including one on his chest, reading 'Liverpool'. You ask him about this and he laughs and says he woke up one morning after partying with his friends and found this on his chest. This was many years ago. You are able to palpate a 2 cm non-tender smooth liver edge below the right costal margin. The rest of the examination is unremarkable.

Q3 What investigations are necessary?

The results shown in Investigation 46.1 are made available.

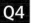
Q4 What do these blood results tell you? What is the most likely diagnosis?

A further radiological investigation is performed. A representative image is shown in Figure 46.1.

Investigation 46.1 Summary of results			
Haemoglobin	109 g/l	White cell count	8.9 x 10⁹/l
MCV	88.6 fl		
MCH	29.5 pg		
MCHC	340 g/l		
Platelets	121 x 10⁹/l		
Sodium	142 mmol/l	Calcium	2.16 mmol/l
Potassium	4.3 mmol/l	Phosphate	1.15 mmol/l
Chloride	106 mmol/l	Total protein	65 g/l
Bicarbonate	27 mmol/l	Albumin	31 g/l
Urea	3.6 mmol/l	Globulins	27 g/l
Creatinine	0.07 mmol/l	Bilirubin	38 µmol/l
Uric acid	0.24 mmol/l	ALT	232 U/l
Glucose	4.4 mmol/l	AST	108 U/l
Cholesterol	3.5 mmol/l	GGT	118 U/l
LDH	212 U/l	ALP	141 U/l
AFP	7891 ng/ml	HBsAg −ve	
Ferritin	341	HCV IgG +ve	
		HCV PCR +ve	

The chest X-ray is normal.

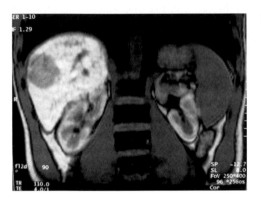

Fig 46.1

Q5 What is this investigation and what does it show? Would a biopsy be helpful?

The diagnosis appears clear and the hepatobiliary surgeons are consulted. They opt to confirm the diagnosis and the operability of the lesion with further imaging.

A view from the investigation is shown (Figure 46.2).

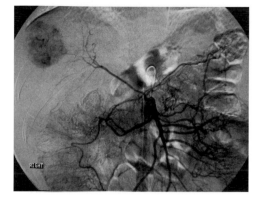

Fig 46.2

Q6 What is this investigation and what does it show?

There were no other abnormalities seen in the abdomen or chest on further CT scanning.

Q7 What would be the next step in this patient's treatment?

A biopsy of the 'normal' left lobe of the liver revealed cirrhosis with chronic hepatitis of moderate activity.

The patient proceeds to surgery. At operation the liver appears cirrhotic with a macronodular appearance. There is mild splenomegaly but no overt varices and the portal vein is patent. There is a large circumscribed tumour in the right lobe of the liver. There is no macroscopic evidence of extrahepatic disease. A subsegmental excision is performed in view of the patient's cirrhosis. Histological examination reveals a hepatocellular carcinoma. The excision margins appear clear.

One year following surgery, the patient is well and there are no signs of recurrence.

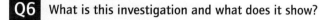

ANSWERS

A1 Ask if he has any risk factors for chronic liver disease. Enquire about previous alcohol intake, risk factors for viral hepatitis, previous episodes of jaundice and family history.

The presence of a mass within the liver is extremely worrying and, although many such lesions are benign, your main concern must be that this represents a malignant process.

You should look especially for:
- Features suggestive of malignancy, e.g. wasting, lymphadenopathy.
- Stigmata of chronic liver disease indicating underlying cirrhosis leading to hepatoma.

- Hepatosplenomegaly.
- Ascites: may suggest chronic liver disease or malignancy.

A2 The differential diagnosis of liver masses is broad:
- Congenital: simple cyst
- Infective: hydatid disease, hepatic abscess
- Vascular: haemangioma
- Regenerative: focal nodular hyperplasia
- Neoplastic: adenoma
            hepatoma
            metastases.

ANSWERS – cont'd

- Congenital cysts: common, usually small and asymptomatic, usually have characteristic ultrasound appearances. This man's liver lesion is highly unlikely to be a cyst.
- Hydatid disease is common in certain sheep-rearing parts of the world. This man could have a hydatid cyst in the liver. The lack of fever and length of history makes an intra-hepatic abscess unlikely.
- Haemangiomas are the most common benign liver tumour with an incidence of up to 20% in some reports. These lesions most often occur in women and present in the 3rd, 4th and 5th decades. Most are small, asymptomatic and occur as incidental findings. Larger lesions may present with abdominal symptoms.
- Focal nodular hyperplasia (FNH) also occurs more frequently in women. The majority are discovered incidentally, although they may very rarely rupture with haemoperitoneum.
- Hepatic adenomas occur almost exclusively in women. The most common cause is the oral contraceptive pill. Patients may present with abdominal pain secondary to haemorrhage within the tumour.
- Primary hepatic tumours occur much less frequently than metastases to the liver. *Hepatocellular carcinoma* (HCC) is associated with cirrhosis in 70–90% of cases. Cirrhosis of all causes can lead to HCC. If the factor causing the cirrhosis is removed, for example alcohol or iron, the high risk of HCC does not decrease.

Up to one-third of all cases of HCC arise within normal livers. This type has distinctive clinical features when compared to HCC arising in cirrhotic livers. The incidence in females is higher, the age of presentation is lower, the tumour is less often AFP-positive, and survival is slightly better.

Although this man has no history of chronic liver disease it will be important to find out if he has any risk factors as HCC can present in patients in whom the cirrhosis has been clinically 'silent'.

Secondary malignant deposits are also a possibility despite his age. Metastases may be the first presentation of colorectal malignancies although the young age would make this unusual. Other sources of metastatic disease include neuro-endocrine tumours (e.g. carcinoid), sarcoma, melanoma and lymphoma.

A3 1 Laboratory investigations
- Complete blood picture looking for anaemia (recent bleeding, chronic disease), leucocytosis (evidence of infection or primary haematological disease) and thrombocytopenia (e.g. chronic liver disease, platelet consumption by haemangioma).
- Check renal and liver function, i.e. bilirubin, enzymes, albumin, INR (evidence of chronic liver disease). If evidence of underlying chronic liver disease should check for viral hepatitis, ferritin, immunoglobulins and autoantibody profile.
- Alpha-fetoprotein (AFP). Serum AFP is raised at presentation in up to 70% of patients with HCC. AFP levels may also be elevated in non-malignant conditions such as acute liver failure and chronic hepatitis.

2 Radiological investigations
- CT or MR scans (with and without contrast) can provide information on liver lesions with regard to the consistency and vascularity of the lesion itself, the presence of other liver lesions, the state of the liver parenchyma and adjacent structures in the abdominal cavity (e.g. portal hypertension or evidence of malignancy elsewhere).
- Arteriography may provide additional information on the vascularity of a tumour as well as providing a route for the administration of chemoembolization agents.
- A chest X-ray may detect the presence of metastatic lung disease.

3 Histology
Histology will confirm the diagnosis of a malignant process and, in the cirrhotic liver, a biopsy away from the focal lesion may help differentiate the underlying cause of the chronic liver disease.

A4 The normocytic anaemia is consistent with a chronic disease picture. The mild thrombocytopenia is consistent with hypersplenism associated with chronic liver disease.

There is an abnormality of liver function consistent with a hepatitic process. The depressed

ANSWERS – cont'd

albumin level could be attributed to poor hepatic synthetic function. To further investigate this it would be useful to have a prothrombin time.

He has antibodies to hepatitis C virus (HCV) and an ongoing viraemia has been confirmed by PCR.

The grossly elevated AFP in the context of a liver mass and positive HCV serology is almost diagnostic of an HCC. The diagnosis is therefore likely to be HCC on a background of previously undiagnosed hepatitis C virus.

A5 This is a T2 weighted MRI scan of the upper abdomen. There is a 6 cm lesion in the right lobe of the liver.

The biopsy of liver lesions is controversial. There is a risk of seeding of tumour along the biopsy tract so, in cases of potentially operable liver malignancies, some surgeons would rely on imaging and a frozen section biopsy taken at the time of laparotomy.

If the lesion is thought to be a haemangioma, it must not be biopsied, as the risk of massive haemorrhage is considerable. Haemangiomas can usually be diagnosed with a high degree of confidence radiologically. They have a characteristic pattern on contrast-enhanced CT.

A6 This investigation is a hepatic arteriogram. The hepatic artery has been cannulated. There is a tumour 'blush' in the top right of the picture confirming that this is a vascular lesion consistent with an HCC.

A7 This man has a single focus of HCC in a cirrhotic liver. His only chance of cure lies with hepatic resection or liver transplantation.

Increasingly, with improving surgical technique and aftercare, liver transplantation is being offered for larger lesions. For those undergoing resection the surgery will depend upon the size and position of the tumour as well as the severity of underlying cirrhosis and subsequent risk of decompensation, should the resected area be too large.

Postoperatively, the patient will need continued surveillance for further HCC as well as treatment for his underlying HCV infection.

REVISION POINTS

Hepatocellular carcinoma

Epidemiology

Sixth most common cancer worldwide but widely varying incidence. Relatively uncommon in developed Western nations (1–2% of all malignancies) where the majority of cases are secondary to alcoholic or HCV-related cirrhosis. However, any form of chronic liver disease (CLD) will predispose to HCC.

Where HBV is endemic, e.g. Africa, Taiwan, Japan, the incidence is much higher. May occur in HBV without cirrhosis due to incorporation of the HBV genome into host DNA.

Other risk factors include the fungus-derived aflatoxins and anabolic steroid use.

Presentation

- Classical triad of right upper quadrant pain, hepatomegaly and weight loss.

- May also present as decompensation or variceal haemorrhage in previously stable CLD.
- Increasingly picked up on screening of CLD patients.

Diagnosis

Ultrasound is the first investigation of choice. CT, MRI and angiography are complementary and will provide extra information about the tumour to allow planning of treatment.

An AFP level above 500 ng/ml in cirrhotic patients, together with a liver mass on imaging, is diagnostic of HCC. Up to 10% of patients who have hepatic metastases have elevated levels. Other tumours (e.g. non-seminomatous germ cell tumours) can express high levels of AFP.

Biopsy is controversial. Therefore, all cases should be referred to a specialist centre if there is a possibility of surgical resection.

continues overleaf

REVISION POINTS — cont'd

Treatment

The only hope of cure is surgical resection or liver transplantation. Contraindications to surgery include extent of tumour, implications of associated liver cirrhosis, extrahepatic metastases and unrelated co-morbidity. Liver transplantation is feasible in patients who have small tumours, irrespective of Child's classification. Approximately 10–15% of patients with HCC will be amenable to resection with a 5-year survival rate of 33–50%.

Chemoembolization under fluoroscopic control is largely of use in the palliation of symptoms of pain. Research therapies include novel chemotherapeutic agents and immunotherapy.

Prognosis

Survival is measured in weeks in high incidence areas from time of diagnosis in the absence of surgical intervention. In low incidence areas this figure is 6–12 months. Large tumours with poor LFTs, vascular invasion and evidence of metastases do very poorly. Small tumours (<3 cm diameter), with good LFTs may survive up to 3 years without treatment

ISSUES TO CONSIDER

- What public health intervention has resulted in a dramatic drop in the incidence of HCC in parts of Asia?

- What are the risks of a percutaneous liver biopsy? How would you obtain informed consent for this procedure?

FURTHER INFORMATION

www.emedicine.com/radio/topic332.htm Another excellent article from emedicine focusing on the radiological investigation of liver tumours.

www.hepnet.com/update17.htm A good overview of screening for HCC from hepnet.com.

Postoperative oliguria in an elderly woman

A 70-year-old woman who lives alone is brought into the emergency department by ambulance. She tripped and fell at home, on to a hard linoleum floor. She lay on the ground for 10 hours before her sister discovered her. She now complains of an acutely painful right arm.

She has a longstanding history of hypertension and had been troubled by shortness of breath and ankle swelling until her local doctor placed her on 'fluid tablets'. She is also troubled with chronic back pain, and arthritic hands and knees. She does not have a history of ischaemic heart disease, diabetes mellitus or cerebrovascular disease. Her medications include:
- frusemide (furosemide) 80 mg daily
- irbesartan 150 mg daily
- aspirin 300 mg daily
- celecoxib 20 mg bd.

On examination she has an obvious fracture with deformity of the right upper arm and a fragment of bone protruding through the skin, and she is distressed by pain. The right hand is neurovascularly intact. She is mildly dehydrated but is afebrile, her pulse is 90 bpm and regular and her blood pressure is 120/60 mm Hg. She has a marked kyphosis and changes of osteoarthritis of her hands and knees. There is mild cardiomegaly, a left ventricular heave and 4th heart sound, but no evidence of cardiac failure.

You give her a small dose of intravenous morphine for pain relief before sending her for an X-ray which shows a displaced fracture of the right humerus. The bones are osteoporotic. The orthopaedic resident reviews the patient and decides the injury requires surgical debridement and stabilization of the fracture.

Q1 What would you like to do for this woman before she goes to the operating theatre?

The patient is taken to the operating theatre, the fracture reduced and stabilized, the wound cleaned and the limb set in a U-slab of plaster. In theatre she is given a dose of 240 mg gentamicin and then prescribed a maintenance dose once-daily gentamicin of 340 mg/day (roughly 5 mg/kg). She is also given flucloxacillin 1 g 6-hourly intravenously.

Postoperatively the patient is cared for in an orthopaedic ward. The intern did not place her on maintenance intravenous fluids for fear of exacerbating her known congestive cardiac failure. She was given frequent narcotic analgesia for her pain and as a result is mildly sedated. All of her usual medications were continued except for the aspirin.

Q2 Which of her medications would you have continued and which would you have stopped? Why?

The injured limb is checked daily and there are no orthopaedic complications. On the second

evening after her admission the intern notes that the patient has only passed 480 ml urine in the previous 24 hours. Review of the fluid balance charts shows that the patient has taken in only modest amounts orally and the urine output had been declining since admission. The patient says she feels thirsty. One litre of 5 per cent dextrose is put up, running over 12 hours with the plan to check the electrolytes the next morning. The intravenous antibiotics and her usual medications are continued.

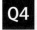

Q3 If you were the doctor on call, would your fluid prescription have been different?

The next morning the patient's urine output for the previous 12 hours is 160 ml. On examination she is afebrile, her pulse rate is 88 bpm and her blood pressure is 120/85 mm Hg. She is mildly dehydrated with dry mucous membranes, but her tissue turgor is normal. Her jugular venous pulse is not visible and there is no evidence of cardiac failure. Her bladder is not palpable. The urinalysis is normal. The intern realizes that on admission blood was taken for electrolytes but the results were not checked. The admission biochemistry results are as follows.

Investigation 47.1 Summary of results			
Sodium	133 mmol/l	Calcium	2.16 mmol/l
Potassium	4.2 mmol/l	Phosphate	1.15 mmol/l
Chloride	97 mmol/l	Total protein	58 g/l
Bicarbonate	24 mmol/l	Albumin	33 g/l
Urea	18.8 mmol/l	Globulins	25 g/l
Creatinine	0.21 mmol/l	Bilirubin	16 µmol/l
Uric acid	0.24 mmol/l	ALT	28 U/l
Glucose	5.5 mmol/l	AST	25 U/l
Cholesterol	3.8 mmol/l	GGT	19 U/l
LDH	245 U/l	ALP	54 U/l

Q4 What are the possible causes of the abnormalities on the admission bloods? What would you like to do?

The patient weighs 60 kg. Her serum creatinine is 0.21 mmol/l and she is 70 years of age.

Q5 What would you have expected this woman's creatinine clearance to be on admission?

Four days after admission her electrolytes are:

Investigation 47.2 Summary of further results			
Sodium	146 mmol/l	Calcium	2.1 mmol/l
Potassium	6.1 mmol/l	Phosphate	1.21 mmol/l
Chloride	99 mmol/l	Total protein	56 g/l
Bicarbonate	17 mmol/l	Albumin	30 g/l
Urea	33.8 mmol/l	Globulins	26 g/l
Creatinine	0.51 mmol/l	Bilirubin	16 μmol/l
Uric acid	0.24 mmol/l	ALT	28 U/l
Glucose	6.7 mmol/l	AST	22 U/l
Cholesterol	3.8 mmol/l	GGT	20 U/l
Creatine kinase	6000 U/l	ALP	59 U/l

Q6 What do these new laboratory results tell you? What are you going to do now? Will any other investigations be helpful?

The woman has no history of renal disease and, apart from twice nightly nocturia, no symptoms attributable to the renal tract.

The patient is catheterized and her medications are stopped. You give her a bolus of 500 ml intravenous isotonic saline over 1 hour. Her mucous membranes return to normal and her jugular venous pressure rises to 2 cm. Her urine output does not increase.

A renal ultrasound shows the kidneys are at the lower limits of normal size with some asymmetry but there is no evidence of obstruction or calculi. A chest X-ray reveals mild cardiomegaly only. A full blood count shows a mild normochromic normocytic anaemia. Coagulation studies are normal. The woman is placed on a regimen of fluid intake being equal to urinary output plus 500 ml/24 h. Despite this, she is now passing less than 10 ml urine per hour.

Q7 Why has the renal function not improved? What would you like to do next?

The woman is given a low protein, low potassium, low sodium diet and oral resonium (a cation-exchange resin). She is placed on prophylactic ranitidine.

Three days later you are called to see her again. She has remained oliguric since you last saw her. She feels generally unwell, anorexic and short of breath. She has developed a tachycardia of 110 bpm and her blood pressure is 150/95 mm Hg. Her jugular venous pressure is elevated 3 cm. She has a third heart sound but has no pericardial rub. She has normal breath sounds but inspiratory crepitations in the lower zones of her chest and dependent oedema with swelling of the ankles. Up-to-date blood results reveal that her creatinine has climbed to 0.85 mmol/l with a potassium of 6.7 mmol/l. A chest X-ray has been performed and is shown in Figure 47.1.

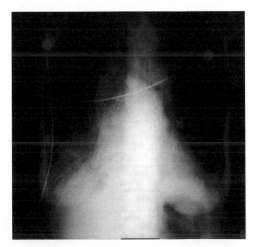

Fig 47.1

Q8 What does the chest X-ray show? What needs to be done immediately? What is the next step in management for this woman?

Following emergency treatment, the patient is transferred to an intensive care unit and continuous veno–venous haemodialysis is started through a double lumen subclavian catheter. Continuous veno–venous haemodialysis is con-tinued for 3 days after which the patient is transferred to the renal unit and intermittent haemodialysis continued on alternate days. Her renal function begins to recover.

Q9 Why may the recovery phase from this illness be dangerous?

Urine output recovers after 3 weeks with a polyuric phase during which time she had a urine output of 3–4 l/day. Her creatinine returned to 0.19 mmol/l.

Q10 What mistakes were made during the management of this case which may have contributed to the patient's illness?

ANSWERS

A1 Elderly people who are unable to get up following a fall can suffer from a high level of morbidity even if the cause of the fall and the injuries sustained are minor. Your job is to make sure she is as fit as possible before she goes to theatre.

Her age, her history of hypertension, probable cardiac failure and the drugs she is taking all predispose her to a degree of renal impairment. In addition, she is likely to have become dehydrated following her fall. Measurement of her electrolytes, urea and creatinine are therefore an essential part of her initial assessment. She is likely to require intravenous fluid replacement and venous access should be established. The exact fluids required will depend partly on your clinical assessment and partly on the results of these blood tests.

An ECG and chest X-ray are essential preoperatively not only because of her past medical history but also to look for possible causes for her fall even though the history sounds like a simple trip.

Her complete blood picture should be checked. She could have lost a significant amount of blood following such an injury.

Her creatinine kinase should be checked. It is likely to be elevated following such an injury. However, after lying on the floor for such a long time, she is at risk of rhabdomyolysis which may further predispose her to the development of renal failure.

You should ensure she has adequate analgesia.

A2 It would have been reasonable to withhold all her medications pending the results of her blood tests and accurate assessment of her fluid status.
- Irbesartan is an angiotensin 2 receptor blocker. It is an excellent antihypertensive but can cause renal impairment in the presence of renovascular disease.
- Celecoxib is a selective COX-2 inhibitor, one of the non-steroidal anti-inflammatory drugs, all of which can worsen renal failure by disabling the prostaglandin-mediated constriction of efferent arterioles in the kidney. Aspirin can also cause renal impairment even at low doses.

A N S W E R S – cont'd

- In the current clinical setting the patient is likely to be volume depleted and her dehydration will be exacerbated by the continued prescription of frusemide (furosemide). This would further impair renal function.
- Gentamicin: she has then been placed on an aminoglycoside antibiotic, well known for their nephrotoxicity, without consideration of renal function. If aminoglycosides are to be used at all, once-daily dosing is recommended for maintenance. The dose must be adjusted for renal function, hydration must be maintained and levels must be monitored. If patients have a history of renal impairment, a non-aminoglycoside antibiotic alternative should be sought.
- This combination of drugs, in the setting of an elderly patient with possible prior renal impairment and volume depletion, is highly likely to be nephrotoxic. The most important issue at this stage is this woman's fluid balance before, during and immediately after operation. Her regular medications can be slowly recommenced over the next few days according to her clinical state, fluid balance and renal function.

A3 Fluid prescription in the postoperative phase must be guided by the patient's clinical status, biochemistry and fluid balance measurements. Inappropriate and non-individualized fluid prescriptions can lead to significant morbidity, especially on surgical wards where dehydration, fluid overload and electrolyte imbalance, especially hyponatraemia, are common problems.

There is a tendency to under-prescribe fluid replacement in these situations, especially in the elderly and in those who have a history of congestive cardiac failure. In these situations, further measures may have to be taken to assess fluid balance such as central venous monitoring.

The key to accurate fluid replacement is close and continuous monitoring with regular reappraisal. In this case, it would be reasonable to prescribe a small volume challenge (250–500 ml) followed by an assessment of response an hour or two later.

A4 She has pre-existing renal impairment. Even relatively healthy elderly patients exhibit a degree of renal impairment if creatinine clearance is measured or calculated. The cause of this patient's chronic renal disease is likely to be multifactorial.

- Ischaemic nephropathy due to atherosclerosis in the small vessels of the kidney.
- Hypertensive nephropathy.
- Drug-induced nephropathy, i.e. NSAIDs, diuretics, irbesartan (may decrease glomerular capillary perfusion pressure in the presence of renovascular disease).

Less likely causes include chronic glomerulonephritis and analgesic nephropathy.

She has, in addition, received a further acute insult to her kidneys from:

- Dehydration after lying on the floor for 10 hours.
- Continuation of nephrotoxic medications.
- Inadequate and inaccurate fluid replacement.
- The prescription of gentamicin.

You should stop all nephrotoxic medications. She needs a fluid challenge: 500 ml isotonic saline over 1–2 hours would be appropriate followed by assessment of response. Her fluid balance should be closely monitored hourly. For this she requires a urinary catheter. If her fluid balance becomes difficult she should have central venous monitoring in a high dependency environment.

A5 Creatinine clearance is a more accurate reflection of renal function, particularly in older smaller patients. The Cockcroft–Gault formula utilizes age, body mass and serum creatinine, and a constant (either 1.23 for males or 1.03 for females):

$$\frac{1.03 \times (140 - \text{age}) \times \text{weight(kg)}}{\text{serum creatinine}}$$

In this patient it gives an estimated creatinine clearance of 21 ml/min. Other equations can be used, which are said to be more accurate than the Cockcroft–Gault equation, such as the Levey equation, which uses age, creatinine, body surface area, albumin and blood urea nitrogen.

A6 The patient has acute renal failure with marked deterioration in her creatinine. Associated with this is hyperkalaemia and metabolic acidosis.

A N S W E R S – cont'd

The elevated creatine kinase raises the possibility of rhabdomyolysis contributing further to her acute on chronic renal failure by causing myoglobin-induced acute tubular necrosis. (It is likely that the creatine kinase level was even higher on admission but the peak was missed as this diagnosis was not considered.)

Management relies on accurate fluid balance as discussed above as well as eliminating precipitating causes such as the nephrotoxic medications. Daily weights may help with fluid balance.

It may well be that her renal function will not recover spontaneously. In this case it is important to involve renal physicians early. A renal ultrasound should be obtained to assess renal size and scarring, and to exclude obstruction. Radiological contrast medium must be avoided as such agents will exacerbate acute renal failure.

Blood should be taken for full biochemical screen, including calcium and phosphate and a complete blood picture.

In this situation urine is often sent for analysis of electrolytes and osmolarity. However, these results would not be meaningful here as the patient has been on a loop-acting diuretic and has probable pre-existent renal impairment. The urine should be examined fresh for the presence of casts and white cells, the latter indicating a possible urinary tract infection.

A7 This woman has developed acute tubular necrosis due to the causes given above. This diagnosis is supported by the production of a small amount of urine in the presence of adequate volume replacement.

If there is no urine output at all renal vascular obstruction should be considered and a renal nuclear perfusion scan may be useful to determining if either kidney is perfused. The early use of dialysis is often instituted to minimize complications.

As all specifically treatable causes have been identified and attempts at establishing urine flow have failed, then conservative therapy for established acute renal failure should be instituted. Fluid input should be equal to urinary output plus insensible losses, which are usually estimated to be about 500 ml per 24 hours in the absence of fever. A high carbohydrate, low protein, low potassium diet should be given. Starvation should be prevented as this promotes catabolism.

Frequent monitoring and daily weights should continue. At this stage electrolytes should be measured twice daily to monitor the progression and treatment of the hyperkalaemia and to assist in the decision concerning commencement of dialysis.

Hyperkalaemia is a constant threat and all attempts should be made to prevent it by withdrawal of all sources of potassium and use of cation exchange resins such as calcium resonium which should be started now in this patient.

Complications such as congestive cardiac failure or infection should be identified early. Any medications used should not be nephrotoxic and be used in decreased doses if excreted in the urine. Some clinicians also use prophylactic histamine-2 antagonists (e.g. ranitidine) in an attempt to prevent gastrointestinal bleeding which is a frequent complication of acute renal failure.

The ultrasound showing small, asymmetrical kidneys is in keeping with ischaemic nephropathy secondary to small or large vessel renovascular disease.

A8 The chest X-ray shows cardiomegaly, plethoric pulmonary vasculature and Kerley B lines. The features are of pulmonary oedema. The patient has congestive cardiac failure secondary to fluid overload, as her kidneys have been unable to regulate her fluid balance. The expansion of extracellular fluid is a consequence of diminished salt and water excretion in the oliguric patient.

Your overriding immediate concern is her hyperkalaemia, which is life-threatening. She should receive a cardioprotective agent such as 10 ml 10% calcium chloride immediately to prevent a fatal dysrhythmia. You need to lower her potassium acutely using an insulin and 50% dextrose infusion (e.g. 20 units fast acting insulin in 50 ml 50% glucose over 30 minutes).

These are only temporary measures and the clinical situation is now such that the patient is

ANSWERS – cont'd

only likely to be saved by dialysis. Absolute indications for dialysis include:

- Severe symptoms of uraemia (neurological such as acute confusion, deteriorating conscious state or seizures, or gastrointestinal such as anorexia, nausea, vomiting or ileus).
- Pericarditis.
- Resistant electrolyte abnormalities such as hyperkalaemia and severe acidosis.
- Fluid overload causing congestive cardiac failure not responsive to conservative therapy.

The decision will need to be made whether or not to embark on acute dialysis.

In the presence of pre-existent renal impairment and gentamicin nephrotoxicity her renal function may not return and the patient could become a chronic dialysis candidate to survive. The decision therefore to start dialysis must be discussed with the family or appropriate carers.

Absolute guidelines are difficult and decisions should made according to the circumstances of each individual case.

In this case it is likely, but not certain, that her renal function will recover but this may take weeks.

Continuous veno–venous haemodialysis (CVVHD) is the preferred technique for acute dialysis in this patient. This modality uses low blood flow and long hours of dialysis, thereby reducing cardiovascular instability. Continuous fluid removal is possible, allowing larger volumes of parenteral nutrition to be given (usually required to maintain nutrition in acute renal failure).

A9 The recovery phase of acute tubular necrosis can involve marked polyuria. As the kidneys recover, the capacity for filtration (GFR) returns, but not the tubular ability to concentrate the urine:

- Life-threatening fluid and electrolyte disturbances can continue to occur due to rapid losses without reabsorbtion, particularly hypokalaemia.
- Intravascular volume depletion may occur due to the high urine output. This may again cause further pre-renal acute renal failure.
- Other complications of acute renal failure such as infections or cardiovascular dysfunction can develop just as they may in the oliguric phase.

The patient therefore needs to be cared for with as much diligence as in the oliguric phase, with scrupulous attention to fluid and electrolyte balance. The patient should be in a high-dependency ward where central venous pressure is monitored and electrolytes taken regularly.

A10 A number of major errors were made in the management of this case, and much of this illness is iatrogenic. This could have had medicolegal implications. The errors included:

- The angiotensin 2 receptor blocker may have controlled this patient's hypertension. However, the combination of an angiotensin 2 blocker and a loop diuretic in an elderly patient may have potentially contributed to renal impairment if there was any pre-existing renovascular disease.
- Admission electrolytes were performed but they were not checked until 4 days later.
- Fluid replacement was inadequate, inaccurate and not based on close monitoring.
- The patient was continued on her usual medications without questioning whether they were appropriate or necessary. For example, the patient was taking in very little orally and yet the frusemide (furosemide) was continued. This exacerbated dehydration and pre-renal failure.
- The deterioration in renal function went unnoticed until days after its onset by which time it was too late to correct without renal replacement therapy.
- Toxic quantities of aminoglycoside antibiotics were prescribed because the renal function was not considered. This patient's creatinine clearance on admission was only 21 ml/min (normal 125 ml/min). Furthermore, the Cockroft–Gault equation can overestimate creatinine clearance in elderly patients, and her renal function may have been worse. The dose of gentamicin should have been no more than 2–3 mg/kg, and the levels monitored carefully. Specialist advice should have been sought. Gentamicin, as well as other nephrotoxic drugs, should have been avoided altogether for this patient.

REVISION POINTS

Acute renal failure

Definition

Sudden onset of renal dysfunction with elevated serum creatinine, reduced creatinine clearance and often hyperkalaemia. Oliguria is usually present (urine output <400 ml/day).

Aetiology

Varied but three main categories:

- Pre-renal: decreased renal perfusion secondary to dehydration, haemorrhage, sepsis or cardiogenic shock.
- Renal: acute glomerulonephritis, e.g. Goodpasture's syndrome, acute interstitial nephritis, acute occlusion of large renal arteries, rhabdomyolysis. Drugs are commonly involved in acute renal failure – particularly ACE-inhibitors, NSAIDs and aminoglycosides.
- Post-renal: obstruction, e.g. prostate disease, pelvic malignancy or calculi.

Pathophysiology

Established acute renal failure in 80% of patients is due to acute tubular necrosis, a spontaneously resolving renal tubular lesion.

Prevention

Recognition of pre-existent renal disease by appropriate testing, avoidance of dehydration and use of contrast media or nephrotoxic drugs, particularly in high-risk patients.

Management

- Reverse remediable factors, e.g. dehydration, hypotension, nephrotoxic drugs, etc.
- Conservative: as outlined in Answer 5. Do not use frusemide (furosemide): a trial of intravenous fluids is recommended. Adequate nutrition must be maintained.
- Dialysis: generally continuous veno–venous haemodialysis followed by intermittent haemodialysis until return of renal function.
- Polyuric phase: intravenous fluids generally required initially with careful attention to electrolytes, particularly potassium loss.

Prognosis

High mortality related largely to pre-existing cardiovascular co-morbidity and severity of underlying cause.

ISSUES TO CONSIDER

- Frusemide (furosemide) is a very commonly used drug. How does it work? What are the complications of diuretic therapy?

- How does the mechanism of haemofiltration differ from that of haemodialysis?

- Why is there a polyuric phase of acute tubular necrosis?

- In what ways can central venous monitoring help in the assessment of intravascular filling? What other ways are there of assessing filling on the intensive care?

FURTHER INFORMATION

www.kidneyatlas.org An extensive web resource covering a wide range of nephrological conditions.

www.studentbmj.com/back_issues/0799/data/0799ed3.htm One of many articles on the studentbmj website, this one covering the management of oliguria on the ward.

A 40-year-old man with lethargy and hypertension

A 40-year-old truck driver presents to the emergency department to have some grit removed from his eye. There is no foreign body on inspection and on fluorescein staining the cornea is intact. The eye is irrigated and the patient claims it now feels better.

In passing he mentions that he has been feeling 'under the weather' lately. You note that he looks ill, and on his observations sheet his blood pressure is 185/110 mm Hg. The man says he cannot recall the last time he attended a doctor and thinks it was years ago. You take some additional history.

He is a single man who spends most of his time on the road. He denies any previous illnesses. He is an ex-smoker and drinks 20–30 grams of alcohol a day. He says that he used to drink more but has been off his food and drink recently. He is on no medication (including over the counter) and uses no street drugs. He admits to feeling unwell and says that he has no energy. He denies any specific cardiac symptoms but has a smoker's cough. He has lost weight and

comments that his jeans are loose. He has not had any vomiting, abdominal pain or change in bowel habit. He has the occasional headache, more frequent recently. He has no pain or difficulty passing his water, but gets up twice during the night to void, even when he hasn't drunk any alcohol in the evening.

On examination he looks unwell. He is afebrile and not cyanosed or jaundiced. He has a ruddy complexion and is not clinically anaemic. He has scratch marks on his arms which he says is 'heat rash'. His pulse is normal and his blood pressure is 185/110 mm Hg. His jugular venous pressure is not elevated. His apex beat is not displaced but there is a left ventricular heave. On auscultation the heart sounds are dual with an added 4th sound. The chest is clear and there is no ankle oedema. The abdomen is unremarkable. The fundi show grade 2 hypertensive retinopathy. There is impaired sensation below the ankles with loss of the ankle jerks but otherwise he is neurologically intact.

 Q1 Which organ systems are you concerned about and why? Although his symptoms and signs are non-specific, what condition could explain these findings? What simple test – which should be part of the general examination – other than a blood test, could provide further information?

The man agrees to stay to have some blood tests. The complete blood picture and biochemical screen are shown in Investigation 48.1.

 Q2 Describe the abnormalities present. How do you interpret these tests?

The urinalysis you ordered reveals moderate proteinuria and microscopic haematuria. Frequent granular, red cell and hyaline casts together with dysmorphic red cells were observed on urine microscopy.

Investigation 48.1 Summary of results			
Haemoglobin	91 g/l	White cell count	4.0 x 10⁹/l
MCV	84 fl		
MCH	30 pg		
Platelets	195 x 10⁹/l		
Sodium	140 mmol/l	Calcium	2.03 mmol/l
Potassium	5.0 mmol/l	Phosphate	1.84 mmol/l
Chloride	98 mmol/l	Total protein	69 g/l
Bicarbonate	19 mmol/l	Albumin	38 g/l
Urea	34 mmol/l	Globulins	31 g/l
Creatinine	0.90 mmol/l	Bilirubin	24 μmol/l
Uric acid	0.63 mmol/l	ALT	44 U/l
Glucose	6.5 mmol/l	AST	45 U/l
Cholesterol	5.0 mmol/l	GGT	46 U/l
LDH	230 U/l	ALP	164 U/l

Q3 What is the first principle in the management of this patient? What non-invasive test would you initially order?

A renal ultrasound was performed and revealed small shrunken kidneys measuring 8.5 cm and 8 cm. The pelvicalyceal systems were not dilated.

A renal biopsy was not performed. You admit this man to hospital for management of his chronic renal failure.

Q4 Outline what is involved in the conservative management of this patient.

You spend some time counselling the patient about his illness, and he slowly improves with conservative measures. He undergoes surgery to construct an arteriovenous fistula in anticipation of the need for haemodialysis in the future.

The man is followed regularly but 3 months later presents to the emergency department unwell and breathless. He states he had been out drinking with friends and eating pizza. On examination he is hypertensive and clinically in left ventricular failure. His electrolytes reveal a metabolic acidosis with a moderate elevation in his serum potassium. His creatinine has deteriorated to 1.10 mmol/l.

Q5 What should be done now?

You admit him to hospital and immediately commence haemodialysis. You discuss renal transplantation, and find that he has only one sister who is ABO mismatched. He is therefore placed on the waiting list for a cadaveric renal transplant, and meanwhile has regular haemodialysis as an outpatient. Figure 48.1 shows the patient's arm 1 year after the commencement of dialysis.

Fig 48.1

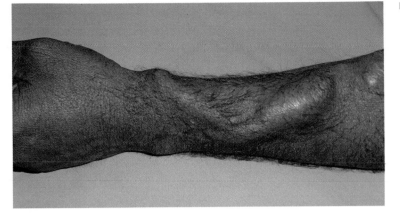

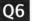 **What does the photograph show?**

ANSWERS

A1 • Cardiovascular: 4th heart sound, hypertension and grade 2 hypertensive retinopathy.
• Renal: his signs and symptoms are consistent with chronic renal failure. He is unwell and lethargic, has lost weight and appetite, has pruritus, evidence of a peripheral neuropathy and a high blood pressure.
• He needs a urinalysis and examination of the urinary sediment. Urinalysis should be part of any clinical examination.

A2 The abnormalities include renal failure, as revealed by the markedly elevated urea and creatinine. Along with the patient's history, the peripheral neuropathy, the biochemical changes reflecting bone disease and the anaemia suggest that the renal failure is chronic.

The blood results show:
• Mild metabolic acidosis.
• Mild hyperkalaemia.
• Raised phosphate, low calcium and raised ALP (this reflects phosphate retention, reduced active circulating vitamin D and secondary hyperparathyroidism).
• Hyperuricaemia (reflects urate retention).
• A normochromic normocytic anaemia. This is secondary to reduced erythropoietin production by the failing kidneys.

A3 Identify and treat any reversible factors which could be causing or exacerbating his renal impairment:
• A drug history is important with particular reference to NSAIDs.
• Fluid status should be assessed and any dehydration (contributing to pre-renal failure) should be corrected if present.
• Infection should be excluded.
An immediate renal ultrasound should be performed to obtain renal size and exclude obstruction:
• Bilateral small symmetric kidneys imply irreversible renal damage, most likely secondary to chronic glomerulonephritis.
• Asymmetric kidney size raises the possibility of renovascular disease, reflux nephropathy or analgesic disease.
• Normal size kidneys may need to be biopsied.

A4 The aim is to prevent further deterioration in renal function:
• Control his symptoms (e.g. anorexia, nausea, pruritus).
• Dietary protein restriction helps to limit the retention of end products of nitrogen metabolism, although this must be balanced against adequate nutrition.

ANSWERS – cont'd

- Potassium accumulation is also prevented by dietary restriction of potassium-containing foods.
- Monitor the patient regularly to prevent life-threatening deterioration.
- Hypertension control is mandatory. Tight blood pressure control slows the progression of kidney failure and prevents end-organ damage (cardiovascular, retinal). ACE inhibitors have been shown to be most effective in reducing proteinuria, slowing disease progression and reducing cardiac remodelling. Hypertension usually requires combination therapy with multiple antihypertensives.
- Renal metabolic bone disease is either prevented or treated with calcitriol (active vitamin D), and phosphate binders (e.g. aluminium hydroxide or calcium carbonate). The aim is to keep calcium and phosphate within the normal range and keep parathyroid hormone levels approximately twice the normal range. The aim is to prevent metastatic calcification and to suppress parathyroid over-activity.
- Atherosclerosis is greatly accelerated in renal failure. It is important to treat hyperlipidaemia – particularly in younger patients.
- Anaemia is managed by replacing lost erythropoietin (EPO) with subcutaneous injections of EPO on a weekly or twice-weekly basis. Iron stores need to be monitored regularly and iron infusions may be necessary to maintain adequate ferritin levels.

The patient should be counselled about the nature of this illness and the necessity of compliance with the above measures. He will also have to be told to come into hospital immediately should he become unwell or develop an intercurrent illness which may lead to decompensation. Future options would need to be discussed with the patient and any family. The issue of transplantation should be broached. The patient should be tissue typed. Any ABO matched sibling who would be willing to act as a live donor should be typed, otherwise the patient should be assessed for placement on a waiting list for a cadaveric transplant.

Conservative treatment is continued only as long as the patient continues to be relatively well. If uraemia cannot be controlled, dialysis should be instituted.

A5 Haemodialysis should be commenced immediately to correct this decompensation. The patient will have to be counselled to prevent future indiscretions with his diet. Support groups may be helpful in coping with renal failure.

A6 Figure 48.1 shows this patient's arteriovenous fistula. This is constructed by anastomosing the cephalic vein to the radial artery in the region of the anatomical 'snuff box', and can be recognized by the presence of a scar over the distal end of the radius and the dilated firm pulsatile forearm veins. A thrill is palpable, and a loud bruit is heard over the anastomosis.

REVISION POINTS

Chronic renal failure

Common causes
- chronic glomerulonephritis
- diabetes
- adult polycystic kidney disease
- reflux nephropathy
- ischaemic renal disease.

Symptoms
- polyuria and nocturia
- lethargy
- pruritus
- weight loss.

Signs
- hypertension
- pallor (anaemia)
- peripheral neuropathy.

Diagnosis
- urinary abnormalities: proteinuria and haematuria
- abnormal renal function tests on biochemistry: hyperkalaemia, hypocalcaemia/hyperphosphataemia
- small kidneys on imaging: if large, consider obstruction, polycystic kidney disease or diabetes.

continues overleaf

REVISION POINTS – cont'd

Management

Conservative

- eliminate reversible factors, e.g. nephrotoxic drugs (especially NSAIDs), volume depletion and urine infection
- slow progression by optimal control of blood pressure to target 130/75 mm Hg if proteinuria present
- control metabolic abnormalities: suppress parathyroid hormone with calcitriol, bind phosphate with calcium carbonate or aluminium hydroxide, correct severe acidosis with sodium bicarbonate and correct lipid abnormalities with statins
- correct anaemia with erythropoietin or analogues
- patient education, particularly in regard to nutrition, vascular access (fistula) for dialysis, dialysis modalities and transplantation options with particular regard to live donors.

Dialysis

Two types:

- haemodialysis (in the main centre, a satellite or at home)
- peritoneal dialysis: continuous ambulatory peritoneal dialysis (CAPD) or automated peritoneal dialysis (APD) using an automatic device which exchanges peritoneal fluid while the patient is asleep.

Dialysis should be instituted before uraemic symptoms become overtly manifest.

Transplantation

This form of treatment offers the best quality of life for end-stage renal failure patients. Donor kidneys may be either cadaveric or from a live donor, not necessarily related.

Contraindications include malignancy, advanced age, severe vascular disease (both cardiac and peripheral), active autoimmune disease and bronchiectasis.

Dual renal/pancreas transplantation should be considered for diabetic patients with end-stage renal failure but with minimal other diabetic complications.

ISSUES TO CONSIDER

- Construct an argument as to why urinalysis should be a routine investigation of all patients who visit a general practice or emergency centre.
- Investigate the costs to the community of long-term dialysis and renal transplantation.

FURTHER INFORMATION

www.merck.com/pubs/mmanual/section17/chapter222/222a.htm A section from the *Merck Manual of Diagnosis and Therapy* on renal failure.

www.emedicine.com/emerg/topic501.htm The emedicine site on chronic renal failure.

A 35-year-old woman with hypertension

A 35-year-old woman presents to the emergency department complaining of 5 days of progressive generalized headache and nausea. Her blood pressure is taken and is recorded at 250/140 mm Hg. The patient states that she has a family history of hypertension and was noted to be hypertensive for the first time 2 years ago. She had no investigations, but was treated with verapamil 80 mg tds. The patient stopped taking this after a few months as it made her constipated.

Q1 From what might this patient be suffering? What further history is required from her?

Q2 What would you look for on examination?

The patient does not have any relevant previous illnesses and had a tubal ligation 6 years ago. She complains of sweating, palpitations and anxiety. She takes no drugs, but smokes 10 cigarettes a day and consumes 100 gm alcohol a week.

On examination the patient is anxious and sweaty, but otherwise appears fit. Her pulse rate is 120 bpm and regular and her blood pressure 250/140 mm Hg. Significant abnormalities include a forceful but undisplaced apical cardiac impulse without evidence of left ventricular failure, and a bruit in the left side of her abdomen. Urinalysis reveals 1+ (0.3 g/l) albumin only. Her retina is shown in Figure 49.1.

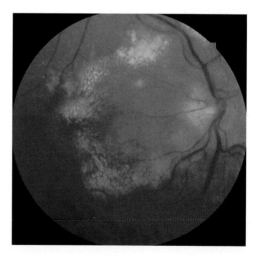

Fig 49.1

Q3 What does this retinal photograph show?

The changes seen on fundoscopy are consistent with the clinical picture of severe hypertension.

Q4 What type of treatment should immediately be instituted?

You insert a radial arterial line for accurate monitoring of blood pressure and admit her to the high dependency ward. Her blood pressure improves with your chosen therapy, and you now have time to think about the possible cause of her hypertensive crisis.

Q5 What are the possible causes of this woman's hypertension and what investigations would you like to organize?

The patient's complete blood picture, ESR, biochemistry, urine microscopy and culture and chest X-ray were normal. The ECG showed a sinus tachycardia and left axis deviation, but was otherwise normal. Urinary catecholamines were within normal limits.

Renal ultrasound is normal. The patient went on to have the investigation shown in Figure 49.2.

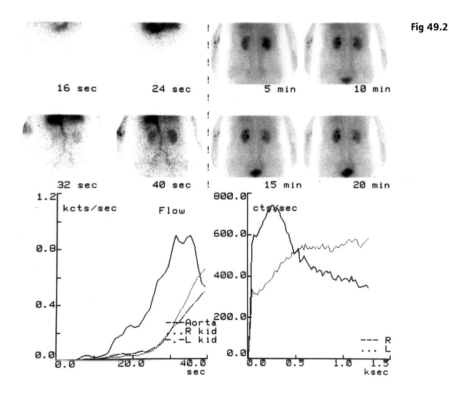

Fig 49.2

Q6 What is this investigation? What does it show?

The patient then had another investigation (Figure 49.3).

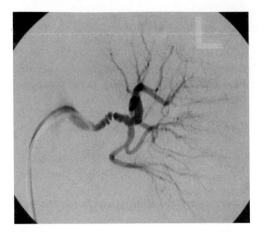

Fig 49.3

Q7 What is the investigation and what does it show? How can this condition be treated?

The patient had the most marked stenotic segment dilated via percutaneous transluminal balloon angioplasty, with a dramatic improvement in her blood pressure.

An important lesson in this case is that the patient was inadequately assessed on her first presentation with hypertension 2 years earlier. At that time the minimum investigation should have included urinalysis, serum biochemical analysis, ECG and possibly echocardiography (to assess for left ventricular hypertrophy), chest X-ray and lipid profile. In addition, there should have been careful follow-up and counselling to stop smoking.

In view of her young age, a specific underlying cause of her hypertension should have been considered. Further, if the abdominal bruit had been listened for (and been present and found) at her initial presentation, her fibromuscular dysplasia may have been diagnosed and the subsequent emergency avoided.

Patient education is vital to prevent loss to follow-up. If unacceptable side effects occur, a switch to an alternative medication will promote compliance. Otherwise, their hypertension may go untreated for long periods.

ANSWERS

A1 She may have poorly controlled essential hypertension or hypertension secondary to underlying kidney disease, and an intercurrent problem such as a viral illness which has produced the headache and nausea. However, she has marked hypertension for a young person and may be in a hypertensive crisis. In this situation encephalopathy can occur which would be suggested by the headache and nausea. Her past medical history will be important as she may give a history of known poorly controlled hypertension or renal disease. You must inquire as to whether she may be pregnant (pre-eclampsia).

You should ask her about the severity of her previously diagnosed hypertension, and whether she knows of her recent blood pressure readings – if it has been progressively increasing over several months the immediate risk is lower than if this has been a sudden rise over a few days or weeks.

Ask her about symptoms associated with hypertensive encephalopathy such as irritability, visual disturbances, confusion, altered consciousness and seizures.

Ask about symptoms that might suggest an underlying disorder to account for her hypertension, such as:

ANSWERS – cont'd

- Renal disease: thirst, polyuria, nocturia, dysuria, haematuria, colic, lethargy and general malaise of uraemia.
- Phaeochromocytoma: sweating, palpitations, anxiety and tremor, particularly occurring in paroxysms.
- Cushing's syndrome: truncal weight gain, thinning of skin, easy bruising, weakness of proximal limb muscles, striae, hirsutism.

You will also need to ask about symptoms suggestive of hypertensive damage to the retina (visual deterioration) or the cardiovascular system, including acute myocardial ischaemia or failure (angina, dyspnoea, orthopnoea, ankle swelling), and aortic dissection (back pain).

A drug history is vital, including past use of analgesics (particularly NSAIDs: analgesic nephropathy), current use of drugs associated with hypertension, e.g. oral contraceptive pill, sympathomimetics (e.g. nasal decongestants), steroids, some antidepressants (including venlafaxine) and combinations of antidepressants associated with a risk of serotonergic syndrome (e.g. SSRIs and monoamine oxidase inhibitors). The patient's use of tobacco, alcohol and other illicit drugs, particularly cocaine and amphetamine derivatives, should also be explored.

A2 On examination you will need to look for evidence of hypertensive damage to:

- The CNS (level of consciousness, visual fields, focal neurological deficits).
- The retina (hypertensive retinopathy, especially haemorrhages, new exudates or optic disc swelling).
- The heart (left ventricular hypertrophy, left ventricular failure).
- The aorta (unequal pulses in aortic dissection).
- The kidney (haematuria or proteinuria on urinalysis).

Note: The presence of any acute features, especially neurological symptoms or signs, retinal haemorrhages, exudates or optic disc swelling, and abnormalities on urinalysis, suggest the presence of accelerated/malignant hypertension requiring emergency treatment.

Features to suggest underlying aetiology:

- Cushingoid habitus.
- Delayed femoral pulses in coarctation of the aorta.
- Palpable hydronephrotic or polycystic kidneys.
- Abdominal bruits.
- Appearance of uraemia.
- Sweating, tremor and tachycardia, and rarely, abdominal masses in phaeochromocytoma.
- Generalized oedema and/or abnormal urinalysis in glomerulonephritis.
- Evidence of a connective tissue disorder such as SLE or skin manifestations of vasculitis.

A3 Figure 49.1 shows:

- Hard exudates.
- Cotton wool spots.
- Flame haemorrhages.

This is grade 3 hypertensive retinopathy. There is considerable hard exudate in the posterior pole with formation of a partial macular star.

In grade 4 retinopathy optic disc swelling would also be present, but there is no evidence that clinical outcomes differ on the basis of the fundoscopic findings and both grade 3 and grade 4 should be regarded as indicators of hypertensive emergency.

A4 This is a medical emergency.

- Her blood pressure should be lowered gradually over several hours, aiming for no more than a 20–25% reduction in mean arterial pressure, or a reduction to no lower than 160/100 mm Hg, over the first 1–2 hours. A careful balance is required between reducing the pressure rapidly enough to prevent or reverse hypertensive encephalopathy and reducing it too rapidly with the attendant risk of cerebral hypoperfusion and infarction (stroke).
- Strict bed rest and intra-arterial blood pressure monitoring are desirable if the facilities are available (e.g. on a high dependency ward).
- Blood pressure reduction using a short-acting parenteral agent such as a sodium nitroprusside or labetalol infusion, titrated according to the blood pressure response, is safer than fixed doses of intravenous, oral or sublingual antihypertensive agents.

ANSWERS – cont'd

- The use of oral nifedipine capsules is no longer recommended because they have a rapid onset of action and reach very high peak plasma concentrations, resulting in the potential for sudden uncontrolled blood pressure reduction and precipitation of stroke.
- Once blood pressure is lowered, a combination of antihypertensive agents will probably be needed to maintain good control, the choice depending on the characteristics of the patient. Nifedipine tablets (not the slow-release OROS or GITS formulations) can be used at this stage in an initial dose of 20 mg, particularly in combination with selective betablockade (e.g. atenolol 50 mg).
- This patient has a renal bruit; in patients with clinical evidence of possible renal artery stenosis, nifedipine and betablockade may be safer and more effective than therapy based on an angiotensin converting enzyme (ACE) inhibitor.
- Note that betablockers can cause a paradoxical and possibly dangerous rise in hypertension in the presence of phaeochromocytoma, while angiotensin converting enzyme (ACE) inhibitors (e.g. captopril) can precipitate a marked deterioration in renal function in patients with bilateral renal artery stenosis.

A5 This woman may have essential (primary) hypertension as she does have a positive family history and the hypertension may be exacerbated by smoking and alcohol. However, the severity of her hypertension at her age suggests a specific underlying cause. The common causes of secondary hypertension include:

- Renal parenchymal disease:
  - Unilateral, e.g. pyelonephritis, obstructive or reflux nephropathy, dysplasia, trauma.
  - Bilateral, e.g. any cause of chronic renal failure, obstructive or reflux nephropathy, diabetes mellitus, analgesic nephropathy, polycystic disease, pyelonephritis, glomerulonephritis, interstitial nephritis.
- Renovascular disease: renal artery stenosis secondary to atheroma, fibromuscular hyperplasia (especially in younger patients), trauma.

- Pregnancy: pre-eclampsia.
- Adrenal disorders: e.g. phaeochromocytoma, Cushing's syndrome, primary aldosteronism (Conn's syndrome).
- Drug associated: e.g. oral contraceptive pill (common), corticosteroids, sympathomimetics, alcoholism.
- Cardiovascular e.g. coarctation of the aorta.

With her anxiety, sweating and resting tachycardia, it is prudent to exclude a phaeochromocytoma, but her abdominal bruit suggests the possibility of renal artery stenosis. Baseline investigations should include:

- Complete blood picture and ESR.
- Electrolytes, including blood glucose, urea and creatinine.
- Urine microscopy (for casts and cells).
- Chest X-ray and ECG (to detect left ventricular hypertrophy).

The next investigation of choice would be a non-invasive screening test for renal artery stenosis. Several different tests can be done, and these include duplex ultrasound scanning, spiral CT angiography and gadolinium-enhanced magnetic resonance angiography (MRA).

Currently, the most commonly available test is a radionuclide scan of the kidneys, which will give data about the blood supply and function of each kidney. The diagnosis of renal artery stenosis can be made with increased certainty by rescanning 1 hour after oral captopril (an ACE inhibitor) is given. This is because when renal perfusion is markedly reduced (as with renal artery stenosis) the glomerular perfusion and filtration is dependent on efferent arteriolar resistance ('back-pressure'). ACE inhibitors reduce angiotensin-mediated post-glomerular vasoconstriction and can cause a dramatic deterioration in glomerular filtration and renal function. Uptake of a radiopharmaceutical (^{99m}Tc DTPA), which is cleared by glomerular filtration, will be reduced. This will be seen as 'blanching' of the affected kidney on the renal scan.

Given the clinical context, this patient should also be screened for a phaeochromocytoma by assessing production of catecholamines. This is usually done by performing a 24-hour urine collection, assayed for excreted catecholamines and their metabolites.

ANSWERS – cont'd

A6 This is a radionuclide scan of the kidneys. It shows (views taken from behind) delayed perfusion and delayed function of the left kidney and then late hyperconcentration of the isotope in the left kidney. The right kidney contributes 65% of total renal function and the left kidney contributes 35%. These results strongly suggest left renal artery stenosis, and the diagnosis should be confirmed by renal angiography, which remains the gold standard for definition of the renal arterial anatomy.

A7 This is a renal angiogram and shows contrast in the left renal artery. There are several narrowed segments in the left renal artery and the origin of the vessel looks normal. This pattern of narrowing is referred to as 'beading'. There are no changes to suggest atheromatous disease of the arterial tree and the cause of the abnormality is fibromuscular dysplasia.

This condition is usually treated by percutaneous balloon angioplasty, or by open surgery.

REVISION POINTS

Hypertensive emergencies

Incidence
Less than 1% of all cases of hypertension; secondary hypertension accounts for about 5% of all cases of hypertension but 25–50% of cases of hypertensive emergency.

Risk factors
- For hypertension: family history, obesity, alcohol abuse.
- For hypertensive crisis: secondary hypertension (esp. renal disease, renovascular disease), oral contraceptive pill, smoking.

Presentation
Headache, visual impairment, dizziness, anxiety, disorientation, tremor, seizures, nausea, vomiting, abdominal pain.

Clinical features
- Usually severe hypertension (diastolic BP > 120) but may occur at moderate BP levels if BP has risen rapidly from a low baseline.
- Grade 3 or 4 retinopathy (haemorrhages, exudates +/− optic disc swelling).
- Proteinuria is common.
- May be focal neurological findings, acute left ventricular failure.

Prognosis
Untreated prognosis is very poor, with 5-year survival about 1%; with antihypertensive treatment 5-year survival is about 75%.

Early management
- Investigations: plasma electrolytes, urea and creatinine, blood picture, ESR; ECG; chest X-ray; urinalysis and urine microscopy.
- Intra-arterial BP monitoring and intensive care, with infusion of sodium nitroprusside or labetalol titrated to response, aiming for no more than 20–25% reduction in BP over first 2 hours.

Later management
Investigations for secondary hypertension as clinically indicated and specific management if a cause is found.

Combination oral antihypertensive drug therapy according to clinical features (usually require at least two drugs for initial control). Captopril, nifedipine (slow release), atenolol, prazosin have all been used successfully. Thiazide diuretics could be used if not volume depleted.

Renovascular hypertension

Epidemiology
- Accounts for approximately 3% of all cases of hypertension and about 15% of cases of hypertensive emergencies.
- Atheromatous renovascular disease is the most common form (seen mainly in elderly men with vascular risk factors).
- Fibromuscular hyperplasia may account for up to one-third of cases and is diagnosed

continues overleaf

REVISION POINTS – cont'd

most commonly in women between the ages of 30 and 50 (bilateral in about 50%).

Diagnosis of renal artery stenosis

- The best method for non-invasive screening is currently controversial.
- The captopril-challenged isotopic renal scan has been the gold standard.
- Newer techniques such as spiral CT angiography, duplex ultrasonography and MR angiography are being evaluated.

All four techniques have reasonable sensitivity and specificity when performed skilfully, but only renal perfusion scanning indicates functional significance of any stenosis.

If non-invasive testing is highly suggestive of renal artery stenosis, then an arterial digital subtraction angiogram, with or without venous renin measurements, should be performed.

Treatment

Indications for treatment are uncontrollable hypertension and deteriorating renal function.

Best treated by balloon angioplasty, or surgery if this is unsuccessful; in fibromuscular dysplasia, 60% of patients treated by percutaneous balloon angioplasty will remain cured at the end of 12 months and long-term prognosis is good.

ISSUES TO CONSIDER

- What non-pharmaceutical methods can hypertensives employ to lower their blood pressure?
- How would you control hypertension secondary to a phaeochromocytoma?
- What problems are associated with continuous infusions of sodium nitroprusside?

FURTHER INFORMATION

www.postgradmed.com/issues/1999/05_01_99/bales.htm Bales, A. Hypertensive crisis: how to tell if it's an emergency or an urgency. *Postgraduate Medicine* 1999.

www.bloodpressure.com An excellent commercial site with information and links for patients and physicians alike.

www.ash-us.org Website of the American Society for Hypertension with lots of links.

Intellectual deterioration in an elderly woman

A 72-year-old woman is brought into your surgery by her daughter. The woman is a widow and lives alone. Her daughter rang the practice yesterday to inform you that she thinks that her mother has early dementia and wants an opinion. She says that her mother had previously been active and fully independent. However, in recent months she has noticed that her mother has become unable to care for herself. She is less well groomed and her house has fallen into disarray. The daughter is concerned that her mother is not eating properly because she no longer prepares meals, but she admits that her mother actually appears to be gaining weight. She says her mother appears much older and is easily distracted, quiet and no longer contributes to conversations like she used to.

The patient is subdued and is slow to respond to questions. She is orientated in time, place and person. Her long-term memory is intact but she has defects in short-term memory and is unable to recite the months of the year backwards or perform calculations. No paranoia is evident in conversation with her. She has some insight into her problems. Her affect is sad, but not labile, and she appears apathetic. The woman denies any physical symptoms but on direct questioning admits to feeling weak and is unable to do anything. She denies being depressed and does not have headache or incontinence.

The patient has a past history of a myocardial infarction at the age of 66. She has infrequent post-infarct angina which is controlled with isosorbide dinitrate 10 mg tds. She is also on enteric-coated aspirin 150 mg daily. There is no history of depression or other psychiatric history and there is no family history of dementia. She does not drink alcohol.

 Q1 What is the aim of investigating this patient?

Figure 50.1 shows the patient.

 Q2 What does the photograph show and what would you look for on physical examination?

Q3 What tests are usually included in a dementia screen? From the history, what test may be particularly relevant in this case?

The woman is mildly obese. She has a pulse rate of 52 bpm and a blood pressure of 165/ 90 mm Hg. There is no clubbing or pallor. The skin is cool and dry. Examination of her cardiovascular, respiratory and gastrointestinal symptoms is unremarkable. There is no papilloedema and the cranial nerves are normal. The limb reflexes are difficult to elicit but the tone and power of the limbs are normal. The plantar reflexes are down-going and tests of cerebellar function and sensation are also normal.

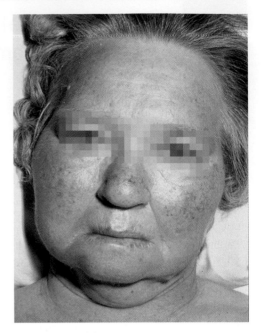

Fig 50.1

Q4   How do your examination findings help you with your diagnosis?

A dementia screen is performed on this patient.
The following results are obtained:

Investigation 50.1 Summary of results			
Haemoglobin	121 g/l	White cell count	4.8 x 10⁹/l
MCHC	330 g/l	Platelets	311 x 10⁹/l
MCV	101 fl	ESR	31 mm/hr
Sodium	126 mmol/l	Calcium	2.17 mmol/l
Potassium	4.2 mmol/l	Phosphate	1.14 mmol/l
Chloride	106 mmol/l	Total protein	62 g/l
Bicarbonate	27 mmol/l	Albumin	35 g/l
Urea	6.8 mmol/l	Globulins	27 g/l
Creatinine	0.10 mmol/l	Bilirubin	16 µmol/l
Uric acid	0.24 mmol/l	ALT	22 U/l
Glucose	4.4 mmol/l	AST	23 U/l
Cholesterol	8.8 mmol/l	GGT	17 U/l
LDH	320 U/l	ALP	50 U/l
Serum TSH	66 mU/l		
Serum T4	5 pmol/l	Serum folate	3.4 µg/l
Serum T3	1.5 pmol/l	Serum B12	612 ng/l

The ECG shows a sinus bradycardia of 50 beats/minute, evidence of an old inferolateral myocardial infarction and non-specific anterior T-wave abnormality. The chest X-ray reveals mild cardiomegaly but is otherwise normal. A CT scan of the brain shows minor age-related atrophy within normal limits.

Q5 What is the diagnosis and how should she be treated. Could there be any hazards of treatment?

The woman is commenced on 25 µg of levothyroxine on alternate days. This is increased to 25 µg daily after 4 weeks and then by 25 µg increments every 6 weeks until a dose of 100 µg is reached. At this dose the metabolic state clinically normalized and the thyroid function (measured 6 weeks after commencing the new dose) returned to normal. The woman did not suffer any exacerbation of her ischaemic heart disease with this replacement regimen. Her mental state improved considerably and she was again able to live independently with the help of her daughter. Her face thinned and after 3 months on treatment she looked younger and more alert.

ANSWERS

A1 This patient appears to have a mild dementia. A small proportion of dementias have a medical cause, and may be partially reversible with treatment of the medical cause. Therefore any patient with dementia requires thorough investigation to identify reversible factors.

A2 The patient's face shows changes characteristic of myxoedema, with puffiness and swelling in the periorbital regions.

A general physical examination should be performed including assessment of the patient's state of hygiene and dress. Evidence for underlying disease of heart, lung, kidney, liver or thyroid should be sought. A thorough neurological examination is necessary. Features of potentially reversible illnesses should be sought, e.g. papilloedema as evidence of raised intracranial pressure, apraxia of gait and incontinence in normal pressure hydrocephalus, posterior and lateral column signs in vitamin B12 deficiency or evidence of liver disease (the dementia being a more subtle manifestation of encephalopathy). The state of vision and hearing needs to be assessed. The mental state and cognitive function should be assessed formally.

A3 The following tests are included in a routine dementia screen:
- Complete blood picture and ESR.
- Biochemistry including renal function and liver function tests.
- Vitamin B12 and folate levels.
- Thyroid function.
- Tests for syphilis.
- ECG.
- Chest X-ray.
- CT scan of the brain.

Sometimes specialized investigations may be appropriate depending on the clinical circumstances. Lumbar puncture, MRI scanning of the brain, HIV serology, SPECT and PET scanning of the brain are sometimes necessary.

The patient's presentation would be consistent with hypothyroidism. Diagnosis is easy with modern assays. T3 and T4 are always low, and a high TSH confirms primary hypothyroidism.

A4 Obesity and signs of recent weight gain, relative bradycardia, cool dry skin and sluggish reflexes (classically slow relaxing) would all support a diagnosis of hypothyroidism. Other features would include weakness and lethargy, cold intolerance, constipation and hoarse voice. These may be accompanied by a myxoedema facies. The disease may also be manifested by a slow insidious intellectual deterioration which is why the tests for thyroid function are included in the dementia screen.

ANSWERS – cont'd

A5 Raised TSH and reduced T4 confirms hypothyroidism. The macrocytosis, mild hyponatraemia, hypercholesterolaemia and elevated LDH, the sinus bradycardia and mild cardiomegaly are in keeping with this.

The patient is likely to have primary idiopathic hypothyroidism. Thyroxine replacement should be commenced. This is complicated by the fact that the patient has ischaemic heart disease. The danger is that too rapid replacement will stimulate the metabolic rate to an extent that myocardial ischaemia or even infarction may be precipitated. Therefore a dose of thyroxine of only 25 µg on alternate days should be started. The dose can then be increased slowly. For example, the dose could be increased to 25 µg daily after 4 weeks and then the daily dose could be increased by 25 µg every 5–6 weeks until normal thyroid function tests are obtained.

This is assessed both clinically and by measuring serum values of TSH, T4 and T3. It must be remembered that once the dose of thyroxine has been changed, you must wait 6–8 weeks before that alteration is reflected in the thyroid function tests. This is because of the long half-life of T4. In view of this patient's confusion, compliance must be ensured and initially she may require supervision until her mental state improves.

REVISION POINTS

Dementia

Definition
A disorder of higher mental functions in which loss of intellectual ability impairs the patient's capacity to continue their usual occupation or function in their usual social environment.

Incidence
10% of persons over 70, and 20–40% of persons over 85 have evidence of cognitive decline.

Aetiology
Multiple, but in practice the vast majority of cases are the result of a few disorders, e.g. Alzheimer's disease and multi-infarct dementia. Can be a manifestation of advanced HIV infection. Investigation is aimed at identifying reversible causes so that dementia can be reversed or its progression halted.

Assessment
Start by interviewing the patient's family.

One of the most important pieces of information is the duration of the illness and how quickly it has progressed. Rapid progression with good previous function implies a potentially treatable underlying cause.

A careful family history should be taken and the patient's medical history should be analysed, e.g. has the patient had uncontrolled hyperten-sion and a stepwise downhill course that would be characteristic of multi-infarct dementia? Ask about:

- The patient's ability to interact with others, function at home or at work, and to self-care should be assessed.
- Change in personality.
- An accurate drug and alcohol history will need to be obtained as well as a history of any head trauma.

A full mental status examination will be needed. This should include assessment of state of consciousness and tests of orientation, speech, short- and long-term memory, calculation and abstract reasoning. The patient's mood will also need to be assessed as the main differential diagnosis of dementia is depression or pseudodementia.

Physical examination is as outlined in Answer 2.

Management
When no reversible factors are found the aim should be to optimize the patient's function, provide a safe environment and support the patient's family. Therapy for Alzheimer's disease with acetyl cholinesterase inhibitors may improve cognitive function or reduce the rate of decline in cognitive function.

continues overleaf

REVISION POINTS – cont'd

Hypothyroidism

- Hypothyroidism in adults is usually primary idiopathic (autoimmune), following thyroid surgery or following radioiodine treatment for hyperthyroidism.
- Typical features of hypothyroidism may *not* be obvious in the elderly (such as weakness and lethargy, weight gain, cold intolerance, constipation, hoarse voice and dry skin and hair).

- Hypothyroidism may also be manifested by a slow insidious intellectual deterioration which is why the tests for thyroid function are included in the dementia screen.
- Thyroxine replacement should be commenced at a low dose in the elderly or those with ischaemic heart disease and increased gradually to avoid precipitating ischaemia.

ISSUES TO CONSIDER

- How can primary hypothyroidism be differentiated from hypothyroidism secondary to pituitary dysfunction? What additional investigations may be helpful? How would management differ?
- What advances have been made in our understanding of the pathogenesis of Alzheimer's disease? What implications may this have in the development of future treatment strategies?

FURTHER INFORMATION

www.emedicine.com/emerg/topic280.htm emedicine article on myxoedema coma and its management.

www.vh.org/adult/provider/familymedicine/ FPHandbook/Chapter06/15-6.html The Virtual Hospital from the University of Iowa contains a vast amount of information on many facets of medicine. This page deals with hypothyroidism.

PROBLEM 51

A young man with depressed conscious state and seizures

A young man is brought into the emergency department early one morning. He was found 'unconscious' in the street and an ambulance called. There were no witnesses. Immediate assessment shows that his airway is intact and patent, he has normal colour and respiratory rate and pulse oximetry, and there is no circulatory compromise. Also, there are no obvious injuries.

He is stuporose and responds with sluggish but purposeful limb movements to painful stimuli. He groans, but does not make any comprehensible sounds. His Glasgow Coma Score is 6 (E1, V2, M3). He has a temperature of 37°C and cardiorespiratory examination is normal. The pupils are mid-position, equal and reactive and the optic fundi are normal. The plantars are downgoing. He has no neck stiffness and Kernig's sign is negative. No focal neurological abnormality can be elicited. The rest of the physical examination is normal.

Q1 What test should immediately be performed on arrival in the emergency department and what else should be sought on examination?

The test does not help elucidate the cause of the patient's collapse. The man is reasonably well kempt but there is a faint smell of alcohol on his breath. On closer inspection there is a superficial laceration over the occiput and bruising of the right lateral aspect of the tongue. The patient's underpants are found to be damp with urine.

Before any further assessment is performed the patient suddenly lets out a grunt, all four limbs extend and his spine arches. He stops breathing and rapidly becomes cyanosed. After 30 seconds, violent rhythmic contractions of the limbs begin.

Q2 What is the diagnosis and what should be done for the patient?

The seizure is aborted after 10 mg intravenous diazepam. At this stage a brother, who had been contacted by the nursing staff, arrives and provides further information. The patient is 24, has had epilepsy since his early teens, and has been on regular anticonvulsant medication although the brother is unsure as to the medication's name.

Q3 What are the causes of this condition? What are the likely causes in this patient?

The brother states that the patient has seizures every few months and his local doctor has told him that it is his legal obligation to stop him from driving. He subsequently stopped seeing that doctor. Over the last few days the patient suffered a 'flu-like illness and had taken a few days off work. Both of them had been out drinking alcohol into the early hours of the morning the night before, but he seemed reasonably well when they left the bar, saying that he would walk home.

The patient slowly regains consciousness over the next 3 hours. He has amnesia for the events of the day and his last recollection was being in a bar with his brother the night before. He confirms his brother's account and admits he has not taken his anticonvulsant medication (carbamazepine) for 5 days.

 How will you manage this patient in the short term?

An electroencephalogram (EEG) is performed, as one had not been done since diagnosis many years ago. This shows a generalized abnormality in keeping with a diagnosis of primary generalized epilepsy.

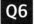 **How are you going to manage his medications?**

You counsel the patient about the medications you feel most appropriate for his needs, and spend some time talking to him about his illness.

 What other advice will you offer him?

Q7 The patient asks you when it is likely he will be able to stop taking anticonvulsant medication. What is your reply?

ANSWERS

A1 Hypoglycaemia should be promptly excluded by blood glucose estimation. Naloxone should be administered in case of opiate overdose.

Further examination should be undertaken for evidence of:
- Drug abuse (needle tracks) and/or drugs or drug paraphernalia on his person.
- Seizure (tongue biting or incontinence).
- Medication usage (medical alert bracelet, personal details in pockets, any information about medications such as sedatives, antidepressants or illicit drugs).
- Signs of chronic liver disease.
- Head injury.

- Assess if the patient is kempt or unkempt and asssess the breath for the smell of alcohol.
- Look for a form of identification or any other personal items that will enable you to contact relatives or friends. Most importantly, these people may be able to give a history.

A2 The initial clinical picture fits a post-ictal state. The subsequent event was a generalized tonic–clonic seizure. He has not regained consciousness between seizures and by definition is in status epilepticus. This is defined as prolonged or recurrent seizures without recovery between attacks. Repeated tonic–clonic seizures are life-

ANSWERS – cont'd

threatening and require prompt treatment to break the seizure cycle.

Management consists of:

- Clear and maintain the airway and call for support.
- Prevent aspiration and nurse the patient on the left lateral position without a pillow.
- Give high-flow oxygen by face mask and connect a pulse oximeter.
- Establish intravenous access with a large-bore cannula.
- Give intravenous diazepam (5–10 mg slowly initially and in repeated dosage up to 20 mg).
- Check for respiratory depression.
- Collect blood for electrolytes, complete blood picture, arterial blood gas and pH estimation.
- If diazepam does not stop the seizure, load with intravenous phenytoin (1 gm given at a rate of 50 mg/min). Ideally, the phenytoin dosage should be calculated according to weight.
- Monitor blood pressure and ECG during drug administration.
- Be prepared to intubate and ventilate the patient should the seizures persist.
- Barbiturates can be used to control refractory seizures and will involve intubation and ventilation.

Only when control of the seizure is obtained can the underlying cause be sought and treated.

A3 Common causes of status epilepticus in adults include:

- Epilepsy exacerbated by non-compliance with medications, intercurrent illness including the 'flu, other lifestyle factors such as alcohol abuse or use of other recreational drugs or sleep deprivation.
- Head trauma.
- Space-occupying lesion, e.g. brain tumour or metastases.
- Cerebrovascular accident including intracranial bleeds.
- Central nervous system infection.
- Metabolic disorders.
- Medication effects including drug withdrawal.

Any of these causes are possible in this patient. Although there are no signs of meningism or focal neurological signs, meningitis, encephalitis or a subarachnoid haemorrhage are still possibilities. Withdrawal from alcohol or sedative medications should also be considered. Further history would be the most helpful in determining the cause and will determine if further investigations such as a CT scan of the brain are necessary.

A4 The additional information from the brother and the rapid recovery diminishes the need for further investigations. The next investigation would be a CT scan. A negative CT would be followed by a lumbar puncture.

In this instance the underlying cause of the status epilepticus was longstanding primary generalized epilepsy exacerbated by:

- Non-compliance with medication.
- Intercurrent viral illness.
- Alcohol abuse.
- Sleep deprivation after a late night.

An EEG may be useful, not to determine whether a seizure has occurred – this will be apparent from the history – but to determine whether there is interictal epileptic activity to suggest a propensity for seizure recurrence. The EEG will also provide information about the type of potentially epileptic activity, guiding further investigation (particularly if a focal discharge is found) and the choice of anticonvulsant (as in this case).

A5 This patient has generalized tonic–clonic seizures and an EEG pattern of primary generalized epilepsy, rather than focal epilepsy with secondary generalization. This diagnosis influences the optimal choice of anticonvulsant. Single drug therapy with sodium valproate (600–1500 mg/day) would be more appropriate than carbamazepine in this instance. The effectiveness of drug therapy, once the patient is compliant, is best assessed by the clinical reduction in seizure frequency. Serum blood levels can be used to monitor compliance and the optimal dose for the patient. If seizures persist, and particularly when there is the suspicion of secondary generalized epilepsy, carbamazepine or phenytoin plus other anticonvulsants (lamotrigine, gabapentin, topiramate or tiagabine) may be indicated. At this stage referral to a neurologist is advisable.

ANSWERS – cont'd

A6 The patient has had a life-threatening exacerbation of his epilepsy. This is a good time to discuss the importance of better illness management with him. You should emphasize that the combination of non-compliance with medications, a viral illness, sleep deprivation and alcohol make a seizure almost guaranteed. Therefore, he must:

- Be compliant with medication.
- Use alcohol in moderation, e.g. 1–2 drinks daily.
- Avoid alcohol excess particularly binges.
- Avoid sleep deprivation and fatigue.
- Give up driving. Poor control of his epilepsy may impose legal as well as medical limitations on his driving.
- Take precautions at work and with recreation.
- Wear a medical alert bracelet and carry information concerning his diagnosis and medication on his person at all times.

A7 Up to 75% of patients with epilepsy will achieve a seizure-free remission of 2 years on anticonvulsant monotherapy in primary generalized epilepsy. If medication is stopped, about 30–40% will have a recurrence of seizures but nearly two-thirds will remain seizure free. The chance of continued remission after anticonvulsant withdrawal is greatest in those who have been seizure free for more than 2 years on anticonvulsants, and have a single seizure type, a normal neurological examination, no underlying structural abnormality of the brain and a normal EEG. Conversely, those with a structural brain abnormality, an abnormal EEG, more than one seizure type and poor seizure control requiring more than one anticonvulsant medication, have a high risk of seizure recurrence if medication is stopped. The risk of having further seizures and the impact of seizures on daily activities (for example driving) should be taken into account before recommending withdrawal of anticonvulsants.

REVISION POINTS

Management of the first seizure

Emergency care
Check ABC: i.e. airway, breathing and circulation. Stop seizure with intravenous benzodiazepine, e.g. diazepam.

Aetiology
The likely cause depends on the patient's age. Primary epilepsy is unlikely to present for the first time in the elderly but is a common cause in young adults as is drug and alcohol abuse. Space-occupying lesions, cerebrovascular events and metabolic disturbance are all more common causes in the elderly but all causes can occur at any age.

History
You are likely to require an eyewitness.
- How did the seizure start?
- Any aura?
- Any focal or lateralizing features at seizure onset?

- Past history of head trauma, neurological illness, other diseases (e.g. cardiovascular or cancer), drug and alcohol consumption.
- Family history.
- Associated symptoms, e.g. recent headaches, fever.

Investigations
Always search for an underlying cause:
- Neurological disorder:
  – meningitis/encephalitis
  – space-occupying lesion (tumour)
  – cerebrovascular event.
- Metabolic disturbance:
  – hypoglycaemia
  – hyponatraemia
  – hypercalcaemia.
- Drug and alcohol abuse.
- Head injury.

Investigations depend on suspected underlying cause but all patients should have complete

continues overleaf

REVISION POINTS – cont'd

blood picture, glucose, electrolytes and CT scan. Further investigations may include LP, MRI, EEG, toxicology.

Management
Depends on underlying cause. All patients should be given strict advice about driving according to national regulations.

ISSUES TO CONSIDER

- What advice would you give about driving to a young man presenting with a witnessed first fit?
- What non-pharmacological treatments are available for the treatment of debilitating epilepsy?
- What are the detrimental effects of long-term phenytoin therapy?

FURTHER INFORMATION

www.e-epilepsy.org.uk A superb resource for professionals interested in epilepsy from the National Society for Epilepsy. Hundreds of articles, references, literature reviews. Requires (free) registration.

www.epilepsy.org.uk A good website from the British Epilepsy Association with lots of information for patients, carers, professionals. Lots of links.

A middle-aged man with sudden visual loss

A 58-year-old obese man presents distressed, after experiencing a loss of vision in the right eye approximately 2 hours ago. He describes the sensation of a black curtain suddenly dropping in front of that eye, lasting just under 5 minutes. There were no associated ocular symptoms, such as eye pain, and his vision is now normal. You have been treating this patient for essential hypertension for approxi- mately 5 years, although he has not been completely compliant with medication and follow-up for blood pressure monitoring. He has no other significant medical history, and his only medication is atenolol 50 mg daily. He is a smoker. He is feeling physically fit, and you are unable to elicit any additional complaints in a review of symptoms.

Q1 What condition is the patient describing? What are the possible aetiologies?

On examination, you measure the blood pressure at 150/95 mm Hg. Visualization of the retina with a direct ophthalmoscope reveals the finding illustrated in Figure 52.1.

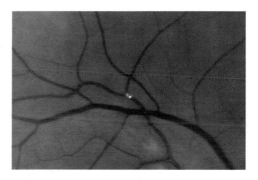

Fig 52.1

Q2 What sign is present in this fundus photograph? What additional physical examination would you perform as part of your initial assessment?

After completing the clinical examination, you arrange carotid Doppler ultrasonography. This indicates a severe (80%) stenosis of the origin of the right internal carotid artery. There is also mild stenosis (no more than 50%) in the region of bifurcation of the left common carotid artery.

What additional investigations would you order at the same time?

After evaluating the results of all investigations, you discuss possible medical treatment and surgical intervention with the patient. The patient tells you that on the evening prior to the review appointment, while he was sitting watching television, his left arm became weak and he was unable to pick up his coffee cup. On trying to stand, he found his left leg was dragging, and he was forced to sit down. The episode lasted approximately 10 minutes.

Q4 What treatment would you recommend to this patient?

The patient decides for the suggested surgical procedure. In preparation for this, the surgeon orders the radiological study illustrated in Figure 52.2.

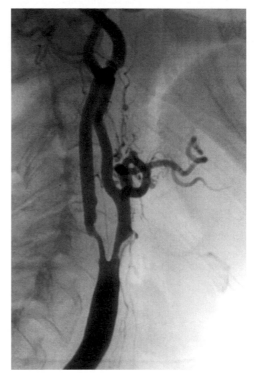

Fig 52.2

Q5 What is this study? Are the findings consistent with the proposed surgical procedure?

The patient undergoes successful carotid surgery. Postoperatively he is maintained on aspirin and vows to get fit. Six months later you hear that he had a cardiac arrest at your local gym.

ANSWERS

A1 This patient has presented with amaurosis fugax, the symptom of sudden-onset transient unilateral visual loss related to an interruption of the ocular circulation. This is a form of transient ischaemic attack (TIA), i.e. a transient cerebral symptom of ischaemic origin, lasting no longer than 24 hours.

Amaurosis fugax, like other TIAs, is most commonly the result of emboli originating from atherosclerotic carotid arteries. Disease is typically located in the region of termination or at the bifurcation of the common carotid artery, or at the origin of the internal carotid artery.

Other sources of emboli include the aortic arch and the heart (mural thrombus, atrial fibrillation and diseased valves). Local thrombosis is a less likely cause of amaurosis fugax.

It is important to consider the possibility of temporal arteritis which may involve the ophthalmic arteries, and has the potential to lead rapidly to arterial occlusion and devastating bilateral blindness. This is most often seen in elderly patients, and other symptoms may include headache, scalp tenderness often apparent when brushing the hair, and jaw claudication, which may occur on chewing food. Polymyalgia rheumatica may co-exist.

Vasculitis or a hypercoagulability state are rare causes, more often seen in younger patients.

A2 Figure 52.1 illustrates an embolus at the branch of a retinal arteriole.

This is most likely a cholesterol embolus or 'Hollenhorst plaque', originating from the carotid arterial system.

When evaluating a patient with amaurosis fugax, a careful cardiovascular examination is essential, including measurement of pulse and blood pressure, examination of carotid and temporal arteries, and assessment of the heart. Remember that the absence of a carotid bruit does not rule out significant carotid disease. Indeed, the most severely diseased carotids often do not have an associated bruit.

This patient has an elevated blood pressure, possibly reflecting poor compliance with antihypertensive medication, which is a risk factor for carotid atherosclerosis.

A3 Other investigations should be chosen for the purposes of excluding risk factors for TIA and stroke. These factors include hypertension, smoking, diabetes mellitus, hyperlipidaemia, cardiac disease and obesity.

Essential investigations should include:
- Urinalysis and fasting serum glucose level.
- Fasting serum lipid profile.
- ECG.

Other investigations:
- Echocardiography is indicated if a significant cardiac abnormality, aortic arch atheroma or mural thrombi are suspected.
- An erythrocyte sedimentation rate (ESR) is an important part of the evaluation for temporal arteritis. The usefulness of the test in this case is debatable. Some would recommend an ESR in any case of retinal arterial ischaemia; others suggest that if a retinal embolus is observed, and there is no clinical evidence of temporal arteritis, determination of the ESR need not be performed.
- When amaurosis fugax occurs in a relatively young person, or if clinical examination suggests an unusual cause, other tests such as autoimmune screening and coagulation studies should be considered to rule out vasculitis and hypercoagulable states.

A4 This patient has suffered a second TIA, perhaps unnecessarily, while awaiting confirmation of the diagnosis. He is at high risk of having a stroke.
- Aspirin has a proven role in reducing the risk of stroke. The exact dose is uncertain, but 300 mg daily is probably appropriate. In the absence of contraindications, this medication can be started immediately if the diagnosis of carotid atheroma is suspected.
- Additional stroke preventative agents such as antiplatelet agents (clopidogrel etc.) have been developed, and in the event that the patient experiences further TIAs after commencement of aspirin, consultation with a neurologist may be advisable.
- Carotid endarterectomy is definitive therapy when performed by a skilled vascular surgeon who has an acceptable complication rate.

ANSWERS – cont'd

Endarterectomy significantly reduces the risk of subsequent stroke for patients with retinal or cerebral ischaemic symptoms related to severe (70–99%) carotid stenotic lesions. Patients with moderate stenoses (50–69%) may benefit from this surgery, but patients with mild stenoses (less than 50%) have no benefit. The role for carotid endarterectomy in the treatment of asymptomatic carotid arterial stenosis is still debated. In this patient, with a high-grade symptomatic right internal carotid arterial stenosis, right carotid endarterectomy would be recommended. However, surgery would not be recommended for the left carotid system. Pharmacological stroke prevention should be continued after the surgery.

- Risk factor reduction is essential. This patient has a number of significant cardiovascular risk factors. Control of blood pressure is important, and tight control will reduce his absolute risk of stroke and of cardiac disease. Cessation of smoking is another important preventative measure. Dietary changes are clearly an issue in this obese patient. If the glucose measurement indicates diabetes mellitus or the lipid profile is abnormal, appropriate dietary and pharmacological measures should be instituted.

A5 This is an intra-arterial digital subtraction carotid angiogram which shows filling of the common carotid, internal carotid and external carotid arteries. This has been the gold standard for evaluating a patient with atherosclerosis of the carotid arterial tree.

This type of study does have a risk of precipitating stroke, and it is reserved for high-risk patients who require surgery. As an imaging tool performed prior to carotid endarterectomy, carotid angiography is being supplanted by spiral CT angiography and magnetic resonance angiography. These latter two procedures are much less invasive. Carotid Doppler examination is still widely used and, in expert hands, remains a sensitive tool for the detection of carotid disease.

In this patient, the angiogram confirms a severe stenosis at the take-off of the right internal carotid artery, consistent with his symptoms of right amaurosis fugax and left-sided weakness. Yet the artery remains patent. This is an important observation, as endarterectomy cannot be performed on a completely occluded vessel. In other words, the angiographic findings are consistent with the proposed surgical procedure.

REVISION POINTS

Amaurosis fugax: carotid atherosclerosis

Definition
Transient ischaemic attack with sudden complete monocular loss of vision due to obstruction of ophthalmic circulation.

Differential diagnoses
- cardiac disease
- aortic arch atheroma
- temporal arteritis
- hypercoagulability syndromes
- vasculitis.

Significance
Increased stroke and cardiac-related mortality.

History focus
- hypertension

- smoking
- diabetes mellitus
- hyperlipidaemia
- cardiac disease.

Examination focus
- pulse
- blood pressure
- carotid arteries
- temporal arteries
- heart.

Investigations
- carotid Doppler ultrasound
- urinalysis
- fasting serum glucose
- fasting serum lipid profile

REVISION POINTS – cont'd

- electrocardiogram
- consider erythrocyte sedimentation rate.

Treatment
- Treat reversible risk factors

- If no contraindications, commence aspirin (300 mg daily)
- Consider carotid endarterectomy.

ISSUES TO CONSIDER

- Revise the anatomy of the cerebral circulation. For each major vessel, what would be the clinical effect of a transient occlusion (TIA) in that vessel?

- How does warfarin compare with aspirin in the secondary prevention of ischaemic strokes?

- What complications of endarterectomy would you warn the patient about when seeking consent?

FURTHER INFORMATION

neurosurgery.mgh.harvard.edu/neurovascular The website of the neurosurgical vascular service at Harvard with lots of information about carotid endarterectomy.

www.pvss.org Website of the Peripheral Vascular Surgical Society with information for patients and professionals including case studies, an atlas and intraoperative photographs.

Hankey G J, Warlow C P. **Treatment and secondary prevention of stroke: evidence, costs, and effects on individuals and populations**. *Lancet* 1999;354(9188):1457–63.

www.emedicine.com/emerg/topic604.htm Transient ischaemic attacks.

A young man in a coma

A young man is brought into the emergency department by ambulance at 9 a.m. He was discovered unconscious in bed by his flatmate that morning. He had been seen at about 10 p.m. the previous evening when he had been well. The flatmate has not accompanied the patient to the hospital but the ambulance officers relate that the flatmate said the patient was previously healthy. The man appears to be in his twenties and is dressed in jeans and a T-shirt. He is still comatose.

Q1 What are you going to do immediately?

Two doctors and two nursing staff attend the patient. Prior to the ambulance officers leaving it is ensured that the patient's personal details are clear and the name of a next of kin is available.

The patient does not respond to pain and has no gag reflex. He accepts a Guedel airway without response. He is breathing spontaneously, his respiratory rate is 14 breaths per minute and he is not cyanosed. There are no obvious signs of external injury. A high-flow oxygen mask is applied and the patient rolled into the coma position.

His pulse is 110 bpm and his blood pressure is 100/60 mm Hg. An axillary temperature is 37°C. An intravenous line is inserted and an infusion of isotonic saline connected. One nurse removes the T-shirt and jeans (the pockets are empty) and applies a cardiac monitor. The other nurse measures his blood sugar, which is 4.9 mmol/l (normal range 4–8).

An intravenous dose of naloxone (0.8 mg) is given and there is no response. Blood is sent for complete blood count, electrolytes, blood alcohol level and a paracetamol concentration. His oxygen saturation is 99% on 8 l/min oxygen.

Q2 Describe and justify what you should look for on examination.

On examination the patient smells of alcohol. He has no spontaneous movements. There are no needle tracks on his arms. His respiration is shallow and regular. He has no gag reflex or response of any of his limbs to painful stimuli. There is no posturing (decorticate or decerebrate) or twitching. His pupils are mid-range, equal and react sluggishly to light. Gaze is conjugate but there are no spontaneous eye movements. The doll's eye or oculocephalic reflex eye movements are absent (i.e. on turning the head from side to side the eyes move with the head as if 'locked with it' rather than moving in the opposite direction by reflex). The corneal reflexes are absent. The patient has no neck stiffness. The limbs are hypotonic and the limb reflexes are difficult to elicit. There is no evidence of trauma to the head. The fundi are normal. The remainder of the examination is unremarkable.

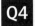

Q3 What are the common causes of coma? What are the likely causes in this patient?

The patient's hospital casenotes are obtained. He is not a known drug abuser. He has made one previous suicide attempt by overdose. On that occasion he took a cocktail of medications and alcohol. He recovered quickly with supportive measures in hospital and was allowed to discharge himself without psychiatric review.

Q4 What substances are of particular concern in this setting?

Soon the patient's flatmate arrives in the emergency department, and brings with him empty medication bottles and tablet foil packaging that he had discovered in the home. He also states that an empty bottle of vodka was next to the patient's bed. From these it is calculated that he may have taken up to 25 x 10 mg tablets temazepam, 25 x 15 mg tablets oxazepam, 40 x 500 mg tablets paracetamol and 30 x 75 mg dothiepin (dosulepin), and half a litre of vodka.

Q5 What is your general management plan at this point?

His serum paracetamol concentrations come back from the laboratory as:
- 700 µmol/l at 9 a.m.
- 500 µmol/l at 11 a.m. (see Figure 53.1).

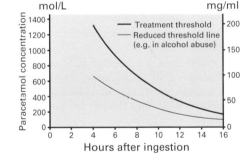

Fig 53.1

Q6 How do you interpret these drug concentrations and what should be done?

A 12-lead ECG shows sinus tachycardia, a QRS complex of 0.12 seconds and non-specific T-wave abnormalities (dimpling). The pCO_2 and pH are within the normal range. The patient is intubated and gastric lavage performed and activated charcoal is given via the nasogastric tube.

A urinary catheter is inserted and urine also saved for toxicology analysis if necessary. A chest X-ray reveals no abnormality.

The patient is cared for in the intensive care unit and given the standard course of intravenous acetylcysteine. Initially he is mechanically ventilated until his conscious state improves, allowing extubation 6 hours later. He continues to have cardiac monitoring for 24 hours by which time the ECG abnormalities resolve.

Q7 What's the next step in management?

He does not suffer any further complications from his self-poisoning and on recovery is transferred to the psychiatry ward for further management.

ANSWERS

A1 This is a medical emergency and the principles of emergency management must be followed. Many of the actions outlined below will be undertaken simultaneously, and ideally by a team of two doctors and two nurses.

A: Check the airway for obstruction, vomitus, etc. Insert a Guedel airway. If the patient accepts the airway without any gag reflex, this provides an objective measure of his neurological state and also tells you that his airway is at risk.

B: Check that he is breathing spontaneously. Apply high-flow oxygen immediately. Measure his respiratory rate.

Now log roll the patient on to his side (the 'coma position'). If there is any possibility of injury the cervical spine must be kept in alignment. Suction equipment should be at the ready in case of vomiting. Monitor oxygen saturation.

C: Measure blood pressure and pulse, assessing him for signs of shock (circulation). Insert a large bore intravenous cannula, noting his response to painful stimuli. Take blood for laboratory analysis.

Commence intravenous isotonic saline. Monitor cardiac rhythm.

Hypoglycaemia is easily treated, easily missed and can be fatal. Perform a bedside glucose test immediately. If there is delay or any doubt, administer 50 ml 50% glucose intravenously. This will not do any harm and, if the patient is hypoglycaemic, may save his life.

- Give 100 mg intravenous thiamine.
- Administer intravenous naloxone. The man is young, apparently previously healthy, and is now deeply unconscious. Opioid drug overdose is a common cause of this presentation (pinpoint pupils and needle tracks on the

arms are not universally present). Naloxone is not harmful and will reverse an opiate coma, but it should be given in small increments (e.g. 200 mg doses) as sudden reversal of an opioid overdose may lead to severe and dangerous withdrawal symptoms and an aggressive, uncooperative and delirious patient.

Note: Administration of flumazenil, a benzodiazepine antagonist, is contraindicated. It may cause intractable seizures in patients who have taken tricyclic antidepressants.

- Call the anaesthesia team as his airway is threatened and he may need intubation.
- Remove the patient's clothing and search for medical details, next of kin contact details and illicit drugs.
- A drug overdose, which is often done together with alcohol, is by far the most likely diagnosis of coma in a previously well young person. Therefore a blood alcohol level, a paracetamol concentration, full blood count, electrolytes, arterial blood gases, and ECG should be performed. Blood can be saved for further toxicology analysis if necessary, although so-called routine 'drug screens' are not useful as they rarely alter management (being qualitative, they are neither sensitive nor specific in making a diagnosis of overdose).
- While all of this is being done a more formal examination of the patient is made by other members of the resuscitation/emergency team.

A2 The degree of unconsciousness should be determined both for initial diagnostic purposes and to act as a baseline for future comparison by calculating and recording his Glasgow Coma Score (GCS), as shown in Table 53.1.

ANSWERS – cont'd

Table 53.1 The Glasgow Coma Score

Eye opening	Motor response	Verbal response
4 Spontaneous	6 Obeys commands	5 Orientated
3 To voice	5 Localizes to pain	4 Confused
2 To pain	4 Withdraws from pain	3 Inappropriate words
1 None	3 Flexion to pain	2 Incomprehensible sounds
	2 Extension to pain	1 None
	1 None	

The patient makes no response to pain or command, either in terms of eye opening or verbal response. His score on GCS is 3 – the lowest possible score.

Look for obvious signs of trauma, especially head injury, the presence of needle tracks, evidence of chronic illness such as a medical alert bracelet and signs of intoxication. Overt skin rashes should be checked for, e.g. the petechial rash of meningococcal septicaemia.

Your respiratory examination should include an assessment of his respiratory pattern. Markedly abnormal breathing patterns are seen in brainstem damage. Compensatory hyperventilation is seen early in metabolic acidosis (e.g. diabetic ketoacidosis, salicylate, methanol, ethylene glycol and other poisonings). Hypoventilation is common in all causes of generalized CNS depression.

Spontaneous movements indicate a lesser degree of unconsciousness. Twitching and jerking might indicate seizure activity or serotonergic toxicity. These should not be confused with muscle fasciculation, which would indicate possibility of organophosphate poisoning. Decorticate or decerebrate posturing or asymmetric responses to pain may indicate neurological injury or dysfunction.

The eyes should be held open and the pupils, oculocephalic reflex (doll's eye movements), spontaneous eye movements and fundi examined. Large pupils are common in overdose of sympathomimetic (e.g. amphetamines) and anticholin-ergic drugs (e.g. antihistamines, tricyclic antidepressants). They also occur with drugs that cause retinal toxicity (e.g. quinine, methanol). Small pupils are common with opioid, anticholinesterase and antipsychotic drug overdose. Both large and small pupils can also occur with midbrain or brainstem damage. A unilateral fixed dilated pupil indicates an ipsilateral third nerve palsy, which occurs when raised intracranial pressure leads to tentorial herniation. In this setting it might indicate an expanding extradural or subdural haematoma.

The limbs should be tested for tone, response to painful stimuli and reflexes. Neck stiffness should be excluded.

A general examination of the rest of the patient is often normal but may reveal evidence of anticholinergic signs or evidence of major organ failure. Regular observations such as respiratory rate, pulse, blood pressure and temperature, as well as pupillary size and reaction and the Glasgow Coma Score should be taken and serially recorded.

A3 The most common causes of coma vary, depending on the initial examination findings. The following list is by no means exhaustive. Whatever the cause, all unconscious patients should receive the same initial emergency management.

1 Localizing cerebral hemisphere signs:
   - closed head injury
   - intracranial haemorrhage (intracerebral, extradural or subdural, subarachnoid)

ANSWERS – cont'd

- raised intracranial pressure due to a space-occupying lesion.

2 Signs of brainstem dysfunction alone:
- brainstem haemorrhage or infarct
- pressure on the brainstem from above (coning) or from the posterior fossa.

3 Meningism:
- subarachnoid haemorrhage
- meningitis or encephalitis.

4 No specific neurological features:
- toxic encephalopathy – poisoning
- metabolic encephalopathy – hypo- or hyperglycaemic coma, hepatic encephalopathy, hyponatraemia.

This patient was apparently well the previous night and has no evidence of major medical disorder. He was found deeply unconscious with evidence of alcohol consumption. A catastrophic intracranial event such as an intracerebral bleed is possible but there are no localizing signs or neck stiffness. This must be excluded, but self-poisoning is the most likely diagnosis. The depressed but symmetrical pupil and tendon reflexes are consistent with this diagnosis.

A4 The main causes of death from poisoning out of hospital include:
- Carbon monoxide.
- Opioids.
- Tricyclic antidepressants (TCAs).
- Alcohol.
- A variety of sleeping tablets.

Many of these respond well to supportive care alone. In hospital the poisons which remain a major concern are those that:
- Are cardiotoxic (e.g. most antiarrhythmic drugs, TCAs, chloroquine).
- Have delayed onset of toxicity (e.g. paracetamol, iron, overdose on 'slow-release' medications).
- Are designed to kill (e.g. pesticides, herbicides, cytotoxic drugs, bleach).
- Frequently lead to long-term morbidity (e.g. heavy metals, carbon monoxide, theophylline).

Note that most of these substances are not detected by the average 'drug screen'.

A5 It should be assumed that the patient has taken an overdose of all these medications.
- Contact your local poisons advice centre if you are not familiar with the management of these drugs in overdose.
- Patients with a GCS <8 usually need to be intubated and admitted to an intensive care unit. This patient cannot protect his airway and will definitely require intubation.
- Gastric lavage is sometimes performed but has little evidence to support its use. In inexperienced hands it can be dangerous.
- Activated charcoal should be given via a nasogastric tube.
- A chest X-ray should be performed to identify evidence of aspiration.
- A 12-lead ECG should be done in all comatose patients suspected to have overdosed. In TCA poisoning, the most common abnormalities include tachycardia, non-specific ST segment and T-wave changes, widening of the QRS complex, an increased QTc and increase in the R/S ratio in aVR (a partial RBBB pattern). The last three abnormalities indicate a greatly increased risk of life-threatening cardiac arrhythmias. If the drug is still being absorbed then a normal ECG on admission may be misleading. The ECG must be repeated after a few hours in all patients with suspected drug-induced coma. If the patient has a suspected or confirmed tricyclic overdose, they should be transferred to an intensive care unit for continuous monitoring.
- An arterial blood gas should also be done to monitor the acid–base status of the patient. Acidosis is associated with hypotension and cardiac complications in TCA poisoning and a pH of about 7.5 should be maintained by mechanical hyperventilation in this patient.
- Salicylate and paracetamol levels should be measured in all patients with a suspected overdose regardless of what they seem to have taken.

Overdoses produce various physiological effects which need to be treated, such as tachycardia, seizures or hypotension. Current emergency medical teaching is to 'treat the patient, not the poison'. Recent thinking employs the concept of

A N S W E R S – cont'd

'toxidromes' which are groups of symptoms and signs producing a clinical picture in different overdose settings. Table 53.2 illustrates the different groups of 'toxidromes'.

Table 53.2 Toxidromes

Stimulant (e.g. amphetamines)	Sedative/hypnotic (e.g. alcohol)	Opiate (e.g. heroin)	Anticholinergic	Cholinergic (opposite of anticholinergic)
Restlessness	Sedation	Pinpoint pupils	Blurred vision	Salivation
Excessive speech	Confusion	Unresponsiveness	Mydriasis	Lacrimation
Excessive motor activity	Paraesthesia	Slow respiratory rate	Dry skin	Urination
Tremor	Diplopia	Shallow respiration	Urinary retention	Defaecation
Insomnia	Blurred vision	Bradycardia	Flushing	Diarrhoea
Tachycardia	Slurred speech	Decreased bowel sounds	Fever	Vomiting
Hallucinations	Ataxia	Hypothermia	Tachycardia	Bradycardia
	Nystagmus		Hallucinations	
	Hallucinations		Psychosis	
	Coma			

A6 Interpretation of the paracetamol nomogram:

- The nomogram indicates the risk of hepatic injury associated with a paracetamol concentration at a known time after ingestion.
- In theory, if the paracetamol concentration lies above the treatment line, N-acetylcysteine should be given. N-acetylcysteine should ideally be started within 8 hours of ingestion.
- In practice, the timing of drug overdose is notoriously unreliable. If the patient has taken a substantial amount of paracetamol (>7.5 gm in an adult) and there is any doubt whatsoever, treatment should be started even if the concentration lies below the treatment line. Always seek expert advice.
- In this patient anywhere between 2 and 12 hours could have elapsed since ingestion. It is impossible to accurately plot this concentration on the nomogram. Treatment with N-acetylcysteine should start immediately.

A7 All patients with deliberate self-poisoning should be assessed by psychiatric services. Self-poisoning is the presentation of an underlying psychiatric or substance abuse problem, which clearly is potentially life-threatening and thus can also be considered a psychiatric emergency to be managed once the acute medical issues have resolved. If these issues are not addressed the patient is likely to present again or successfully commit suicide.

It is useful to classify episodes of attempted self-harm by lethality and by intent, depending on the method used and the patient's intentions. A paracetamol overdose may be a low intent but often high lethality overdose, as patients may not realize how dangerous large quantities of paracetamol can be. This patient must be seen by the psychiatric service prior to discharge. It is not usually necessary to detain all overdose patients under the Mental Health Act; however, this may be required to allow safe treatment and follow-up by appropriate services.

REVISION POINTS

Coma

Definition

Coma is a state of deep unconsciousness where the patient does not wake up with external stimuli.

Emergency care

Airway, Breathing and Circulation: i.e. secure the airway and ensure adequate respiration, check pulse and blood pressure, insert an intravenous line and connect to a cardiac monitor so as to identify arrhythmias.

Risk factors

Examples of coma which lead rapidly to very different pathways of investigation and management include patients who:

- have severe medical disorders (e.g. chronic obstructive airways disease with respiratory failure, chronic liver disease or uraemia, diabetes)
- collapsed after suffering a sudden onset severe headache (subarachnoid haemorrhage)
- have pinpoint pupils and needle tracks (narcotic overdose)
- are found surrounded with empty pill bottles
- have localizing neurological signs, necessitating emergency CT scan of the brain and neurosurgical review.

Self-poisoning is a very common cause of coma and two-thirds of patients ingest more than one substance, and may manifest confusing signs from the combined effects of multiple drugs.

Routine screening for drugs is rarely useful and is expensive.

Management

The management of the comatose patient due to a drug overdose is largely supportive. Some specific measures to consider include:

- early consideration of intubation to prevent aspiration and manage airway
- gastric lavage only if seen soon after drug ingestion
- administration of activated charcoal if possible within a few hours of paracetamol ingestion
- exclude and treat hypoglycaemia
- naloxone is routinely given, but should be titrated slowly in a known opioid overdose.

Features to look for in examination of the comatose patient and the classification of causes of coma accordingly are outlined in Answers 2 and 3.

Paracetamol overdose (POD)

Epidemiology

- paracetamol is the most frequently ingested drug in the Western world
- POD is the most common drug overdose in the UK and if untreated can be lethal.

Pharmacology

Overdose saturates the normal metabolic pathways of conjugation by the hepatocytes. Paracetamol metabolism is then diverted to the oxidative pathway (CYP450) leading to toxic intermediate metabolites which accumulate to cause lethal hepatotoxicity.

Treatment

The use of the paracetamol nomogram is important in determining the need for N-acetylcysteine therapy. The nomogram indicates the risk of hepatic injury associated with a paracetamol concentration at a known time after ingestion.

Adequate history to establish time of ingestion is therefore very useful. If in doubt, treat as the 'worst-case scenario'.

N-acetylcysteine is an effective antidote, which should ideally be given within 8–10 hours of ingestion. It is still helpful in overdoses presenting late and in patients with established hepatotoxicity. It works by liberating cysteine allowing for resynthesis of hepatic glutathione. In patients intolerant of N-acetylcysteine, oral methionine is a less effective alternative.

Peak hepatotoxicity may not occur for some days. Following a significant overdose, the INR should be monitored for 24–48 hours. Patients with signs of significant hepatotoxicity should be discussed early with a liver unit. These signs include a worsening coagulopathy, rising creatinine, acidosis and the development of hepatic encephalopathy. A small proportion of patients will develop acute liver failure and some come to liver transplant.

Follow-up of patients with deliberate self-poisoning and attempted suicide is an important area, and coordination of mental health and support services is essential to prevent the patient undergoing further self-harm, and to treat the underlying causes.

ISSUES TO CONSIDER

- Identify the formal steps that you would need to taken to arrange the detention of a patient with an acute psychiatric illness
- How would you treat a carbon monoxide poisoning?
- What are the criteria for liver transplantation in paracetamol overdose? What other factors would need to be taken into consideration if this situation arose?

FURTHER INFORMATION

www.hypertox.com Downloadable toxicology software.

www.pharmweb.net Excellent UK site; follow the links to the paracetamol information service with detailed info on all aspects of the drug.

A 31-year-old woman with vertigo

A 31-year-old teacher presents to your general practice with a 2-day history of a sensation of the room spinning and unsteadiness while walking. The sensation is continuous and partially relieved by lying down. These symptoms have prevented her from going to work. There are no obvious precipitating factors. She otherwise feels well, is not nauseated and does not have a headache. She feels her hearing is normal and she has no tinnitus. She does not complain of any other neurological symptoms. Her only medication is the oral contraceptive pill.

Q1 What are the principles of assessing a patient with vertigo?

Q2 How do you differentiate central from peripheral causes of vertigo? What are some causes of each?

On examination she appears fit and well. She is afebrile and her cardiovascular examination is normal. The ear canals and tympanic membranes appear normal. There is no evidence of hearing impairment on clinical testing. Visual acuity testing reveals 6/6 vision on the right but 6/9 on the left. The pupils are symmetrical, but there is an afferent pupillary defect on the left. On fundoscopy the left optic disc appears pale compared to the right.

On testing the external ocular movements there is nystagmus on looking to the right and on vertical gaze. The nystagmus is independent of head position and is not fatigable. The remainder of the cranial nerve examination is intact. On examination of the limbs the tone, power and reflexes are normal. However, on finger-nose testing there is an intention tremor of the right arm and rapid alternating movements are performed less well with the right hand compared with the left. Otherwise coordination is intact, as are the sensory modalities.

On further questioning the patient recalls that she had problems in taking a photograph using her left eye while on holiday 3 months previously. This had resolved spontaneously over 1 week and she did not pursue the matter. She had also recently noticed a mild tremor of her right hand particularly when dressing, but this had not disturbed her greatly as she is left-handed.

There is nothing else in the history and from the examination that helped elucidate the cause of the patient's current problem.

Q3 How do you interpret this woman's neurological signs?

Given the probable site of the problem, the patient is referred to a neurologist. Her vertigo had improved but has not resolved completely.

Various tests were performed. Figures 54.1 and 54.2 were taken from one of the tests.

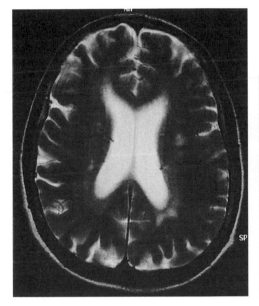

Fig 54.1   **Fig 54.2**

Q4 Name the investigation and describe the abnormalities.

Q5 What is the likely diagnosis and what other tests could be done to further support the diagnosis?

The cerebrospinal fluid showed a moderate elevation of mononuclear cells and protein and was positive for oligoclonal bands.

After the diagnosis is made, the patient returns to see you. Her symptoms have largely resolved. She asks what her prognosis is and if any treatment is available.

Q6 What is your reply?

ANSWERS

A1 Vertigo is a sensation of movement, typically spinning or rotating, either of the environment or the patient in relation to the environment. This spinning sensation distinguishes vertigo from pre-syncopal 'dizziness' which occurs in cardiac arrhythmias, postural hypotension, anaemia or hypoglycaemia. A history of loss of consciousness suggests syncope or epilepsy.

The major task in the assessment of vertigo is to decide whether the cause is peripheral (related to the vestibular apparatus) or central (vestibular nuclei and connections). Central causes of vertigo may be more sinister, and a thorough neurological examination is required in patients presenting with new-onset vertigo.

On examination attention should be paid to a full neurological examination looking for focal signs suggesting a central cause. In particular:

- examine the eyes looking for nystagmus
- examine the external ear, including the tympanic membrane and hearing.

You will also need to perform a screening general physical examination.

A2 Signs suggesting central nervous system involvement include:

- vertical nystagmus
- internuclear ophthalmoplegia
- facial sensory loss
- upper motor neurone signs and limb or gait ataxia.

Examples of central lesions causing vertigo include:

- vertebrobasilar ischaemia
- demyelination (e.g. multiple sclerosis)
- cerebellar disease
- basilar migraine
- temporal lobe epilepsy (rare)
- cerebellopontine angle tumour. The most common is a schwannoma of the vestibular nerve, but these typically produce progressive deafness rather than vertigo, and may be associated with ataxia and other neurological signs such as facial sensory loss.

Examples of peripheral causes of vertigo include:

- benign paroxysmal positional vertigo
- vestibular neuronitis
- Ménière's disease
- middle ear disease.

A3 This woman has multiple signs of CNS pathology supporting a central cause of vertigo. The vertical nystagmus suggests brainstem dysfunction. The pale left optic disc suggests optic nerve disease and intention tremor of the right arm suggests a disorder of the right cerebellar hemisphere or its connections.

She has no tinnitus, deafness or nausea and does not find that head turning precipitates vertigo. She is otherwise well. This would be unusual for any of the common peripheral causes of vertigo.

A4 These are T2-weighted MRI scans of the brain. They show multiple high T2 and FLAIR signal foci throughout both corona radiata and the corpus callosum white matter. The morphology and distribution of these white matter plaques are non-specific, but in a young patient are quite consistent with demyelination, particularly with this clinical presentation.

A5 This woman has a number of features in her illness that point to central nervous system disease:

- left optic atrophy (previous optic neuritis)
- vertigo and nystagmus (brainstem dysfunction)
- poor control of right arm movement (cerebellar disturbance)
- multiple white plaques on MRI.

The presence of multiple symptoms, occurring over time, related to different sites within the central nervous system, and the finding of multiple demyelinating lesions within the central nervous system make multiple sclerosis (MS) the most likely diagnosis.

Vertigo is an unusual presenting symptom in MS, though one-third of patients will experience this symptom during the course of the illness.

Cerebrospinal fluid (CSF) obtained at lumbar puncture could be examined. The most characteristic finding in MS is an increase in CSF IgG, which fractionates into oligoclonal bands on electrophoresis. Evoked visual response testing would not be relevant in this case because the

ANSWERS – cont'd

patient has optic atrophy. Therefore we know already that this is a site of disease.

A6 It is too early to say what her prognosis is since the course of the disease is often unpredictable. Multiple sclerosis can vary from a relapsing and remitting pattern with near complete recovery after each relapse, to those who are left with permanent residual deficits after each relapse. Approximately half of the latter group will develop progressive disease. In a further group, predominantly aged over 40, the disease is slowly progressive from the outset with spinal cord dysfunction being the major feature. Currently, the average survival is at least 30 years from the diagnosis.

There is no curative treatment for the disease. Acute episodes can be treated with oral glucocorticoids or high-dose intravenous methylpred-

nisolone. This hastens recovery of function but does not alter the degree of recovery from acute relapses or the longer term prognosis. In established relapsing-remitting MS, immunomodulation with interferon beta has been shown to reduce the rate of clinical relapse by 30%. The severity of relapse and number of lesions on MRI are also reduced. Glatiramer acetate produces a similar effect. Immunosuppression with azathioprine, methotrexate, cyclophosphamide or ciclosporin A in progressive MS may reduce the rate of progression, but this benefit needs to be balanced against the toxic side effects of these drugs. Supportive treatment particularly for spasticity (e.g. baclofen and physiotherapy) and urinary dysfunction are important. Psychological support is also vital and patients may benefit from involvement with national MS societies and support groups.

REVISION POINTS

Multiple sclerosis

Definition
A demyelinating disease of the central nervous system.

Aetiology
The aetiology is uncertain although autoimmunity or infectious precipitants have been proposed.

Clinical features
The disease is characterized by plaques of demyelination scattered throughout the central nervous system 'disseminated in time and space'. It often begins in early adult life and is more common in women.

Symptoms and signs correspond to involvement of cerebral hemispheres, brainstem, cerebellum or spinal cord.

Diagnosis
- Multiple symptoms and lesions within the CNS need to be demonstrated occurring over time. If the symptoms and signs can be accounted for by a single lesion then the diagnosis cannot be made.

- Visual and somatosensory evoked response testing may reveal subclinical conduction defects.
- Plaques on MRI scanning will provide evidence of additional lesions that enable the diagnosis to be made.

Optic neuritis
- Presents as unilateral partial or complete central visual loss associated with pain on eye movement.
- In the acute phase the optic disc will appear normal. Subsequently optic atrophy will occur as evidenced by disc pallor as in this case.
- It is reversible in two-thirds.
- However, in women, 75% of those with optic neuritis will go on to develop MS.

Vertigo

Clinical symptoms to assist in deciding whether vertigo is of central or peripheral origin are shown in Table 54.1.

continues overleaf

REVISION POINTS – cont'd

Table 54.1 Clinical symptoms of vertigo

	Peripheral	Central
Characteristics	Severe, episodic	Mild, semicontinuous
Precipitants	Head movement, typically turning, lying down in bed	May be exacerbated by movement
Exacerbating factors	Head movement	Head movement
Interval after movement	Few seconds	Immediate
Duration	Several seconds	Continuous
Nystagmus	Mixed horizontal/torsional suppressed by fixation	Horizontal, vertical, gaze provoked, not suppressed by fixation
Associated features	Deafness, tinnitus	Brainstem signs, e.g. facial numbness, diplopia, ataxia, weakness
Causes	Vestibular neuronitis, Ménière's disease, benign paroxysmal positional vertigo, middle ear disease	Ischaemia, demyelination

ISSUES TO CONSIDER

- What other conditions may cause disc pallor and optic atrophy?
- Sudden unilateral loss or diminution of vision has a number of causes – what are they?

FURTHER INFORMATION

www.nejm.com Noseworthy J et al. **Multiple sclerosis**. *New England Journal of Medicine* September 2000: 938–52.

www.msfacts.org The multiple sclerosis website with information for patients and health professionals. Many links.

Headache in a middle-aged woman

A 48-year-old woman comes into the emergency department with an 8-hour history of headache. The headache came on suddenly while she was playing tennis at a friend's house. It started at the back of her head on both sides and radiated down her neck. It was severe, and is the worst headache she has ever had. It forced her to stop playing and lie down for 2 hours. During that time she felt nauseated and vomited once.

By the time she arrives in the emergency department she feels considerably improved, although exhausted. She then waits 2 hours before being seen by a doctor by which time she wants to go home. She has no significant past medical history, is on no medications, is a non-smoker and drinks about 100 grams of alcohol a week. She does not usually suffer with headaches and has never had one like this before. She did not strain her neck in any unusual way while playing tennis.

The examination is normal and the patient is discharged home with a provisional diagnosis of musculoskeletal strain and a viral illness with a differential diagnosis of migraine.

Q1 What important diagnosis should have been considered and excluded in this patient?

Twenty-four hours later the patient is brought into the emergency department by ambulance. She collapsed suddenly at home and was unconscious for approximately 15 minutes. She began to regain consciousness in the ambulance.

Q2 What will you look for on your examination?

On examination her blood pressure is 130/70 mm Hg and her pulse rate is 90 bpm. Examination of the rest of the cardiovascular system is unremarkable.

She can be roused and responds to commands, but is confused. She has evidence of meningeal irritation including neck stiffness and limitation of straight leg raising.

On neurological examination there is a partial right ptosis and the right pupil is larger that the left. The right eye does not adduct fully on looking to the left. Otherwise there are no other focal neurological signs. Fundoscopy shows the abnormality depicted in Figure 55.1.

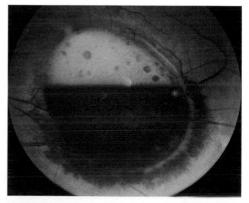

Fig 55.1

Q3 What is the abnormality and what is its significance?

An emergency investigation was performed. Two of the images are shown (Figures 55.2 and 55.3).

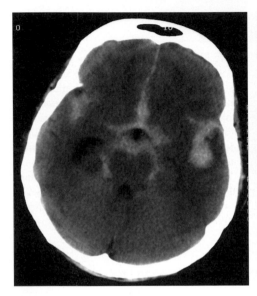

Fig 55.2

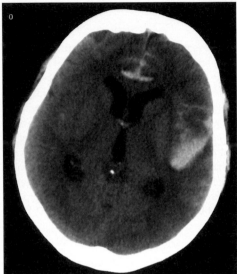

Fig 55.3

Q4 What abnormalities are shown on these images?

The patient immediately went on to have a further investigation. One view from this study is shown (Figure 55.4).

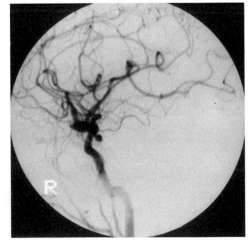

Fig 55.4

What does this investigation show? How does the finding relate to her symptoms?

The patient went on to have immediate emergency neurosurgery. The aneurysm was clipped to prevent further haemorrhage.

 What is a potential major complication of her condition and how can it be prevented?

She was kept well hydrated and placed on the calcium channel antagonist nimodipine from the time of admission in an attempt to reduce the severity of cerebral vasospasm. She was also placed on the anticonvulsant phenytoin postoperatively to prevent seizures.

 What options, other than surgery, exist for preventing rupture of cerebral arterial aneurysms?

Her neurological state gradually improves and 2 weeks after the operation the right third cranial nerve palsy resolves. She subsequently makes a full recovery and is able to return to playing tennis.

ANSWERS

A1 Headache is a common presenting complaint for emergency departments and in general practice. The majority of these have 'benign' causes. It is important to be able to recognize symptoms and signs that signify more serious pathology.

This woman's history is classic of a 'warning leak' of a cerebral aneurysm, i.e. a subarachnoid haemorrhage (SAH). The particular features that suggest this are:
- severe pain: 'the worst headache ever'
- sudden onset: 'like being hit over the back of the head'
- nausea and vomiting
- uncharacteristic for this patient
- spontaneous improvement.

Patients presenting with severe migraine or tension headache have nearly always had a similar type of headache before. In addition these types of headache are usually not sudden in onset and migraine and tension headaches do not improve quickly.

The patient should have been admitted and an emergency CT scan performed. If this was negative a lumbar puncture should have been performed looking for the presence of red blood cells and xanthochromia.

Even if these studies were negative, in a patient with a 'good' history some clinicians would have recommended cerebral angiography to exclude an aneurysm. The reason for this is that early surgery for subarachnoid haemorrhage in patients with no neurological deficit has excellent results. If an initial small bleed is missed the patient is likely to suffer a further bleed. The greatest risk of this is within the first 24 hours after a warning bleed. The sequelae of a second or third haemorrhage are frequently disastrous.

A much less invasive investigation than angiography is CT or magnetic resonance angiography (MRA). Figure 55.5 is an MRA and shows an aneurysm of the right middle cerebral artery. Although these investigations do not as yet provide sufficient information for surgery, they will usually detect aneurysms greater than 2 mm in diameter and are often used for screening in cases where the clinical

ANSWERS – cont'd

suspicion of SAH is not high enough to warrant angiography but not low enough to ignore completely.

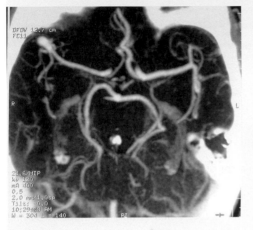

Fig 55.5

A2 You should assess her Glasgow Coma Score (see p. 313) and her ability to protect her own airway. If there is any doubt, an anaesthetist should be called for possible intubation.

She should have a full neurological examination looking for evidence of focal neurology such as cranial nerve palsies and pyramidal signs. You must examine her fundi looking for evidence of papilloedema and subhyaloid haemorrhage. You should look for evidence of meningism such as neck stiffness, photophobia and a positive Kernig's sign (back and neck pain limiting her straight leg raise).

She should have a full general examination looking for evidence of infection or other causes for her collapse.

A3 The retinal photograph shows a large subhyaloid haemorrhage at the posterior pole, overlying the fovea. This shows a classic 'inverted D' appearance and is pathognomonic of subarachnoid haemorrhage. This physical sign is not common.

A4 These are plain CT scans of the brain. There is evidence of subarachnoid blood (which is white) in the basal cisterns, the interhemispheric fissure (anteriorly) and is most prevalent in the left Sylvian fissure. There is no evidence of infarction.

A5 This is a lateral view of a cerebral angiogram. A saccular aneurysm is visible at the take-off of the right posterior communicating artery from the internal carotid artery. The posterior communicating artery itself is not seen. An aneurysm in this position explains her partial right oculomotor nerve palsy.

A6 Cerebral vasospasm is a complication of subarachnoid haemorrhage which can occur from the end of the first week to 14 days after a bleed. It is a constriction of cerebral arteries which can result in infarction (stroke) and death and is thought to be triggered by breakdown products of red blood cells in the subarachnoid space causing cerebral vessels to spasm.

Untreated, about 30% of patients will die and a similar number will suffer permanent neurological deficit. It is thought that the likelihood of the complication occurring is proportional to the amount of blood in the subarachnoid space.

Traditionally this is prevented by maintaining high cerebral perfusion pressure. To do this, intravenous fluid hydration and vasopressor agents (dopamine, ephedrine) may be required. More recently, the calcium channel blocker nimodipine has been used to decrease vasospasm. Nimodipine is a peripheral vasodilator although the exact mechanism of action on cerebral circulation is unclear. It is used for both prevention and treatment of cerebral spasm, but hypotension must be avoided as it may precipitate cerebral infarction.

Hyponatraemia is also a common complication due to inappropriate release of ADH, and may cause a 'cerebral salt-wasting syndrome'. Close monitoring of serum sodium is required.

A7 Endovascular coiling techniques (GDC coils) are a major recent change in the management of aneurysmal subarachnoid haemorrhage. These platinum metal coils are introduced under radiological control through a catheter inserted

ANSWERS – cont'd

into the femoral artery and guided to the neck of the aneurysm. As the coils are released they fold in upon themselves. Multiple coils are used to pack the aneurysm and exclude it from the circulation.

Not all aneurysms are amenable to coiling but the most suitable are often those that are the most difficult to treat surgically (e.g. basilar aneurysms). In some centres there are now more aneurysms being coiled than clipped but this is highly dependent on local experience. The decision about how to treat an individual case is made jointly between neurosurgeons and neuroradiologists.

REVISION POINTS

Subarachnoid haemorrhage

Epidemiology
- 50% mortality rate
- 70% are caused by rupture of saccular ('berry') aneurysms
- 70% of patients will have a 'warning leak'
- many rebleeds occur within 24 hrs of warning bleed
- the rebleed may be catastrophic
- patients with minimal neurological deficits tend to fare better.

Clinical features
- sudden severe headache
- 'never had headache like this before'
- examination may be normal but look for photophobia and neck stiffness
- have high index of suspicion and low threshold for ordering a CT scan
- if CT is normal and the history is convincing, a lumbar puncture should be done

- further imaging will be with angiography (or CTA/MRA)
- emphasis on early diagnosis and early surgery to minimize the risk of a rebleed and improve prognosis.

Treatment
- surgery or endovascular coiling to exclude the aneurysm from the circulation
- complications include rebleeding prior to clipping/coiling, vasospasm, hydrocephalus, electrolyte disturbances and pulmonary oedema.

Advances in the management of the condition have focused on:
- early surgical intervention
- strategies to reduce the risk of cerebral vasospasm
- use of minimally-invasive imaging techniques
- endovascular coiling techniques.

ISSUES TO CONSIDER

- How would you advise a patient who had an asymptomatic saccular aneurysm noted incidentally during cerebral imaging?
- What other medical conditions are associated with an increased incidence of cerebral arterial aneurysms?
- What are other common causes of headache and how are they treated?

FURTHER INFORMATION

www.neurosurgery.org The official website of the American Association of Neurological Surgeons with lots of excellent articles, links and images.

www.headaches.org Website of the National Headache Foundation. Patient centred but with links to research, pharmaceutical companies and patient support groups.

Back pain in a 50-year-old woman

A 50-year-old waitress complains of several weeks of increasingly severe mid and low back pain. Apart from an episode of low back pain following heavy lifting 10 years ago, she has no significant past medical history. She cannot recall any precipitant for the pain. She has been taking paracetamol and naproxen with minimal relief. Although the pain is worst on movement, it is also present at rest and has now started to wake her at night. She has smoked over 20 cigarettes daily for 30 years. She also states she has become more lethargic recently.

On examination she moves slowly due to pain, and is pale. Examination of her cardiovascular system is unremarkable. Similarly, there is nothing abnormal to find on abdominal examination. Her spine is tender to palpation at T5, T10 and the lumbar region. There are several areas of rib tenderness bilaterally. There are no neurological signs in the lower limbs.

Q1 What are the possible causes of this woman's back pain? What initial investigations should be requested?

Plain X-rays of the chest and thoracolumbar spine are performed. The thoracolumbar spine X-ray shows generalized osteopaenia, mottling of the bones and erosion of several vertebral pedicles. The chest X-ray is shown in Figure 56.1.

Results of the complete blood picture, ESR and biochemistry include:

Investigation 56.1 Summary of results			
Haemoglobin	91 g/l	White cell count	4.1 x 10^9/l
MCV	86 fl	ESR	130 mm/hr
MCH	29 pg		
MCHC	340 g/l		
Platelets	211 x 10^9/l		
Sodium	130 mmol/l	Calcium	2.8 mmol/l
Potassium	4.1 mmol/l	Phosphate	0.45 mmol/l
Chloride	106 mmol/l	Albumin	38 g/l
Bicarbonate	27 mmol/l	Bilirubin	15 µmol/l
Urea	20.1 mmol/l	ALT	18 U/l
Creatinine	0.21 mmol/l	AST	20 U/l
Uric acid	0.24 mmol/l	GGT	30 U/l
Glucose	4.6 mmol/l	ALP	90 U/l
LDH	188 U/l		

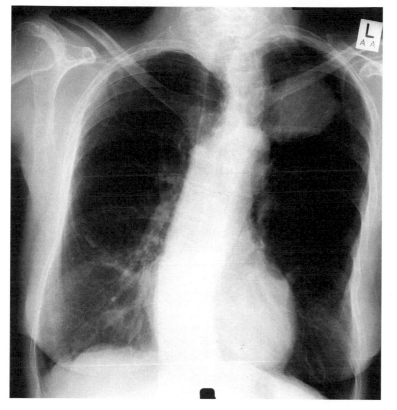

Fig 56.1

Interpret the chest X-ray and blood test results. What investigations and management should now be arranged?

The woman is admitted to hospital for emergency treatment of her hypercalcaemia and investigation of the cause of the back pain. Regular analgesia is started using twice daily oral slow-release morphine with rapid acting morphine every 2–4 hours for breakthrough pain. The narcotic analgesia is supplemented with paracetamol and laxatives (senna and a stool softener) are given twice daily. The patient is aggressively hydrated to treat the hypercalcaemia and renal impairment. A CT chest is performed. One of the axial slices (taken at T5) is shown (Figure 56.2).

Serum immunoglobulin studies and a serum protein electrophoresis are performed.

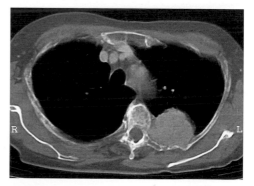

Fig 56.2

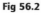

Investigation 56.2 Summary of results		
Total protein	94 g/l	(R 65–81)
IgG	2.3 g/l	(R 8.5–16.0)
IgA	48.5 g/l	(R 1.0–4.0)
IgM	0.2 g/l	(R 0.7–4.0)
Serum electrophoresis	Paraprotein detected	
Paraprotein immunofixation	IgA λ, 40 g/l	

Q3 What does the CT scan show? What diagnosis do these investigations point to? What other tests should be performed?

A core biopsy of the chest lesion is performed under CT guidance, and reveals a plasmacytoma. A bone marrow biopsy is performed, and shows an extensive infiltrate of immature plasma cells which overall comprise 60% of the marrow cellularity. A smear from the aspirate (Figure 56.3) and a heavily involved area of the trephine core are shown (Figure 56.4).

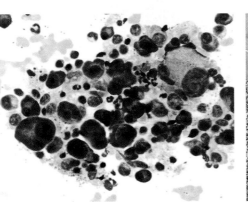

Fig 56.3

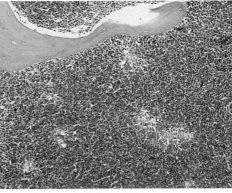

Fig 56.4

Electrophoresis of a urine sample shows the presence of free immunoglobulin lambda light chains in the urine (Bence-Jones protein). This is quantified in a 24-hour urine collection at 1.70 g/l. A radiological skeletal survey is performed. The skull X-ray is shown in Figure 56.5. The patient is given a dose of an intravenous biphosphonate to assist in treatment of the hypercalcaemia.

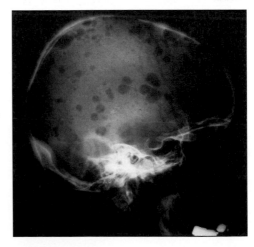

Fig 56.5

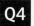 **What is the diagnosis?**

Following admission, the patient has several episodes of epistaxis on the ward. Two days after admission, she complains of headache and visual loss. She becomes progressively confused, and has a tonic–clonic seizure. You are called to see her urgently.

Q5 **What investigation(s) should be performed?**

A CT scan of her head is performed, and is normal. A lumbar puncture shows normal opening pressure, protein and glucose concentration, and is acellular. CSF Gram stain and viral antigen testing are negative. Electrolytes and calcium are normal. A plasma viscosity is performed, and is 6.0 centipoise (R 1.1–1.7)

Q6 **What is the cause of her deterioration, and what is the treatment?**

With treatment the patient recovers from the complication described above.

Q7 **In brief, describe the possible treatment options for this patient in the future.**

ANSWERS

A1 Back pain is one of the most common disorders in the community.

Degenerative disease and soft tissue injuries are common causes, and usually respond to simple measures without further investigation. However, several features of this case suggest a serious cause requiring further action:

- The characteristics of her pain, particularly the progressive nature and the fact that it is present at rest and waking her at night are worrisome. This, her lethargy and the examination findings of point tenderness at multiple levels, accompanying rib tenderness and pallor, all suggest serious underlying pathology (i.e. possibly malignancy).
- Possibilities include metastases (e.g. breast or lung carcinoma) or a haematologic malignancy (e.g. myeloma).

- Plain radiographs of the chest, ribs and spine are required. A complete blood picture, ESR, CRP and full biochemistry are also warranted.

A2 The most striking abnormality on the chest X-ray is the opacity in the left upper zone. Possible causes include a primary lung lesion, loculated fluid, collapse/consolidation or a mass arising from the vertebrae or ribs. More subtle features are erosion of the ribs. The presence of multiple bony lesions suggests a malignant process.

Key blood abnormalities are a normocytic, normochromic anaemia, a grossly elevated ESR, renal impairment and hypercalcaemia.

The bony erosions, osteopenia and blood abnormalities are highly suggestive of underlying malignancy. The extent of elevation of the ESR and the normal ALP favours myeloma bone disease,

ANSWERS – cont'd

whereas in other malignancies metastatic to bone the ALP is often elevated.

- Further investigations should include protein electrophoresis of serum and urine, measurement of serum immunoglobulins and a bone marrow biopsy.
- The mass lesion requires further investigation with a CT scan of the chest.
- The hypercalcaemia is a medical emergency and requires immediate treatment starting with aggressive hydration.

A3 The CT scan shows a large paravertebral mass lesion with associated destruction of the rib. There is a mottled appearance of the adjacent vertebral body.

- The IgA concentration is markedly increased, and IgM and IgG reduced.
- The serum electrophoresis shows a monoclonal band ('M-band') or paraprotein, of IgA lambda type.
- It is important to note that the presence of a serum paraprotein is not diagnostic of myeloma, and further investigations are required. These include a bone marrow biopsy, urine electrophoresis for free light chain (Bence-Jones protein), and radiographs of the skeleton for lytic lesions. Biopsy of the mass lesion is also required.

A4 The marrow smear shows a collection of plasma cells, many of which demonstrate abnormal features (increased size, bizarre or multiple nuclei, prominent nucleoli) (Figure 56.3). The histological section shows marked hypercellularity with diffuse infiltration by plasma cells and a bony trabeculum, which is thinned (Figure 56.4). The skull X-ray shows multiple 'punched-out' lytic lesions in the skull. This patient fulfils the three diagnostic criteria of myeloma:

- Monoclonal paraprotein.
- Bony lytic lesions of the skeleton.
- Bone marrow plasmacytosis.

Soft tissue plasmacytomas, such as seen in this woman, are less common and can be solitary, multiple or part of the presentation of myeloma.

A5 This is an emergency.

A clinical diagnosis of hyperviscosity can be made (due to the magnitude of the paraproteinaemia and the associated symptoms) and the plasma viscosity can be measured to support this diagnosis.

Additional tests to exclude other diagnoses include:

- CT scan of the head.
- Lumbar puncture with an urgent CSF Gram stain (meningitis).
- Urgent electrolytes and calcium.

A6 The patient has hyperviscosity syndrome, a complication of high levels of paraprotein, (usually IgA or IgM), marked polycythaemia and leukaemias with extreme leucocytosis. IgA and IgM immunoglobulins may polymerize and markedly increase blood viscosity. Clinical features are visual changes, lethargy, confusion, heart failure, a variety of central nervous system phenomena and retinal changes such as venous engorgement and haemorrhages. The diagnosis is primarily clinical in the setting of the above diseases and consistent symptoms. The clinical diagnosis can be supported by a whole blood or plasma viscosity although often this is not necessary. Treatment for paraprotein-related hyperviscosity is hydration, urgent plasmaphoresis, and treatment of the underlying condition (e.g. with chemotherapy).

A7 Multiple myeloma has a median survival of 3 years with standard chemotherapy. Treatment options include:

- Oral corticosteroids (e.g. pulsed dexamethasone).
- Chemotherapy (e.g. melphalan and prednisolone or combinations such as VAD).
- Stem cell transplantation.

A standard transplant approach is to initially treat with non-stem cell toxic chemotherapy (e.g. vincristine, adriamycin and dexamethasone or VAD) and then mobilize peripheral blood stem cells and proceed with high dose conditioning and autologous stem cell rescue. This approach is not curative but can be seen as an 'aggressive palliation'. Allogeneic transplantation can be associated with prolonged disease-free survival in some

ANSWERS – cont'd

patients but has a substantial risk of transplant-related mortality. New approaches include:

- Evaluation of such agents as thalidomide.
- Treatment of minimal residual disease after autologous transplantation (to prolong the disease-free interval).
- Allogeneic transplantation after non-myeloablative preparative regimens.

For all patients aggressive supportive care is necessary which includes prevention and treatment of infections, renal impairment and bone disease. Treatment with intravenous biphosphonates is now routine therapy for myeloma bone disease.

REVISION POINTS

Multiple myeloma

Multiple myeloma is:
- A malignancy of plasma cells.
- A disease of middle age and the elderly.
- Incurable in most patients.

Clinical features

These include:
- Bony lytic lesions and osteoporosis, resulting in bone pain and pathologic fractures, which may cause spinal cord compression.
- Anaemia.
- Infections (due to depressed levels of normal immunoglobulin, defects in cell-mediated immunity and neutropenia).
- Renal failure (multifactorial).
- Hypercalcaemia.
- Abnormal bleeding (due to thrombocytopenia and abnormal platelet function, and paraprotein interference with coagulation factors).
- Amyloidosis due to deposition of light chain (macroglossia, heart failure, neuropathy, etc.).

- Plasmacytomas: soft tissue masses of plasma cells.
- Hyperviscosity syndrome.

Diagnosis

A diagnosis of myeloma requires that at least one major and one minor, or three minor, criteria be present from Box 56.1.

Management

Specific treatment for myeloma:
- Oral chemotherapy (e.g. melphalan and prednisolone).
- Fit patients under 70 may receive an autologous stem cell transplantation.
- Other drugs, e.g. pulsed dexamethasone, thalidomide or experimental approaches.

Good supportive care is vital:
- Treatment of reversible causes of renal failure.
- Transfusion or erythropoietin for anaemia.
- Good analgesia essential (narcotics often needed).
- Plasmapheresis for hyperviscosity.
- Prompt identification and treatment of infection.

Box 56.1 Criteria of myeloma	
Major criteria	Minor criteria
Bone marrow plasmacytosis >30%	Marrow plasmacytosis 10–30%
Plasmacytoma on biopsy	Paraprotein less than for major criteria
Paraprotein	Lytic bone lesions
serum IgG >35 or IgA >20 g/l	Normal immunoglobulins <50% normal
urine >1g/24hour Bence-Jones protein	

continues overleaf

REVISION POINTS – cont'd

- Hypercalcaemia is prevented with bisphosphonates such as zoledronic acid and pamidronate, which have also been shown to reduce the incidence of skeletal complications such as fractures.

- Radiotherapy and surgical intervention (internal fixation or spinal cord decompression) may be required for lytic lesions, pathologic fractures and spinal cord compression.

ISSUES TO CONSIDER

- What are the most common causes of back pain in the community? How are they treated?

- What signs/symptoms associated with back pain require further investigation for serious underlying causes such as in this case?

- What other malignancies affect bone and may present with back pain?

- Renal failure is a common feature of multiple myeloma – what factors may influence its development?

FURTHER INFORMATION

British Committee for Standards in Haematology. Diagnosis and management of multiple myeloma. *British Journal of Haematology* 2001;115(3):522–40.

www.myeloma.org Website of the International Myeloma Foundation with links to sites giving updates on current trials and other aspects of management of myeloma.

www.multiplemyeloma.org The Multiple Myeloma Research Foundation. Information on clinical aspects of the disease and current research.

A woman with a lump in the neck

A 62-year-old woman is referred to hospital for investigation of a neck mass. She has a past history of hypertension for which she has been prescribed felodipine 5 mg twice a day. She is a non-smoker and drinks alcohol occasionally.

She has noticed an enlarging lump in her left neck over the last 6 weeks. There is no pain associated with the mass. Over recent weeks she has also been feeling tired and generally unwell and has lost 3 kg in weight.

On examination the woman is afebrile. She is not pale or jaundiced, her blood pressure is 170/105 mm Hg and she has a prominent but undisplaced apex beat. The remainder of her cardiorespiratory examination is normal and she has no peripheral oedema. There is left supra-clavicular, firm, non-tender lymphadenopathy with the nodal mass measuring approximately 3.5 x 4.5 cm in diameter. Her abdomen is unre-markable with no organomegaly or palpable abdominal masses. She has two enlarged nodes in the left groin measuring 2 cm and 2.5 cm in diameter. Urinalysis showed 1+ protein (300 mg/l) on dipstick testing.

Q1 What further information should be obtained from the history and what else should be looked for on examination?

The patient had no other symptoms of note except she has started sweating at night suffi-cient to dampen her pillow. Further examination was normal.

Q2 What is the differential diagnosis? Overall, what is the most likely diagnosis?

Q3 What initial investigations would you perform on this patient?

Some investigations are performed and the results shown in Investigation 57.1.

Investigation 57.1 Summary of results				
Haemoglobin	100 g/l	White cell count		3.2 x 10⁹/l
RBC	4.39×10^{12}/l	Neutrophils	61%	2.0×10^9/l
PCV	0.38	Lymphocytes	28%	0.9×10^9/l
MCV	86.9 fl	Monocytes	6%	0.3×10^9/l
MCH	29.5 pg	Eosinophils	3%	0.1×10^9/l
MCHC	340 g/l	Basophils	2%	0.1×10^9/l
Platelets	102×10^9/l			
Sodium	136 mmol/l	Calcium		2.16 mmol/l
Potassium	4.0 mmol/l	Phosphate		1.15 mmol/l
Chloride	98 mmol/l	Total protein		65 g/l
Bicarbonate	22 mmol/l	Albumin		28 g/l
Urea	6.1 mmol/l	Globulins		27 g/l
Creatinine	0.19 mmol/l	Bilirubin		16 µmol/l
Uric acid	0.65 mmol/l	ALT		22 U/l
Glucose	7.0 mmol/l	AST		23 U/l
Cholesterol	3.5 mmol/l	GGT		17 U/l
LDH	654 U/l	ALP		54 U/l

A CT scan of the chest, abdomen and pelvis is performed. One of the images from the abdomen is shown (Figure 57.1).

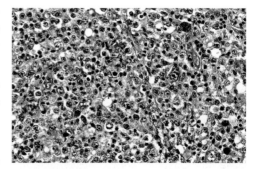

Fig 57.1

Q4　What do the laboratory results and the scan show?

One of the enlarged neck nodes is excised for histological examination. It shows a diffuse large B-cell (CD20+) non-Hodgkin's lymphoma, intermediate grade (Figure 57.2).

The patient is well hydrated and allopurinol is given to treat her hyperuricaemia. Over the next 2 days her creatinine improves to 0.12 mmol/l.

Staging is completed by performing a bone marrow biopsy and another imaging study. A view from the latter is shown (Figure 57.3).

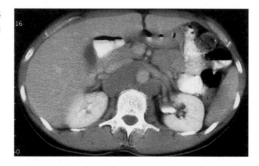

Fig 57.2

Fig 57.3

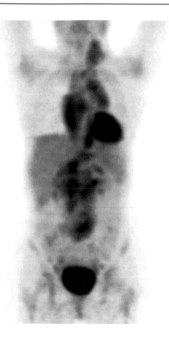

 Q5 What is the investigation and what does it show?

The bone marrow biopsy reveals bone marrow involvement with lymphoma accounting for her mild pancytopaenia. As the patient has advanced stage disease, a lumbar puncture is done to exclude CNS involvement. The investigation is negative. The patient has no neurological symptoms or signs, and no CNS imaging is done.

 Q6 Describe the pathological classification used for classifying non-Hodgkin's lymphoma.

Q7 List the staging procedures routinely performed on patients with non-Hodgkin's lymphoma. What stage is this patient?

 Q8 What are the next considerations in this patient's management?

A gated blood pool scan shows a left ventricular ejection fraction at the lower limit of normal. The patient is treated with combination chemotherapy, namely cyclophosphamide, doxorubicin, vincristine and prednisolone (CHOP) and rituximab (monoclonal anti-CD20 antibody). Chemotherapy is delivered in full dose and on time with no major complications. She achieves a complete response but relapses 8 months after completion of therapy. She has a complete remission to salvage chemotherapy and undergoes autologous transplantation using high dose chemoradiotherapy and mobilized peripheral blood stem cells. She subsequently remains disease free.

ANSWERS

A1 The patient has constitutional symptoms associated with bulky neck nodes and likely additional pathological adenopathy in the groin. Therefore, she probably has a lymphoproliferative malignancy.

You should ask about her past medical history as any co-morbidity may have an impact on current management. Do a general review of systems. Specifically you will want to know about constitutional symptoms such as fever, sweats, loss of appetite/weight and any symptoms that could be related to malignant involvement of specific structures, e.g. bone pain, shortness of breath, cough, back pain (can be presentation of retroperitoneal disease) and neurological symptoms.

Other lymph node groups should be examined, i.e. axillae, elbow for epitrochlear nodes and popliteal regions. The tonsils should also be examined, these being part of Waldeyer's ring. Do a full neurological examination.

A2 The differential diagnoses of lymphadenopathy:

1 Inflammatory
   - local, regional or systemic infection
   - autoimmune disease, e.g. systemic lupus erythematosus.
2 Granulomatous
   - infective, e.g. tuberculosis
   - non-infective, e.g. sarcoidosis.
3 Malignancy
   - primary: lymphoproliferative malignancies (e.g. lymphomas, chronic lymphocytic leukaemia) more likely generalized
   - secondary: (e.g. melanoma or carcinoma) more likely localized.

In the context of constitutional symptoms and neck and inguinal lymphadenopathy, a lymphoproliferative malignancy is the most likely diagnosis.

A3 Initial investigations should include:
- Complete blood picture.
- Biochemical screen including uric acid, albumin, total protein, calcium, liver function tests and LDH.
- Chest X-ray.

- Excisional lymph node biopsy sent for histology and special studies (immunohistochemistry and molecular studies).
- CT scan of chest, abdomen and pelvis.

A4 The laboratory results show a mild pancytopenia including a normocytic anaemia. The albumin is low, the uric acid is raised and the creatinine is mildly elevated. The LDH is elevated but the liver enzymes are normal. These abnormalities in conjunction with the CT scan showing extensive retroperitoneal lymphadenopathy support the diagnosis of lymphoma. The cytopenia suggests the possibility of bone marrow involvement. The LDH is a tumour marker for lymphoma and is a marker indicating worse prognosis. There is no obvious hydronephrosis on the CT although this patient would be at risk of renal tract obstruction. The elevated creatinine is likely contributed to by the high uric acid.

A5 This Positron Emmission Tomogram (PET) scan shows extensive increase in activity due to lymphomatous involvement of nodes in the left side of the neck, the mediastinum, the retroperitoneum and there is minor activity in the left groin.

A6 The Working Formulation has been used to classify non-Hodgkin's lymphoma into low, intermediate or high-grade disease on the basis of histology and clinical behaviour. In general, low-grade lymphomas have a more indolent clinical course but are not cured with conventional therapy. In contrast, intermediate and high-grade tumours have a much more aggressive clinical course, but are responsive to chemotherapy and potentially can be cured.

More recently the World Health Organization (WHO) classification has been introduced as a more sophisticated classification of haematological malignancies. It characterizes all of the currently recognized lymphomas as distinct entities based on morphology, immunophenotype, genetic and clinical features.

Pathologists now describe a lymphoma in terms of the WHO classification and correlate this with a grade according to the Working Formulation.

ANSWERS – cont'd

Treatment decisions are based upon the histological diagnosis. Thus, adequate biopsy of involved tissue allowing demonstration of node architecture and fresh samples for immunophenotyping and molecular studies is crucial. Fine needle aspirates of a lymph node are never satisfactory for diagnosis of lymphoma.

A7 In staging the patient, decide from the history if constitutional B symptoms (i.e. fever, night sweats, weight loss greater than 10% of body weight in the last 6 months) exist. On clinical examination document the size and extent of involved nodes and other organs. Then undertake the following:

- Laboratory tests: complete blood picture, biochemical screen (including lactate dehydrogenase), electrophoretogram to document presence of paraprotein.
- Chest X-ray.
- CT scan of chest, abdomen and pelvis.
- Bone marrow biopsy.
- Gallium or positron emission tomography (PET) scanning can be useful in some patients.
- For high-grade disease and some other lymphomas, assessment of other areas can be necessary including Waldeyer's ring and the CNS and sometimes the gut and other organs.

Hodgkin's and non-Hodgkin's lymphoma are staged according to the Ann Arbor staging system as shown in Box 57.1.

The Ann Arbor staging system was originally developed for Hodgkin's disease and is more relevant to the contiguous spread of that disease.

Most patients with NHL present with widespread (stage III/IV) disease.

This patient is stage IVB as she has bone marrow involvement and B symptoms.

A8 This patient has a disseminated, aggressive malignancy and therefore death will be rapid without treatment with cytotoxic chemotherapy. However, she is in her sixties with longstanding hypertension and may have left ventricular dysfunction. She needs a gated blood pool scan prior to administration of an anthracycline-containing chemotherapy regimen such as CHOP. The principles of treatment include:

- Administration of repeated cycles of combination chemotherapy.
- Supportive care attending to issues such as prevention and management of the tumour lysis syndrome, prevention and treatment of infection, monitoring of cytopaenia and administration of growth factor and/or transfusions as necessary.
- Documentation of response to chemotherapy both clinically and using imaging (CT scans in all patients and sometimes either gallium or PET scans can be useful).

This patient has poor prognosis disease according to the International Prognostic Index and therefore she is at increased risk of either primary resistance to chemotherapy or subsequent relapse of her disease. If possible, she should be enrolled in a randomized study to evaluate novel treatment strategies for such patients, such as combined modality treatment or elective high-dose therapy as primary treatment.

Box 57.1 Staging of Hodgkin's and non-Hodgkin's lymphomas	
Stage I	confined to a single nodal region
Stage II	involvement of two or more nodal regions on same side of diaphragm
Stage III	involvement of nodes on both sides of the diaphragm
Stage IV	disseminated nodal involvement or one or more extra lymphatic organs (e.g. bone marrow, ascites)
A	no systemic symptoms
B	fever >38°, sweats, loss of 10% of body weight

REVISION POINTS

Non-Hodgkin's lymphoma

Definition

- Tumours arising from the lymphatic system.
- More common than Hodgkin's lymphoma.
- 85% from mature B cells: minority from T cells.

Incidence

NHL increases with age (although important between 20–40 years).

Risk factors

- None identified in majority.
- Higher incidence in autoimmune disease (Sjögren's, rheumatoid, SLE, coeliac).
- Immunodeficiency (congenital, acquired or drug-induced, e.g. post transplant).
- Epstein–Barr virus (EBV).
- 100% of endemic Burkitt's lymphoma (B cell).
- 40% sporadic/HIV associated.

Genetics

Cytogenetic abnormalities in majority leading to activation of proto-oncogenes and inactivation of tumour suppression genes. Identification has allowed better disease classification, prognosis prediction and treatment selection.

Clinical features

- Two-thirds present with painless lymphadenopathy. Persistent lymphadenopathy (>4 weeks, no infection, >1 cm diameter) should be biopsied.
- Adequate tissue sample to allow accurate histological classification and special studies is mandatory.
- Spreads haematogenously therefore usually advanced at presentation.
- May present with extranodal involvement, e.g. bone, gut, CNS.

Staging

See Answer 7.

Prognosis

The International Prognostic Index assigns 1 point for each of the following factors: age >60, performance status >2, raised LDH, involvement of >1 extranodal site, Stage III or IV disease. Score >2 indicates a poorer prognosis.

Grade

Low grade/indolent 75% of all cases. Slow course, survival 8–10 years. Using traditional therapy cure possible only in localized (stage I or II) disease. Treatment involves radiotherapy and/or chemotherapy. Treatment of widespread disease is commenced when the disease becomes symptomatic and involves systemic chemotherapy. New approaches include monoclonal antibodies either alone or conjugated to radioisotopes. Allogeneic haematopoietic stem cell transplantation after non-myeloablative preparative regimens is another exciting new therapy being investigated for selected patients with low and intermediate grade disease.

Intermediate/high grade require immediate combination chemotherapy, as untreated they are rapidly fatal. Standard treatment of intermediate grade NHL involves CHOP (cyclophosphamide, doxorubicin, vincristine and prednisolone) chemotherapy. 60% achieve a complete response, 30% achieve long-term disease-free survival. Recently, improved results have been seen with the addition of rituximab to the CHOP regimen. Young patients with poor prognosis disease or patients who have relapsed may be considered for high-dose therapy and autologous (from self) stem cell transplantation.

High grade require treatment with intensive combination chemotherapy regimens similar to those used in acute lymphoblastic leukaemia. Also require intrathecal chemotherapy (into the cerebrospinal fluid) to prevent CNS relapse. 50% of treated patients will be disease free at 3 years.

Gallium and PET scanning

Gallium and PET scanning may identify sites of disease not detected on CT scanning, which may upstage the disease and alter management. They are also very useful as an adjunct to CT in assessing tumour response following treatment. Patients with bulky baseline disease may be left with a residual mass post treatment and gallium or PET can assist in delineating residual lymphoma from necrotic or scar tissue.

Gallium scanning involves the injection of Gallium-67 and scans are then performed at 48 and 72 hours. The gallium binds to transferrrin receptors which are over-expressed on tumour cells.

continues overleaf

REVISION POINTS — cont'd

PET scanning involves the injection of fluoro-18-deoxyglucose (FDG), a glucose analogue labelled with a short-lived positron emitter. This tracer is taken up by actively metabolizing cells and thus is preferentially taken up at sites of inflammation or malignancy. The patient must lie still for 1 hour (to reduce the activity of skeletal muscle which may interfere with the scan) before the scan is performed. PET scanning is likely to replace gallium scanning as a more sensitive and less time-consuming investigation although currently it is very expensive.

ISSUES TO CONSIDER

- What are the hazards of the administration of chemotherapy? How does the treatment of Hodgkin's lymphoma differ?

- By what mechanisms could a virus such as EBV be implicated in the production of tumours?

FURTHER INFORMATION

www.cancernet.nci.nih.gov Lots of information on lymphoma on the website of the National Cancer Institute in the USA.

www.lymphomafocus.com An excellent site with information and links for professionals and patients alike.

Severe dehydration in a young woman

An 18-year-old girl is brought into the emergency department by ambulance from a youth hostel. She is a backpacker and has been travelling around the country. She is drowsy and unable to give any history. Her airway is clear and her breathing is unhindered. She reacts purposefully to painful stimuli, moving all limbs and grunts but does not speak. She opens her eyes briefly in response to you shouting her name.

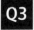

Q1 What is her Glasgow Coma Score?

She is of normal build and is well kept. Her temperature is normal, her pulse rate is 135 bpm and her supine blood pressure is 95/60 mm Hg. She has deep sighing respirations with a respiratory rate of 25 breaths/minute. Her mouth is extremely dry and her tissue turgor is reduced. She has no other abnormalities on cardiac and respiratory examination, and she has no focal neurological signs. Her abdomen is not distended and is soft to palpation, but there is widespread tenderness. Bowel sounds are present.

Another girl appears who says she is a companion from the hostel. The two have only known each other for 2 weeks and agreed to travel together. The girl claims her friend became unwell over the last week, particularly over the last 2 days. She complained of being very tired. The patient had become lethargic and listless. She has not wanted to eat, but has complained of extreme thirst and has been drinking large amounts of water. Today she stayed on her bunk and was unable to get up. She complained of abdominal pain and vomited three times. The friend had gone out for a few hours and on her return found the patient looking very unwell and an ambulance had been called. The patient is not known to have any major medical problems or to take medications or drugs of any kind.

Q2 Provide a differential diagnosis.

There are a number of possible causes for this woman's comatose state.

Q3 What should be done immediately?

A finger-prick blood glucose measurement has been obtained using a bedside glucose meter and reads 'high'. A urinary catheter drains 50 ml urine which when tested with a strip, registers ketones as ++++. After initial resuscitation, results of the preliminary blood tests come back as follows:

Investigation 58.1 Summary of results			
Haemoglobin	151 g/l	White cell count	18.6 x 10⁹/l
Platelets	289 x 10⁹/l	Neutrophils 57%	10.6 x 10⁹/l
PCV	0.38	Lymphocytes 27%	5.0 x 10⁹/l
MCV	86.9 fl	Monocytes 11%	2.0 x 10⁹/l
MCH	29.5 pg	Eosinophils 3%	0.6 x 10⁹/l
MCHC	340 g/l	Basophils 2%	0.4 x 10⁹/l
Sodium	140 mmol/l	Calcium	2.16 mmol/l
Potassium	6.0 mmol/l	Phosphate	1.15 mmol/l
Chloride	109 mmol/l	Total protein	67 g/l
Bicarbonate	7.0 mmol/l	Albumin	38 g/l
Urea	6.1 mmol/l	Globulins	29 g/l
Creatinine	0.13 mmol/l	Bilirubin	16 μmol/l
Anion gap	28.5	ALT	24 U/l
Glucose	30 mmol/l	AST	28 U/l
Cholesterol	3.8 mmol/l	GGT	19 U/l
LDH	202 U/l	ALP	52 U/l

Arterial blood gas analysis on room air			
pO₂	99 mm Hg	pCO₂	15 mm Hg
pH	7.0	Calculated bicarbonate	7.0 mmol/l

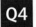

Q4 What are the abnormalities? How do they help in clarifying your differential diagnosis?

You have a working diagnosis for this patient who is critically ill.

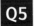

Q5 What is your acute management plan?

You institute emergency management. A central line is inserted, and she is managed in the high dependency ward with close nursing care to monitor all vital signs and to keep the airway clear. The patient's urine output is regularly charted to establish that renal function is normal and urine production is taking place.

In addition to your fluid replacements, the electrolytes are checked after 2 hours to measure the potassium concentration. It is now 3.6 mmol/l and you begin to add potassium supplementation to the intravenous infusion at 13.6 mmol (1 gm KCl) per hour. You check her potassium level again at 4 hours and 8 hours. A chest X-ray is performed and urine microscopy sent off to look for any intercurrent infection.

After 12 hours the patient's blood glucose is down to 15 mmol/l. The intravenous fluid is changed to 5% dextrose 1 litre over 6 hours with 2 gm KCl added to each litre of fluid.

24 hours later your patient's condition has significantly improved. She is fully conscious, no longer vomiting or nauseated and is allowed to start eating. The urine shows only a trace of ketones.

Q6 How will you change her insulin therapy now?

She responds well to your insulin regimen, and is stable for discharge. Further history establishes that she has previously been healthy: now she has a diagnosis of diabetes. She is frightened by what has happened, and anxious about her diabetes management.

Q7 Describe your ongoing management plan for this patient while she is in hospital and prior to discharge.

The patient decides to curtail her backpacking holiday and return home.

ANSWERS

A1 Her Glasgow Coma Score is 11 (E4, V2, M5).

A2 Given her young age, history of polydipsia and clinical evidence of dehydration and hyperventilation, the most likely diagnosis is diabetic ketoacidosis. Abdominal pain is quite common in this condition and does not indicate any acute abdominal problem (although intra-abdominal problems must be considered in the differential diagnosis). Other diagnoses to consider include poisoning (alcohol, food or drug-related, particularly street drugs) and infection (e.g. meningitis).

A3 As part of the immediate management, the following must be undertaken:
- Protect the airway.
- Insert an intravenous cannula and take blood for electrolytes, blood glucose, complete blood picture, lipase.
- Collect a finger-prick blood sample for glucose estimation.
- Perform an arterial blood gas assay to obtain the pH and ascertain if patient is acidotic.
- Insert a urinary catheter and check for urinary ketones and measure the urine output.
- Commence emergency resuscitation with intravenous infusion of isotonic saline. At least 1–1.5 litres should be given over the first hour.

A4 The patient has a severe metabolic acidosis as characterized by the low serum pH and low bicarbonate level. The low pCO_2 is due to respiratory compensation for the metabolic acidosis. This accounts for the hyperventilation.

The increased anion gap is due to the presence of anions not measured when the anion gap is calculated. This 'hidden' anion here is the ketone bodies.

Metabolic acidosis can be divided into:
- High anion gap acidosis (addition of anions to the blood, e.g. ketoacidosis, lactic acidosis and salicylate or alcohol poisoning).
- Normal anion gap acidosis with a high chloride level, usually as a result of loss of alkali (bicarbonate), for example from the gut with severe diarrhoea or in renal tubular acidosis.

The apparent hyperkalaemia is due to the shift of potassium from the intracellular space to the extracellular space caused by the acidosis (potassium in exchange for hydrogen ions). In spite of the elevated serum potassium, these patients are usually depleted of total body potassium. This is an important point to grasp. Large amounts of potassium are lost via the kidneys as a result of the glucose diuresis and also through vomiting. The serum potassium level will need careful monitoring as it will drop rapidly when treatment is commenced and the acidosis starts to correct, placing the patient at risk of hypokalaemia and arrhythmias.

Hyperglycaemia is consistent with the diagnosis of diabetes and is a marker of insulin deficiency. The glucose level, though usually

ANSWERS – cont'd

elevated in patients with ketoacidosis, may not be particularly high nor at the levels generally seen in patients with hyperosmolar non-ketotic coma.

Leucocytosis is seen quite commonly in association with ketoacidosis and does not necessarily indicate infection. Infections are common triggers for ketoacidosis, and patients should be checked for septic foci once their resuscitation has started.

The combination of the clinical picture, hyperglycaemia, metabolic acidosis with high anion gap and ketones in the urine confirms the diagnosis of diabetic ketoacidosis.

A5 Diabetes ketoacidosis is an acute medical emergency, requiring rapid diagnosis and treatment. These patients are critically ill and need specialized care and close monitoring. The patient's vital signs must be observed regularly, and recorded along with fluid input and output and bedside blood glucose monitoring. If the patient's potassium concentrations are significantly abnormal cardiac monitoring may be needed. Ketoacidosis may induce gastroparesis and the patient should be kept fasted to minimize the risk from gastric aspiration.

Principal steps in management
Urgent:
- Fluid and sodium replacement.
- Correction of the acidosis and hyperglycaemia with insulin.
- Monitoring and replacement of potassium.

Then:
- Diagnosis and management of precipitating events.
- Prevention of complications of ketoacidosis.

Once patient is better:
- (Re)establishment of ongoing diabetes management plan.
- Prevention of recurrence of ketoacidosis.

Fluid and sodium replacement
- Severe dehydration is common. This is secondary to the osmotic diuresis (hyperglycaemia and ketonuria) compounded by vomiting and hyperventilation. The degree of dehydration needs to be assessed both clinically and biochemically.

- Sodium depletion is common. This is consequent on the diuresis (although the serum sodium level may appear normal).
- Rehydration is started with isotonic saline. For example, give 1 litre/hour for 2 hours then a third litre over the following 4 hours. The severely dehydrated patient may need 6–8 litres of fluid in the first 24 hours.

After 12 hours (or once the blood glucose has dropped to 15 mmol/l), fluid replacement can be changed to 5% dextrose.

Urine output should be monitored (an indwelling bladder catheter can be placed as part of the initial resuscitation). Hypovolaemia and the risk of acute renal tubular necrosis must be minimized. During the osmotic diuresis, the urine output must be matched on a regular basis with intravenous fluid replacement. Once the dehydration has been corrected, an output of at least 30 ml/hour must be maintained.

Correction of acidosis and hyperglycaemia with insulin
Insulin therapy will correct both the acidosis and hyperglycaemia.

Continuous intravenous infusion of insulin using an insulin pump at 4–8 units per hour is the best method of delivering insulin Rapid changes in pH, glucose and potassium are thus avoided, thereby preventing complications such as cardiac arrhythmias and cerebral oedema.

If infusion is not possible hourly intramuscular doses may be used; subcutaneous insulin therapy should *not* be used in the acute treatment of diabetic ketoacidosis because of the unreliable rate of absorption.

Blood glucose must be monitored frequently using a bedside glucose meter while patient is receiving intravenous insulin infusion.

The use of bicarbonate is generally not required in the treatment of diabetic ketoacidosis. The metabolic acidosis is corrected by rehydration and by cessation of ketogenesis with the use of insulin.

Potassium replacement
Rapid shifts in potassium will occur once treatment for ketoacidosis is started. Correction of the acidosis will cause shift of potassium back from the extracellular to the intracellular space.

A N S W E R S – cont'd

Insulin therapy will drive potassium into the cells. As the patient is also depleted of total body potassium, the drop in serum potassium can be potentially life threatening.

- Replacement potassium can commence with the second litre of saline – provided the initial serum potassium was in the normal range.
- If the initial potassium level is high, recheck the potassium after 2 hours of intravenous saline infusion and commence potassium replacement as soon as the serum potassium is in the normal range (do not wait till hypokalaemia has occurred to start potassium replacement).
- Potassium replacement in range of 10–20 mmol/l/hour (1 gm KCl = 13.6 mmol). This rate is likely to be required for the first 12 hours.
- Check serum electrolytes every 2–4 hours for the first 24 hours. Insertion of a central line allows repeated drawing of blood without venepuncture as well as monitoring of central venous filling.
- Ensure adequate urine output has been established. If the patient is not producing urine they may be in acute renal failure, and potassium replacement may need to be modified.

Diagnosis and treatment of precipitating events

Once resuscitation of the acute metabolic state is underway it is important to look for any precipitating event that may have triggered the onset of ketoacidosis. In this patient's age group the commonest causes are either infection or omission of insulin. Investigations should be performed for chest, urinary tract and gastrointestinal infections.

Prevention of the complications of ketoacidosis

- Cerebral oedema is a rare but dangerous complication; it can be prevented by careful fluid balance and avoiding dramatic drops in blood glucose levels.
- Aspiration of gastric contents can be prevented by careful nursing and keeping the patient fasting until she is fully conscious and has bowel sounds.

- Thrombosis is a relatively common complication; anticoagulation until the patient is mobile may need to be considered.

A6 You are now able to change the patient to subcutaneous insulin using a bolus of short-acting insulin with each main meal and intermediate acting insulin at bedtime.

Insulin infusion is ceased 1 hour after the first dose of subcutaneous insulin given.

A7 Once the acute event of the ketoacidosis is over a long-term management plan for the ongoing treatment of the patient will need to be developed. In this patient the ketoacidosis was the mode of first presentation of her diabetes. During hospitalization she might not be able to fully comprehend the diagnosis and its implications. She would not be reasonably expected to assimilate all the information that she needs to manage her diabetes. Therefore she should only be given the necessary information to enable her to manage her diabetes in the immediate future with further education to occur as an outpatient.

In hospital:
- She needs to be commenced on a basal/bolus insulin regimen using short-acting insulin before each main meal and intermediate acting insulin at bedtime. She should be taught the action of the different insulins that she will be using. (A starting dose of insulin may be estimated using the calculation of 0.5 to 1 unit insulin per kg of body weight per 24 hours split evenly into the 4 doses.)
- She needs to understand that she should never omit her insulin therapy.
- She should be taught how to self-administer insulin using syringes or an insulin pen device. Diabetes nurse educators and support groups will be important in helping her cope with these and other issues.
- She should be taught how to use a personal blood glucose monitor and how to interpret the readings that she obtains. She needs to understand what factors affect blood glucose levels, e.g. food, exercise, insulin dose. She should learn to keep a record of her blood glucose.

ANSWERS – cont'd

As an outpatient:

- A simple diet plan is important with some basic knowledge on the appropriate food types. 50% of her total daily caloric requirement should be as carbohydrates (complex carbohydrates should be encouraged and simple sugars avoided) and less than 30% as fat. Most importantly she should understand the necessity to eat regularly with an even spread of carbohydrates over the day and not to miss meals. Between-meal snacks and supper will need to be taken.
- She should be advised to be very moderate with alcohol consumption and to ensure that she eats adequate carbohydrate type food when she drinks alcohol.
- She should be taught how to recognize the symptoms of hypoglycaemia and what the appropriate treatment is.

- She should be given information on how travelling can affect diabetes and what steps she needs to take.
- The patient needs to understand that diabetes is a life-long disease that needs to be managed well to prevent long-term complications. However, details of long-term treatment and prevention and monitoring of long-term complications can be given at a later date when she is getting used to her condition.
- She should be strongly advised to seek referral to a specialist diabetes centre on her return to her home country to continue her diabetes management and education.
- If she drives a car, her licence may be affected and she will need to contact the appropriate authority.

REVISION POINTS

Diabetes ketoacidosis

Diabetic ketoacidosis is an acute medical emergency that is potentially life threatening but completely reversible if diagnosed and treated rapidly.

With aggressive and early management of ketoacidosis in recent years the mortality rate from ketoacidosis has been markedly reduced to less than 5%.

Ketoacidosis can occur as the first presentation of a patient developing type 1 diabetes or as a complication in a patient known to have the condition. It occurs in type 1 diabetics when there is absence or insufficiency of insulin due to:

- failure to administer insulin; or
- an increased need for insulin at times of physical stress (e.g. an intercurrent infection, trauma, surgery, etc.).

Aetiology

Insufficient insulin leads to uncontrolled gluconeogenesis and impaired peripheral glucose utilization, both of which result in hyperglycaemia and glucosuria. A severe osmotic diuresis results leading to loss of fluid and electrolytes. Insulin deficiency also leads to the formation of ketone bodies which are strong acids leading to a metabolic acidosis.

Clinical features

- polyuria
- polydipsia
- anorexia, nausea and vomiting
- long sighing respiration (Kussmaul breathing)
- sweet-smelling ketotic breath
- clinical signs of dehydration
- coma (in severe cases).

Treatment

Intravenous insulin infusion allows a gradual and steady correction of the metabolic abnormalities.

Complications

- electrolyte disturbances as indicated above (particularly hypokalaemia)
- hypoglycaemia
- infections such as aspiration or stasis pneumonia and urinary tract infection from indwelling catheters
- thrombosis risk may require short-term anticoagulation
- gastric dilatation and haemorrhage

continues overleaf

REVISION POINTS – cont'd

- ominous but fortunately rare complications include adult respiratory distress syndrome and the cerebral dysequilibrium syndrome from cerebral oedema.

Follow-up

Patients must be encouraged to learn and perform regular home blood-glucose monitoring for day-to-day adjustment of their insulin regimen, while their longer term glycaemic control can be monitored by measuring the glycosylated haemoglobin (HBA1c).

Macrovascular complications leading to ischaemic heart disease, cerebrovascular disease and peripheral vascular disease can also be significantly reduced by concomitantly treating hypertension and hyperlipidaemia and urging patients to stop smoking.

Patients with type 1 diabetes should be followed in specialized diabetes centres if possible, where multidisciplinary care is available from endocrinologists, diabetes nurse educators, dieticians and podiatrists.

The achievement of optimal control of diabetes is especially important in young patients with type 1 diabetes such as this patient as there are now impressive data to show that the long-term microvascular complications (retinopathy, nephropathy and neuropathy) are significantly reduced with good blood glucose levels.

Young women such this patient should be counselled in avoiding unplanned pregnancy as it is important for the diabetes to be optimally controlled prior to conception to achieve the best outcome for both mother and baby. Contraception should be encouraged if the patient is sexually active and not planning pregnancy. Patients with diabetes may face restrictions with their driving licences and need to apply annually for licence renewal.

Future developments in the management of diabetes range from glucose-monitoring devices which do not require finger punctures, new insulin analogues, new insulin delivery methods such as inhaled insulin, pancreas transplantation and recent advances in islet cell transplantation. The more distant future will see the use of gene therapy to replace insulin-producing cells in patients with type 1 diabetes. However, the current imperatives remain to assist patients in achieving the best control of diabetes to prevent both short-term problems like ketoacidosis and long-term complications such as blindness, renal failure, etc.

ISSUES TO CONSIDER

- How do you manage a type 2 diabetic patient in hyperosmolar non-ketotic state?
- What new drugs are becoming available for the treatment of type 1 and type 2 diabetes?

FURTHER INFORMATION

www.emedicine.com/emerg/topic135.htm A tutorial on the emergency management of diabetic ketoacidosis.

www.diabetesnet.com A patient-focused website dealing with many of the practical aspects of living with diabetes, including information on the newer insulins.

PROBLEM

59

A 22-year-old woman with palpitations and anxiety

A 22-year-old woman presents with a 3-month history of frequent episodes of rapid regular palpitations. On questioning, you discover she is pleased she has lost weight despite eating a lot but says she feels 'weird', as if she has 'drunk too much coffee'. She also complains of sweating despite cool weather and has been increasingly irritable. She has no other complaints. On mental state examination she appears anxious but is otherwise normal.

Q1 What further information would you like from the history and why?

As you talk to the patient, you observe a physical sign (Figure 59.1).

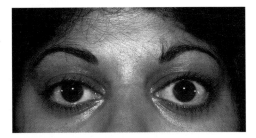

Fig 59.1

Q2 What abnormal physical sign can you see in Figure 59.1? What else would you look for on physical examination and why?

A more extensive history from the patient seems to give you no further additional clues.

On examination she is slim and easily distracted. She has warm moist hands and a fine tremor when the arms are outstretched. There is lid lag when she is asked to look down from an upward gaze. She has an obvious goitre which is soft, smooth and slightly asymmetrical, but has no bruit. She has a regular tachycardia of 120 bpm but no other cardiovascular abnormality.

Q3 What would you like to do now?

Some blood test results are shown in Investigation 59.1.

Investigation 59.1 Summary of results	
Free T4	66 pmol/l
Free T3	18.7 pmol/l
TSH	<0.01 mU/l

Q4 What is the diagnosis?

Q5 What are the treatment options available to you?

ANSWERS

A1 This clinical picture of tachycardia, weight loss with a normal appetite, sweating and anxiety all suggest a diagnosis of hyperthyroidism. As such, you should enquire about:

- A family history of autoimmune disease, especially of the thyroid, e.g. Graves' disease.
- Has the patient noticed a swelling in the neck, consistent with a goitre as seen, for instance, in Graves' disease?
- A recent history of an upper respiratory tract infection with sore throat, fever and muscle aches and pains may indicate viral thyroiditis. Ask about a painful region in the lower neck.
- Recent pregnancy. Autoimmune thyroid disease has a propensity to occur in the post-partum period (e.g. 3–6 months after pregnancy).
- Has the patient been exposed to X-ray contrast agents containing iodine, an iodine-rich diet, e.g. kelp, or drugs that predispose to hyperthyroidism, e.g. amiodarone?
- Where is the patient from? Certain geographical locations have a greater frequency of multinodular goitre.

It is also important to think of other possible causes such as anxiety and depression, abuse of sympathomimetic drugs, e.g. amphetamines, 'diet pills' and even excessive caffeine intake. Enquire about:

- The duration and nature of the palpitations. Do they occur at night? Do they disappear on exercise or with alcohol?

- The presence of other symptoms suggestive of a psychological cause such as low affect, sleep disturbance, poor concentration and reduced libido although all these may be seen in hyperthyroidism. Ask also about a history of depression and anxiety.
- Drug use and caffeine consumption.

A2 The patient has proptosis. There is left-sided 'scleral show' superiorly – i.e. lid retraction. The proptosis is predominantly left sided.

You would also look for:

- Systemic features of hyperthyroidism such as sweating, tremor, sinus tachycardia and rarely atrial fibrillation, high cardiac output state with bounding pulses, hyperreflexia, emotional lability, nervousness, proximal myopathy and muscle wasting.
- Uncommon signs of autoimmune thyroid disease (Graves' disease) include pretibial myxoedema and clubbing.
- The eye signs of hyperthyroidism relating to
  - sympathetic overactivity, i.e. lid-lag and lid-retraction ('thyroid ophthalmopathy')
  - autoimmune thyroid disease (e.g. Graves' disease and Hashimoto's disease) including subconjunctival injection, chemosis, proptosis, ophthalmoplegia and rarely papilloedema.
- The presence of a goitre. It will be typically smooth in Graves' disease, nodular in a multinodular gland, painful and tender in

ANSWERS – cont'd

thyroiditis (in particular viral thyroiditis). There maybe an associated bruit in Graves' disease.

- Skin changes can include palmar erythema and sweating.

A3 Clinically this patient has thyrotoxicosis and the diagnosis can be confirmed with thyroid function tests, including direct assays of TSH, free T4 and free T3.

Thyroid autoantibodies, in particular thyroid peroxidase antibody, would confirm the diagnosis of autoimmune thyroid disease. Thyroid-stimulating autoantibody will be positive in Graves' disease but does not contribute to the management.

A radioisotope thyroid scan would confirm the diagnosis of Graves' disease by demonstrating homogeneous increased uptake throughout the gland but is not necessarily required in this patient.

In addition, the history of palpitations warrants an ECG.

A4 The blood tests confirm your suspicions of hyperthyroidism with a raised free T4, free T3 and suppressed TSH to an undetectable level.

It is almost certain the patient has Graves' disease, which is an autoimmune disease with diffuse hyperplasia and associated hyperthyroidism. Alternative diagnoses (which are less likely) include:

- Single toxic autonomous functioning nodule.
- Multinodular thyroid gland with a dominant functional nodule.
- Thyroiditis, either autoimmune or viral.
- Iodine-induced hyperthyroidism: e.g. following intravenous contrast or oral iodine and usually associated with a multinodular goitre.
- Factitious hyperthyroidism which typically has the signs of hyperthyroidism, but no goitre.

A5 There are three treatment options available. No single approach is optimum and some patients will require a combined approach to their management. Patient preferences must be taken into account, depending on their views on

radiotherapy, lifelong medications and the risks of surgery.

1 Antithyroid medication (carbimazole or propylthiouracil).
   Patients can be treated with a course of antithyroid medication for a period of 6–12 months, rendering them euthyroid. This form of treatment would be appropriate in women of childbearing age, those with small goitres and as pretreatment for radioiodine. These drugs have potentially serious side effects. The long-term remission rate is low and if relapse occurs, then the patient may be considered either for radioiodine therapy or surgery.

2 Radioiodine therapy.
   Radioiodine (131-I) causes direct destruction of thyroid cells. There are no known serious long-term side-effects from radioiodine therapy (e.g. thyroid cancer or other malignancies) although eventually hypothyroidism will occur. Many American physicians would treat this patient with radioiodine as their first option, without first rendering the patient euthyroid. Radioiodine can be administered as an outpatient and is a safe procedure if some simple precautions are taken. The results of therapy are predictable.
   Radioactive iodine cannot be administered if the patient is pregnant, breast feeding or contemplating pregnancy within the next 6 months of the administration of the dose.
   Side-effects of radioiodine include:
   - radiation-induced thyroiditis (uncommon and can be prevented with glucocorticosteroids)
   - a thyrotoxic storm may be (rarely) precipitated by radioiodine and is prevented by pretreating with antithyroid drugs
   - hypothyroidism occurs in most patients within 10 years of therapy (especially in Graves' disease) and thyroxine supplements will be required
   - thyroid eye disease may progress.

3 Surgery.
   Surgery is primarily reserved today for patients in whom there is a very large thyroid gland,

A N S W E R S – cont'd

often associated with significant thyroid ophthalmopathy. In these circumstances, drug treatment and radioiodine therapy will be ineffective in the long term. The advantage of surgery is that it is immediately curative. Current practice advocates a near-total thyroidectomy to minimize recurrence of hyperthyroidism, which was as high as 30% in the past. The risk to the patient of hypoparathyroidism and recurrent laryngeal nerve palsy is less than 2% when performed by experienced thyroid surgeons.

Betablockers can be used to control the symptoms of hyperthyroidism especially related to the sympathetic overdrive. They can be used in combination with antithyroid drugs, prior to surgery and/or radioiodine.

R E V I S I O N   P O I N T S

Graves' disease

Incidence
- 80:100 000 women per year (new cases)
- <10:100 000 men per year (new cases).

Risk factors
- other autoimmune disease
- family history of autoimmune thyroid disease
- adults aged 20–50 years
- possible role of stress-inducing hyperthyroidism.

Pathology
- Diffuse hyperplasia and hypertrophy of the thyroid
- TSH-receptor stimulatory autoantibody.

Presentation
- weight loss
- tachycardia
- eye signs.

Prognosis
Tendency to remission and relapse.

Treatment
- antithyroid drugs:
  - potential side-effects
  - usually able to avoid lifelong medications
  - suitable for use in pregnancy, young patients and those with small goitres
- radioiodine:
  - definitive, easy to use, safe, predictable
  - will require lifelong thyroxine replacement
  - suitable for most patients
- surgery:
  - definitive and rapid resolution of the problem
  - good for large goitres
  - may need lifelong thyroxine
  - more costly than the other options
  - best suited for young patients with autonomous toxic nodules, large goitres, goitres with low avidity for radioiodine, allergy to antithyroid drugs or continuous requirement for drugs, or if suspicion of malignancy.

ISSUES TO CONSIDER

- How would you manage a patient who presented with a unilateral proptosis?
- How do drugs such as amiodarone cause hyperthyroidism?
- What other causes should be considered in cases of weight loss in the presence of a normal appetite?

FURTHER INFORMATION

www.emedicine.com/radio/topic315.htm A comprehensive, didactic chapter on the diagnosis and management of thyrotoxicosis.

www.aace.com Excellent website of the American Association of Clinical Endocrinologists with management guidelines and links to a thyroid awareness programme.

A 21-year-old woman with fever, lethargy and painful joints

A 21-year-old newly married woman presents to her general practitioner with a complaint of generally feeling unwell for 3 months. She has had intermittent fevers and sweats, anorexia and weight loss of 4 kg. Her joints and muscles ache and her hands are painful and clumsy with stiffness in the mornings for about 1 hour. She has no cardiac or respiratory symptoms. She was diagnosed as having migraine 5 months ago by another doctor and was told to take a combination of aspirin and codeine and

metoclopramide as necessary for the attacks. The patient has no other past medical history and was previously fit. She is on no medications (including the oral contraceptive pill). She and her husband use condoms and spermicide for contraception and are considering a pregnancy in the near future. Her mother has a history of an 'under-functioning thyroid'.

On examination, the patient looks flushed. She has a fever of 38.6°C. You note the changes shown in Figure 60.1.

Fig 60.1

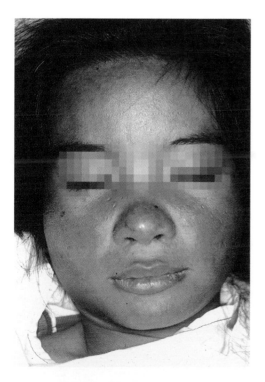

Q1   What is the abnormality shown in the photograph?

Her pulse is 95 bpm and regular and her blood pressure is 110/65 mm Hg. Multiple aphthous-like ulcers are present on her buccal mucosa. The cardiac and respiratory systems are normal. Examination of her abdomen reveals that her spleen is enlarged one finger's breadth below the left costal margin. Her proximal interphalangeal joints are swollen and tender.

Neurological examination of cranial nerves and upper and lower limbs is normal. Her urinalysis shows a trace of protein (0.3 g/l).

Q2   What are the possible causes of her fever? What additional information should be sought on history and examination and why?

Blood is taken for some routine screens and the results are shown below.

Investigation 60.1 Summary of results

Haemoglobin	101 g/l	White cell count		4.9 x 10⁹/l
RBC	4.39 x 10¹²/l	Neutrophils	57%	6.0 x 10⁹/l
PCV	0.30	Lymphocytes	27%	2.9 x 10⁹/l
MCV	81.9 fl	Monocytes	11%	1.2 x 10⁹/l
MCH	27.5 pg	Eosinophils	3%	0.3 x 10⁹/l
MCHC	340 g/l	Basophils	2%	0.2 x 10⁹/l
Platelets	85 x 10⁹/l			
Biochemistry	normal			
Blood cultures	negative			
ESR	55 mm/hour			
C-reactive protein	5 mg/l			
Viral serology:				
– Epstein–Barr virus	previous infection indicated			
– parvovirus B19	previous infection indicated			
– Ross River virus	negative			
– hepatitis B and HIV	negative			

Plain radiology of the hands demonstrates soft tissue swelling and there is no bony abnormality such as erosions. A chest X-ray is normal.

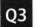

Q3   Which tests would assist in making the diagnosis and why?

Further results are as follows:

Investigation 60.2 Summary of results	
Rheumatoid factor	<20 kIU/l (normal <20)
Antinuclear antibody	positive titre 1:2560 (speckled pattern) (<1:160 is unlikely to be clinically significant)
Antibodies to extractable nuclear antigens	anti-SSA (anti-Ro) +ve
Double-stranded DNA antibody	21 units/ml (normal <3 units/ml)
Complement C3	0.83 g/l (0.6–1.2)
Complement C4	0.14 g/l (0.12–0.35)

Iron studies are normal apart from an elevated ferritin. A haemolysis screen (peripheral blood film, reticulocyte count, a Coombs' test, serum haptoglobin, unconjugated bilirubin, and lactate dehydrogenase) is negative. A urinary sediment is unremarkable.

 Q4 What is the likely diagnosis?

 Q5 What drugs are used in the management of this condition and how should this patient be managed?

The patient's arthritis, fever and lethargy are managed with non-steroidal anti-inflammatory agents and, because of an inadequate response, hydroxychloroquine is added with good effect. As part of your counselling, you discuss long-term management strategies with the patient. At initial interview she expressed a desire to conceive in the near future.

Q6 What is your counsel?

Three months later, she presents with painful fingers (Figure 60.2).

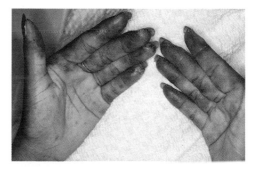

 Fig 60.2

Q7 What does the photograph show and how will this alter your management?

In addition to the changes in her fingers, the patient has similar changes to her toes. She had more extensive maculopapular eruption, alopecia and pleuropericarditis. She was put on a course of oral prednisolone, 15 mg daily, and weaned over 2 months. She is monitored closely thereafter.

ANSWERS

A1 There is facial erythema extending over the bridge of her nose and on to her cheeks.

A2 Many of the symptoms are non-specific but the presence of fever with true synovitis narrows down the differential diagnosis. A full review of systems and physical examination is essential.

- Non-specific constitutional symptoms (fever, lethargy, arthralgia and myalgia) suggest possible viral or bacterial infections. Symmetrical small joint arthritis may occur in hepatitis B, parvovirus B19, Ross River and human immunodeficiency viruses, but is unusual in infectious mononucleosis and subacute bacterial endocarditis although arthralgias may occur. Specific information that should be sought includes history of intravenous drug use, unsafe sex, exposure to children with 'slapped cheek syndrome' (due to parvovirus B19), mosquito bites, sore throat, valvular heart disease, lymphadenopthy and jaundice (develops after resolution of arthralgias in hepatitis B).
- Other possibilities are malignancy, vasculitis, granulomatous diseases (e.g. sarcoidosis, Crohn's disease) and miscellaneous causes (e.g. drug fever). The following additional information should be gathered: evidence of ocular pain, redness and loss of vision (uveitis of sarcoidosis), palpable purpura of vasculitis, diarrhoea and abdominal pain.
- Given this patient's history of lethargy, weight loss, myalgia, arthralgias and her examination findings of fever, malar rash, oral ulceration, and symmetrical small joint polyarthritis, a connective tissue disorder, in particular systemic lupus erythematosus (SLE), is likely. The patient should be examined for Raynaud's phenomenon and dilated nailfold capillaries (SLE, scleroderma, dermatomyositis and mixed connective tissue disease), alopecia and asked about exacerbation of symptoms by sun exposure (SLE), dry eyes and mouth (Sjögren's syndrome), dysphagia and gastro-oesophageal reflux (myopathies, scleroderma) and muscle weakness (polymyositis). Rheumatoid arthritis is less likely because of the rash and high fever.

A3 Investigations for evidence of multisystem disease in connective tissue diseases include CBE (haemolysis, pancytopenia), biochemistry (renal and liver function, creatine kinase), chest radiographs and urinalysis.

Investigations that indicate generalized systemic inflammation include erythrocyte sedimentation rate, C-reactive protein and globulins.

A number of auto-antibodies should be measured:

- Rheumatoid factor and antinuclear antibodies (ANA) are not specific for rheumatoid arthritis or SLE respectively, but a high titre in the appropriate clinical setting suggests an underlying autoimmune disease.
- Antinuclear antibodies are positive in 98% of SLE patients and are the best screening test for SLE.
- Anti-double stranded DNA and anti-Sm antibodies are less sensitive (being present in 80% and 30% of SLE patients respectively), but are relatively specific for SLE.
- Other antibodies to extractable nuclear antigens such as anti-SSA may occur in SLE, but if found with anti-SSB antibodies, suggest Sjögren's syndrome.

Complement levels of C3 and C4 are reduced in active SLE and can be used to follow the course of the disease in conjunction with clinical indices (e.g. severity of joint inflammation, presence of proteinuria or active sediment).

A4 According to the revised American College of Rheumatology criteria this patient can be diagnosed with SLE. The diagnostic features include malar rash, oral ulceration, non-erosive arthritis, thrombocytopenia (likely to be auto-immune), strongly positive antinuclear antibody and elevated anti-ds DNA. The anaemia is likely to be an anaemia of chronic disease.

A5 NSAIDs are an appropriate initial treatment. Your patient's main complaints are constitutional (lethargy, anorexia, fever) and musculoskeletal symptoms (myalgia, arthralgia, arthritis). NSAIDs are effective in reducing these symptoms in SLE.

A N S W E R S – cont'd

Hydroxychloroquine (e.g. 200 mg twice daily) may be added if NSAIDs are ineffective. As this drug has the potential for retinal toxicity, ophthalmological reviews should occur regularly (at least 6-monthly).

Corticosteroids should only be used if these drugs fail to control her symptoms, and only in low dose (e.g. prednisolone 15 mg mane). The patient's migraine headaches are likely to be secondary to her SLE but should be managed in the usual way.

Education is important. Autoimmune disorders are hard for patients to understand and accept, and lifestyle measures play an important part in improving quality of life. You should talk to her about general measures, e.g. an exercise plan to maintain activity level, avoidance of ultraviolet light exposure and use of 'block-out' sunscreen to prevent precipitating a flare of her disease (photosensitivity). The prospects for future pregnancy will need to be considered (see below).

It should be explained to the patient and her husband that SLE is a chronic disease which is very variable in expression that may remit and relapse and requires close monitoring. Additional advice and support from the local Arthritis Foundation may be helpful.

A6 Her fertility should be normal. It is only reduced in very active SLE such as with nephritis. The timing of the pregnancy should be planned as the risks to mother and fetus are least if the disease is inactive at the time of conception. Adequate contraception is necessary until the disease becomes inactive. Oestrogen-containing contraceptives are not advisable as they may exacerbate the disease, but progesterone-only oral contraceptive agents are acceptable.

- 10–30% of women will have an exacerbation of SLE during pregnancy. This patient has the advantage that she does not have severe disease.
- Overall, there is about twice the normal risk of fetal morbidity and mortality through miscarriage, intrauterine growth retardation and premature labour. She should be referred to a specialist obstetric hospital for advice prior to conception, and for close monitoring during pregnancy in a high-risk pregnancy clinic.
- Anti-SSA and anti-SSB antibodies are associated with fetal heart block and neonatal lupus. As she is contemplating pregnancy, it is reasonable to screen for the anticardiolipin antibody (an antiphospholipid antibody) which is associated with a high risk of arterial and venous thrombosis and increased fetal loss. Pregnancy is a hypercoagulable state and if anticardiolipin antibodies are positive in moderate to high titre, consideration should be given to the use of prophylactic treatment (e.g. combinations of corticosteroids, aspirin and subcutaneous low molecular weight heparin) during the pregnancy.

A7 Figure 60.2 shows changes of digital ischaemia. She has had a flare-up of her SLE and now needs to be urgently treated with steroids; depending on the response additonal agents may be necessary. The severity of her disease in regard to organ involvement, e.g. the kidney, will also need to be reassessed.

R E V I S I O N   P O I N T S

Systemic lupus erythematosus

Definition
A chronic autoimmune, multisystem disorder of uncertain aetiology. Genetic and environmental factors contribute.

Pathogenesis
Polyclonal B lymphocyte activation and hyperactivity, and defective T-cell function and immunoregulation result in deposition of pathogenic autoantibodies and immune complexes which mediate tissue damage.

continues overleaf

REVISION POINTS – cont'd

Incidence

40–50:100 000, increased in certain races, e.g. Afro-Americans and Asians.

Epidemiology

90% of cases are women, with onset typically in the reproductive years. The sex difference becomes less marked over the age of 60.

Clinical features

Constitutional symptoms of fever, lethargy, malaise and weight loss are almost universal. Musculoskeletal manifestations including arthralgias, myalgias and a non-erosive (mainly small joint) symmetrical polyarthritis occur in the vast majority. Skin lesions are also very common, the most frequent being photosensitivity, oral ulcers, a malar rash and alopecia.

Complications

Cardiopulmonary involvement includes pleurisy, pneumonitis, pleural effusions and pericarditis. Anaemia (chronic disease or haemolytic), leucopaenia and thrombocytopaenia can occur. Venous and arterial thrombosis are associated with the presence of anticardiolipin antibodies.

The most serious manifestations are renal and neurological. A variety of glomerular lesions can occur and the renal interstitium is also affected. 50% of patients will have renal involvement which may manifest as an abnormal urinalysis with an active sediment or nephrotic syndrome. A variety of neurologic syndromes can occur, ranging from migraines to seizures, organic brain syndromes to cord lesions and peripheral neuropathy. Some complications of pregnancy are mentioned in Answer 5.

Investigations

See Answer 2.

Diagnosis

A combination of characteristic clinical manifestations and laboratory findings. The American College of Rheumatology revised classification criteria for SLE require four of 11 criteria. However, these criteria were designed to classify patients for clinical studies, and in clinical practice, a diagnosis of SLE may be made even when four criteria are not present.

Management

See Answer 4. Severe major organ involvement, such as CNS and renal disease, usually requires high-dose steroids including intravenous methylprednisolone, often with immunosuppressive agents such as cyclophosphamide, azathioprine, ciclosporin A and mycophenolate mofetil.

Clinical course

A chronic disease with exacerbations and remissions, requiring close monitoring of disease activity and for drug toxicity.

Prognosis

Major organ involvement, particularly CNS and renal disease, has a poorer outcome. Mortality may be due to the disease or complications of therapy such as infection.

ISSUES TO CONSIDER

- What support groups and community information are available for patients with SLE and other autoimmune diseases in your region?

FURTHER INFORMATION

www.lupus.org The website of The Lupus Foundation of America. Information on education, support and research, with many links.

A collapsed, breathless woman

An ambulance arrives at the emergency department with a middle-aged woman, who collapsed in a Thai restaurant, and now has difficulty breathing. The triage nurse brings the patient directly from the ambulance to the resuscitation bay, having alerted the resuscitation team.

The history from the ambulance officer is one of a previously healthy mother of two, who was at lunch at a restaurant with her friends when she began to feel unwell and complained of tingling around her mouth and lips, and of tightness in her chest. An ambulance was called.

The patient is in obvious respiratory distress despite high-flow oxygen by mask. She has an externally audible wheeze and stridor. She is unable to speak clearly.

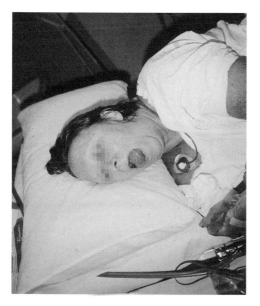

Fig 61.1

Q1 What does Figure 61.1 show? What is the likely diagnosis and prognosis?

The ambulance officer tells you her pulse is 130 bpm and her blood pressure 70/50 mm Hg.

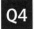 **What is your immediate management?**

The patient responds well to your treatment and does not require intubation. She is now stable. You now have time to examine her further.

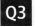 **What do you look for on specific examination and why?**

By this time, you have been able to talk with the patient. She has a past history of mild eczema, but takes no medications, and she has no cardiovascular risk factors which would complicate management.

She says that when she was a child she had an allergic reaction to peanut butter, and has avoided peanuts ever since. She says the dish she was eating did not appear to have any nuts according to the menu.

 How long will you keep her in hospital, and why? What was the likely cause of her anaphylactic reaction?

You admit your patient to the ward for observation. She complains of an itchy sensation on her torso, and a headache with some mild nausea.

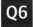 **What other medications could be used in the management of this acute allergic reaction? What will you tell her prior to discharge, and what important arrangements must be in place before she leaves hospital?**

Your patient recovers well and is grateful for your treatment. You see her on the ward the next morning, and make arrangements for her discharge.

The patient tells you that her daughter has

eczema, and is known to be allergic to bees. She wants to know if anything can be done for her daughter to prevent something similar happening if she was stung by a bee.

Q6 **What is your advice?**

You discharge your patient, armed with an adrenaline (epinephrine) pen and the knowledge of how to use it, letters to her local doctor and her

immunologist, and a shiny new medical alert bracelet.

ANSWERS

A1 Her lips, face and tongue are acutely swollen. She has the classical presentation of a severe anaphylactic reaction, with the sudden appearance of:

- Facial and tongue swelling.
- Bronchial oedema and airway restriction.
- Collapse (due to hypotension).
- A rapid rate of deterioration.

This is a life-threatening emergency. The patient has airway obstruction and cardiorespiratory arrest may be imminent unless you take immediate action.

A2 Immediate management:

- Call for immediate assistance from additional staff (an arrest code would be appropriate).
- Give adrenaline (epinephrine) intramuscularly: 0.5 mg adrenaline (0.5 ml of 1:1000 adrenaline which should be readily available in any resuscitation bay).
- Maintain the airway.
- Administer high-flow oxygen and add a nebulized beta agonist or adrenaline (epinephrine).
- Insert an intravenous catheter and start high-flow intravenous fluids.
- Attach the patient to a cardiac monitor.
- Attach a pulse oximeter.
- Reassure the patient.

A team approach is critical in the management of this medical emergency. Remember the ABC of resuscitation:

Airway

The patient has stridor and this suggests imminent airway obstruction. The facial and tongue oedema may make endotracheal intubation extremely difficult. Be prepared to intubate the patient before the obstruction worsens and intubation becomes impossible. Alert the staff (and yourself) that the patient may require a cricothyroidotomy or emergency tracheostomy. Give 100% oxygen through a non-rebreathing mask.

Breathing

- Bronchoconstriction, when present as in this case, is indicative of potentially life-threatening allergy/anaphylaxis.

- Remember that severe bronchoconstriction may not have a loud wheeze, as airflow is so severely restricted.
- Adrenaline (epinephrine) treats both bronchoconstriction and oedema via beta-1 adrenergic effects.
- Beta agonists such as continuously nebulized salbutamol should be administered.

Circulation

Profound hypotension (due to acute vasodilatation and increased capillary permeability) is common in anaphylactic shock. In addition to its effects on the respiratory tract adrenaline (epinephrine) acts as a peripheral vasoconstrictor via alpha-receptors and is a positive inotrope and chronotrope.

Intravenous fluids should be given immediately and titrated to blood pressure and urine output. In severe anaphylactic shock the patient may require:

- A urinary catheter to guide fluid therapy.
- A central venous line and arterial line to closely monitor blood pressure and ventricular filling.

Specific causes should be treated, including removal of the venom sac from bee or wasp stings.

Do not induce emesis even if the causative agent (e.g. medication or food) is in the gut.

A3 A complete physical examination is carried out specifically looking for:

- A cause not immediately evident, e.g. a sting or a bite.
- Distribution, nature and evolution of any skin lesions, such as macular, papular, erythemata or urticarial lesions.
- Concomitant conditions such as trauma sustained after collapse.

The quicker the progression of signs, the more severe the anaphylactic reaction and the more urgent the need for treatment. It is important to monitor her closely for any further progression of the anaphylactic reaction.

A4 This patient has had a life-threatening anaphylactic reaction, and must be closely observed until completely symptom free.

Up to a third of patients with anaphylaxis have a biphasic reaction, in which symptoms resolve with adrenaline (epinephrine), only to recur later with sudden bronchoconstriction. The biphasic reaction usually occurs within 4 hours of initial treatment and is more difficult to treat, often requiring intubation and mechanical ventilation.

This woman should therefore be observed for an absolute minimum of 4 hours, but given the severity of her reaction she should ideally be admitted overnight for observation on the ward.

The patient has a known allergy to peanuts, and this is the most likely trigger for her allergic reaction. Peanut allergy is highly specific, and tiny trace amounts of peanut protein in foods can trigger anaphylaxis. It is likely that the meal she ate contained some trace of peanut protein, either in the ingredients or possibly the pans used to cook her meal may have had contact with peanuts or peanut oils. It is estimated that a person with peanut allergy will have an allergic reaction once every 3–5 years, despite being fastidious about avoiding foods containing peanuts and other nuts.

A5 With her present symptoms, you might want to consider the following medications:
- Histamine 1(H1) antihistamines for rash and pruritus (e.g. phenergan or diphenhydramine).
- H2 receptor blockers (e.g. ranitidine) can also be given to complete the histamine blockade.
- Paracetamol for mild headache.
- Oral steroids are often given for a 3–5 day course, although there is evidence to suggest that they do not actually prevent recurrences in the 24–48 hours after the initial event.

Most symptoms such as diarrhoea and nausea resolve quickly and spontaneously.

Anaphylaxis is very frightening experience, and the intravenous adrenaline (epinephrine) can contribute to feelings of fear and 'impending doom'. Several discussions with patient and family will be necessary to talk about anaphylaxis and to establish emergency plans should it happen again. An anaphylaxis management plan should be constructed (much like the asthma management plan outlined in Chapter 43).

Adrenaline (epinephrine) pens for self-injection can be life saving. Many patients find the con-cept of self-injecting difficult to face. Involvement of a diabetes nurse educator may be useful as they have experience in teaching self-injection techniques. The adrenaline (epinephrine) pen is most useful as it is preset and does not require any specific technique; however, it must be made clear that the patient needs to have one readily accessible at all times.

A medical alert bracelet or wallet-card should be organized. Do not leave it up to the patient's GP to organize this after discharge: it could happen again on the way home! It is your responsibility to ensure that this patient leaves the hospital safely, with a good understanding of her illness and with contingency plans in place.

At least two letters should be provided to the patient: one for her GP, and one for the patient to keep for her own records.

Referral to a specialist immunologist can be organized for identification of further allergens, possible desensitization and future follow-up.

A6 A history of eczema, asthma and allergy should alert you to the possibility of atopy – a familial disorder of high circulating levels of IgE which predispose to immune hypersensitivity reactions.

Her daughter could be referred to an allergy clinic where an immunologist can measure her IgE levels and can perform specific antigen testing for bee allergy:
- RAST (radio allergoabsorbent test) testing, which measures specific anti-bee venom IgE.
- Skin prick intradermal tests can be performed with dilutions of bee venom.

If the tests are positive, immunotherapy to bee antigen can be offered to desensitize the immune system and prevent anaphylaxis. The patient receives repeated injections of the venom extract starting in minuscule dilutions and gradually increasing the dose. These are performed in hospital, with resuscitation equipment easily at hand. Once the dose of one bee sting is reached the patient is protected. Desensitization to bee stings is effective in about 95% of cases if the protocol is followed. The maintenance injections are given for 5 years.

REVISION POINTS

Anaphylaxis

Aetiology

- Anaphylaxis is due to immediate hypersensitivity mediated by specific antigen-antibody reaction.
- It occurs in a presensitized subject after administration of a specific antigen to which antibodies have already been developed.
- It is a systemic reaction.
- The antigen interacts with pre-formed antigen-specific IgE which triggers the release of inflammatory mediators such as histamine and prostaglandins (PGD_2).

Triggers

Food allergies are the most common form of anaphylaxis presenting to emergency departments, and peanut allergy accounts for the majority of life-threatening anaphylactic reactions. However, many antigens cause anaphylaxis. These include:

- Exogenous proteins (insulin, vasopressin, parathormone).
- Enzymes (streptokinase, trypsin).
- Foods (nuts, egg, milk, seafoods, gelatin in medicine capsules).
- Anaesthetic muscle relaxants are an important cause in hospital anaphylaxis.
- Antibiotics (penicillin, cephalosporins, quinolones).
- Intravenous dextrans (e.g. haemaccel/ gelofusine).
- Insects (bees, wasps, etc., with *Hymenoptera* venom).

- Aspirin and NSAIDs, other drugs and radio-contrast media can induce 'anaphylactoid' reactions which are similar in all respects to anaphylaxis, but are not mediated by specific antigen-antibody interaction, e.g. direct action on mast cells causing degranulation and histamine release.

Symptoms

- Bronchospasm due to histamine and leukotriene release.
- Oedema due to 'leaky capillaries': laryngeal oedema, airway oedema, facial oedema.
- Hypotension due to sudden systemic vasodilatation.
- Rash – usually urticarial.

Management

- Adrenaline (epinephrine) and oxygen.
- Airway: intubation may be necessary.
- Breathing: bronchodilators and adrenaline (epinephrine).
- Circulation: rapid fluid resuscitation, cardiac monitoring, and if necessary vasoconstrictor infusion (e.g. isoprenaline).

Prevention

- Identification of allergens.
- Patient education and awareness: medical alert bracelets and adrenaline (epinephrine) pens. Counselling the patient and family is important, and having a clear emergency anaphylaxis plan is essential.
- Immunologist referral and identification of specific allergens may allow immunotherapy and desensitization.

ISSUES TO CONSIDER

- How do you perform an emergency cricothyroidotomy or tracheostomy?
- How else could you deliver oxygen to a patient with an obstructed upper airway?
- What is meant by the term 'atopy'? Do atopic people have a higher incidence of anaphylactic reactions?
- If someone is allergic to penicillin, is it safe to give them a cephalosporin?

FURTHER INFORMATION

Long, A. **The nuts and bolts of peanut allergy**. Editorial. *New England Journal of Medicine* 2002; v346:1320–1.

www.foodallergy.org Food Allergy and Anaphylaxis Network.

www.jcaai.org Joint Council of Allergy, Asthma and Immunology.

A 32-year-old unemployed man presents for a check-up. He and his partner have recently moved from another city 'for personal reasons'. He claims he has no major health problems and takes no medications. He smokes about 30 cigarettes a day and drinks 30–70 grams of alcohol daily. Sensing that there is more to the story, you spend some time talking to the man in an effort to establish the true reason for his visit. During the course of the conversation he reveals that just prior to leaving the city he used to live in 2 weeks ago he had a blood test and this showed that he was human immunodeficiency virus (HIV) antibody positive.

Q1 What further information should be gained from the history and what should be sought on examination?

The patient reveals that previously he and his partner were involved with a group of intravenous drug users and shared needles for about 5 months. He denies any homosexual contacts and states he has had no other sexual contacts other than his partner for 8 months. He has never had a blood transfusion. On direct enquiry he recalls a severe 'flu-like illness about 4 months ago which involved headache, fever, weakness and muscle aches and pains and lasted about 10 days. The patient explains that he and his partner have definitely ceased intravenous drug use and limit their drug use to marijuana. She has not had an HIV antibody test as she is 'too scared'.

Currently, the patient's health is good. His weight is stable, he has no fevers or sweats and his systems review is unremarkable. The patient is examined and nothing is found that might be attributable to his recent diagnosis.

Q2 What investigations should be performed?

Blood screens show a complete blood picture within the normal range, a CD4 lymphocyte count of 800/μl (RR 405–2205 cells/μl) and an HIV viral load of 4000 copies/μl. He is hepatitis B surface antigen negative and hepatitis C antibody positive.

Q3 What may the 'flu-like illness 4 months ago have represented? At what stage of infection is this man currently?

This patient appears to have seroconverted and is now asymptomatic.

What else needs to be done?

The partner is also found to be HIV antibody positive and has similar hepatitis serology. Counselled together, they are told that under no circumstances should they have unprotected intercourse or share needles with any other persons. The prospects of a future pregnancy are discussed and the couple decide against child-bearing. She therefore continues her usual contraceptive pill and the necessity of strict compliance is emphasized. They are offered vaccination against hepatitis B given their recent history of injecting drug use. The patient and his partner decline to identify any of their contacts. They are followed every 3 months with a full review of symptoms,

examination findings and blood screens for 12 months but then they stop returning for appointments and are lost to follow-up.

Four and half years later the man presents with a 3–4-week history of feeling unwell. He is tired and lethargic and has lost 6 kg in weight. He has also had a sore mouth. He denies any other gastrointestinal symptoms including diarrhoea and there are no other significant symptoms on systems review.

On examination he appears thinner than previously and looks depressed. He is afebrile. His oral mucosa is as illustrated in Figure 62.1.

Fig 62.1

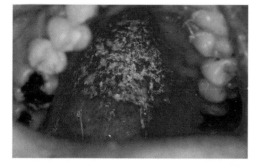

He has generalized lymphadenopathy, the nodes being 1–2 cm in size. He is referred to a hospital infectious diseases clinic. Infective screens fail to reveal any additional infectious cause for his deterioration other than the condition in his

mouth. His blood screens reveal his haemoglobin has dropped to 112 g/l but his complete blood count is otherwise normal, his CD4 lymphocyte count has dropped to 110/µl and the HIV viral load is now >200 000 copies/µl.

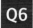

What does the figure show? What has happened? In brief, what are the principles of management now?

The patient is offered and commenced on antiretroviral therapy with zidovudine 250 mg bd, lamivudine 150 mg bd (both nucleotide-analogue reverse transcriptase inhibitors) and indinavir 800 mg tds (a protease inhibitor). His oral candidiasis is treated with fluconazole 100 mg daily and prophylaxis against pneumocystis pneumonia with co-trimoxazole 160–800 mg daily is begun. He is reviewed monthly.

Q6 The patient asks if this treatment will cure his HIV infection and if not, whether he will develop AIDS. What would be an appropriate reply?

ANSWERS

A1 The following history should be obtained:

- The patient's understanding of the meaning of a positive HIV antibody test. There is much misunderstanding in the community about HIV and AIDS. If he does not understand the implications of this they should be carefully explained.
- A sexual history, history of intravenous drug use and history of blood transfusions. Knowledge of how the infection was contracted should be obtained and whether unsafe sex or needle use is still putting others at risk. These questions will give information about potential contacts who should be traced. It may also identify drug addiction which may need to be dealt with separately.
- Enquiries must be made to determine if the partner knows and whether he or she has been tested.
- The patient should be asked if he is positive for other infections which may be spread by similar mechanisms as HIV (e.g. hepatitis B and C), and whether the man has been vaccinated against hepatitis B.

A systems review is needed with emphasis on constitutional symptoms such as lethargy, weight loss and sweats and gastrointestinal symptoms (sore mouth, dysphagia, abdominal pain, diarrhoea), respiratory symptoms (exercise intolerance and dry cough), skin eruptions, lymph node enlargement, bleeding or bruising and neurological symptoms (e.g. headache, visual symptoms, confusion, weakness or numbness of the limbs).

As part of the physical examination, particular attention should be paid to:

- Evidence of obvious ill health, fever, weight loss, anaemia.
- Skin eruptions, e.g. Kaposi's sarcoma, seborrhoeic dermatitis or cutaneous candidiasis.
- Oral lesions, e.g. candidiasis, Herpes simplex, hairy leukoplakia.
- Lymphadenopathy and hepatosplenomegaly.
- Abnormalities in specific systems, e.g. respiratory or neurological signs.
- Perianal disease, e.g. warts due to papilloma virus or vesicles or ulcers consistent with Herpes simplex.

A2 Investigations include a complete blood picture, biochemistry and liver function tests, CD4 count and CD4/CD8 ratio and HIV viral load. The patient should also have his hepatitis B and C and syphilis serology checked. Baseline serology for cryptococcus antigen, toxoplasma antibodies and CMV serology can be useful for diagnosing future opportunistic infections.

A3 Patients with HIV progress through four stages of infection.

1 *Seroconversion illness* includes fever, lymphadenopathy, rash and malaise occurring at the time of seroconversion to anti-HIV antibody positivity. Not all patients experience these symptoms.

2 *Asymptomatic HIV infection* where the patient feels well, but is infectious and has slowly falling CD4 counts.

3 *Symptomatic HIV infection* with lymphadenopathy, low CD4 counts, some generalized symptoms and minor opportunistic infections.

4 *Advanced HIV infection* or AIDS. A patient is said to have AIDS if they suffer so-called 'AIDS defining' conditions, such as opportunistic infections or certain secondary neoplasms, e.g. Kaposi's sarcoma. However, severe constitutional illness or neurological disease (e.g. AIDS related dementia) will also place the patient in the AIDS category.

This patient's 'flu-like illness sounds characteristic of a seroconversion illness, although it is not specific and could therefore be attributed to something else. He is currently in the asymptomatic stage of his infection.

A4 The patient should be counselled together with his partner. She will also need to be tested and it can be explained that knowledge of her antibody status can enhance their management. If she were negative the antibody test would need to be repeated at 3-monthly intervals for 6 months after her last 'unsafe' exposure (to ensure she was not a late seroconverter). In the meantime they would need to engage in 'safe' protected sexual intercourse in an effort to

ANSWERS – cont'd

prevent her from becoming infected. If she is already infected this is obviously less of an issue.

The prospects of future pregnancy should be discussed, pointing out the significant risk of the child being infected. Transmission of HIV from mother to child can be greatly reduced with the use of antiretroviral medication during pregnancy. It should be ensured that the patient knows not to engage in unprotected intercourse or share needles with any other person because of the risk of infecting them. The issue of contact tracing will also need to be discussed.

It should be explained to the patient that he will require regular medical follow-up to monitor the status of his disease. In this way, when the disease progresses medication can be started in an effort to keep him healthy for as long as possible. The patient should be made aware that HIV is a lethal condition, but with the introduction of therapies such as Highly Active Anti-Retroviral Therapy (HAART), long-term survival is possible.

A5 The figure illustrates white plaques of oral candidiasis on the hard palate. The patient's CD4 count is now below 200/µl which suggests severe immune compromise, and consistent with this he has developed constitutional symptoms (lethargy and weight loss), generalized lymphadenopathy and an opportunistic infection – oral candida. This is in keeping with his degree of immunodeficiency as measured by his CD4 count.

He has uncontrolled viral replication as demonstrated by his high HIV viral load. He now has symptomatic HIV infection (stage 3 above). Management should now be in conjunction with a specialist hospital clinic.

1 Control the HIV viral replication with antiretroviral therapy (ART). This slows the rate of damage to the immune system and allows the CD4 count to recover and 'immune reconstitution' to occur. His constitutional symptoms will improve with this treatment. ART consists of at least three or four drugs used in combination, which target HIV replication at least two points in the cycle. Classes of available drugs include the nucleotide analogue

reverse transcriptase inhibitors (e.g. zidovudine and lamivudine), non-nucleotide analogue reverse transcriptase inhibitors (e.g. nevirapine) and the protease inhibitors (e.g. indinavir and saquinavir). HIV replicates very rapidly and mutates frequently and unless the patient is extremely compliant with his medications, his virus will quickly become resistant to therapy. The importance of not missing his tablets must be reinforced at each visit. ART has side-effects and these should be discussed with the patient before commencing therapy.

2 Treat and prevent opportunistic infections until immune recovery has occurred. He has oral candidiasis, and this will respond to fluconazole 100 mg daily. Given that his CD4 count is 110 cells/µl, prophylactic therapy for *Pneumocystis carinii* pneumonia (PCP) with co-trimoxazole (160/800 mg daily) should be given. If his CD4 count falls to below 50 cells/µl then prophylaxis against *Mycobacterium avium* complex infections with azithromycin 1.2 g weekly is indicated.

3 Monitor for the development of malignancies such as non-Hodgkin's lymphoma, carcinoma of the anal canal (especially if he has perianal warts) or Kaposi's sarcoma.

A6 Explain to the patient that antiretroviral therapy does not cure HIV and, that once acquired, the HIV virus cannot be eradicated from the body. However, ART does successfully control HIV replication and provides relief from the constitutional symptoms of advanced HIV. The immune recovery protects against superimposed opportunistic infections. With ART, the patient can expect to have a further 3–5 years or more of good quality life. Without treatment, he will develop AIDS within 2 years with a progressive decline in health to death.

He will need to have ongoing monitoring during ART for complications of the therapy and development of viral resistance (indicated by rising HIV viral load) and the need for change in therapy.

The role of support groups and counselling for patients with HIV should be discussed.

REVISION POINTS

HIV infection

Aetiology

- It is estimated that more than 40 million people are infected with HIV worldwide. The majority live in sub-Saharan Africa.
- HIV is an RNA virus, with rapid rates of replication and frequent replication errors leading to high mutation rates. It infects lymphocytes and monocytes using the CD4 receptor and causes destruction of these cells resulting in failure of the immune system.
- The HIV virus is spread through contact with blood (transfusion and recreational intravenous drug use) and body fluids (semen, vaginal secretions, breast milk) and vertical transmission from mother to child.
- Immune failure is followed by disease due to opportunistic infection (e.g. oral candida, *Pneumocystis carinii* pneumonia, cytomegalovirus, *Toxoplasma*, *Mycobacterium avium* complex infection), malignancies (cerebral lymphoma, Kaposi's sarcoma) and disease due to HIV itself (e.g. HIV encephalopathy and wasting syndrome).

Treatment

- Antiretroviral therapy (ART or HAART): antiviral drugs used in combination which prevent replication of the HIV virus and thus infection of new CD4$^+$ cells. This allows restoration of immune function.
- Prophylaxis and treatment of opportunistic infections and malignancies.
- Supportive care during the terminal phases of the disease.

ART is effective over a period of 2–5 years. It cannot cure HIV infection but immune recovery occurs with return of general health status and protection against opportunistic infections. The virus mutates after exposure to antiretroviral therapy and eventually becomes resistant to treatment with reactivation of viral replication, return of symptoms, progressive immune failure and death.

Monitoring of HIV infection includes CD4 lymphocyte counts to monitor the degree of immune damage and HIV viral loads on plasma to assess the rates of viral replication which estimates the risk of progressing to AIDS and the effectiveness of ART. With effective ART, CD4 counts rise towards normal and the HIV viral load should become undetectable.

ISSUES TO CONSIDER

- What is the risk to healthcare workers of accidental transmission of HIV? What policies exist in your hospital to address this and how can risks be reduced?
- What measures do you know of to deal with the global AIDS epidemic by the world community? What ideas do you have?
- What are the risks of an HIV-infected mother passing the virus on to her child?
- Are we any nearer to finding a vaccine? What are the hurdles?

FURTHER INFORMATION

Palella F J, Delaney K M, Moorman A C et al. **Declining morbidity and mortality among patients with advanced human immunodeficiency virus infection**. *New England Journal of Medicine* 1998;338:853–60.

Mindel A, Tennant-Flowers M. ABC of AIDS: **Natural history and management of early HIV infection**. *British Journal of Medicine* 2001;322:1290–94.

Weller I V D, Williams I G. ABC of AIDS: **Antiretroviral drugs**. *British Journal of Medicine*. 2001;322:1410–12.

Mofenson L M, McIntyre J A. **Advances and research directions in the prevention of mother-to-child HIV-1 transmission**. *Lancet* 2000;355;2237–44.

www.aidsinfo.nih.gov An excellent AIDS and HIV resource from the US Department of Health.

Back and leg pain in a middle-aged man

A 50-year-old man experiences a sudden onset of back and leg pain while walking. The pain radiates from the left buttock to his knee and as far as his ankle. There is no recent history of trauma. He has no significant past medical or surgical history. He has been bedbound for 3 days.

Q1 What key features need to be sought from the history?

On specific questioning, there is a similar pain which radiates down his right leg although this is of a lesser intensity. The patient has noticed that the pain is aggravated when he coughs or strains. He has noticed some numbness over his buttocks. This is associated with some difficulty in voiding. Prior to the onset of this pain, the patient had not experienced any urinary symptoms. There has been no alteration in bowel function. His general health is good and he has not lost any weight recently. He is not on any medications.

Q2 What specific features should be sought on physical examination?

A general physical examination is unremarkable. His blood pressure is 130/90 mm Hg and his heart rate is 90 bpm. The rest of the cardiovascular system is normal, and in particular all his peripheral pulses are present and of good volume. Abdominal examination is unremarkable except for some dullness to percussion in the suprapubic region. Digital examination of the rectum suggests a rather lax anal sphincter. Examination of his back reveals no significant spinal tenderness. Straight leg raising is restricted to 30° in both legs, with reproduction of leg pain. The power and tone of both legs are normal to testing in the bed but he is unable to stand on his toes, indicating plantar flexion weakness. The ankle jerks are bilaterally absent and his plantar responses are flexor. Hypoaesthesia is present in the lateral and plantar aspects of both feet. In addition, sensory testing to pin-prick reveals some numbness over the buttocks and reduced sensation in the perineum.

Q3 What is the diagnosis?

The clinical picture fits for an acute neurological problem.

Q4 How should the patient be investigated?

An investigation is performed (Figures 63.1–63.3).

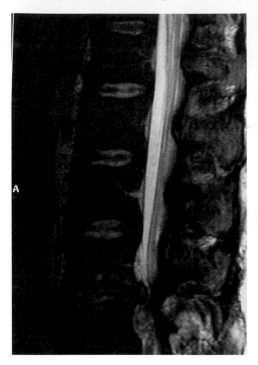

Fig 63.1

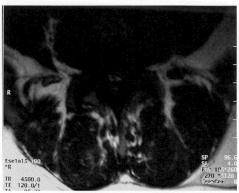

Fig 63.2

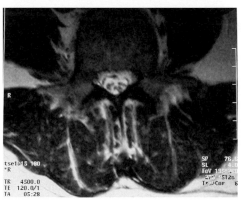

Fig 63.3

Q5 What is the investigation and what do the three images show?

The patient underwent a microdiscectomy as an emergency procedure. This gave him relief of his pain and his symptoms of cauda equina compression resolved over the next week.

ANSWERS

A1 The first aim of the history is to try to distinguish between the major causes of limb pain. These include:
- Vascular:
  - intermittent claudication
  - chronic venous insufficiency.

- Musculoskeletal:
  - joint disease
  - muscle/ligament injury
  - stress fracture.
- Neurogenic:
  - sciatica

ANSWERS – cont'd

- spinal canal stenosis
- cauda equina syndrome.

This patient gives a typical account of 'sciatica' (which often arises from lumbar disc herniation). It is important to distinguish between radiculopathic pain ('sciatica') and non-specific lumbar pain. Radiculopathic pain refers to pain which radiates into the limb in a dermatomal distribution. It arises from compression or compromise of particular nerve root(s). This is typically exacerbated by coughing, sneezing or straining. Surgery to relieve nerve root compression (e.g. lumbar discectomy in the presence of a significant disc prolapse) is generally performed with the key aim of improving radiculopathic pain. Non-specific lumbar or back pain may radiate to the buttock and thigh but not usually beyond the knee. It is usually not helped by surgery.

The clinician may also use the patient's description of radiculopathic pain to deduce the possible nerve roots affected in the majority of patients. For example, an L3 radiculopathy typically results in pain which radiates to the knee. In contrast, an S1 radiculopathy usually causes pain which is felt as far as the ankle/foot. Asking specific questions about the pattern of any sensory changes may further point to specific dermatome(s).

Further history should be directed towards excluding:
- Serious ('red flag') underlying conditions, e.g.
  - tumour
  - infection
  - coagulopathy.
- Severe neurological compromise, e.g. evidence of:
  - lower limb weakness
  - sensory changes
  - bladder or bowel symptoms.

A2 On physical examination evidence should be sought of overall state of health, e.g:
- Fever.
- Recent weight loss.
- Disseminated malignancy (e.g. cachexia, pallor, lymphadenopathy, pleural effusions, breast lumps, hepatomegaly, prostatic enlargement, bone tenderness, unexplained bruises).

Specific features referable to the symptoms and the need to be excluded:
- Peripheral vascular disease (check pulses).
- Musculoskeletal disorders (examine joints).
- Neurological disorders (the examination must focus on the trunk and lower limbs, including the perineum, ensuring that no sensory level is missed).

A3 This patient has evidence of cauda equina compression. This is judged by symptoms of acute bladder paralysis and buttock numbness. The clinical examination has revealed a distended bladder, reduced anal tone and numbness in the perineal and buttock regions (S2,3,4). There are also signs consistent with S1 nerve root compression (absent ankle reflexes and plantar flexion weakness).

A4 This is a neurological emergency and any delay in treatment may compromise neurological recovery and result in permanent paralysis. An urgent MRI scan of the lumbosacral spine is the investigation of choice, but may not always be available. A CT scan is the more often performed procedure. In the absence of MRI or CT, a lumbar myelogram can also point to the diagnosis. Plain X-rays are generally unhelpful. Lack of appropriate radiological facilities and neurosurgical expertise should prompt an urgent transfer of the patient to a centre where these are available. Cauda equina compression requires prompt surgery to optimize the chances of neurological recovery.

Blood tests should be done but must not delay emergency treatment. They are of lesser importance in those patients who otherwise appear in normal health, making a benign aetiology more likely. They can be very important in those with presentations suspicious of a sinister underlying problem, e.g. malignancy. An elevated white cell count or inflammatory markers (ESR, CRP) may suggest infection. Other abnormalities in blood counts, liver function tests, total protein or calcium levels could suggest underlying malignancy. Tumour markers (e.g. PSA) may be helpful. Coagulation studies (INR, APTT) should be performed when there is clinical suspicion of a bleeding diathesis.

ANSWERS – cont'd

A5 These are MRI scans, with focus on the spinal canal. T2 weighted images show cerebrospinal fluid (CSF) contained within the thecal sac as hyperintense (bright) material. A compressive lesion (e.g. disc prolapse) is easier to recognize on this sequence. It will also demonstrate any abnormalities involving the vertebral body (e.g. osteomyelitis, metastatic disease) or disc (e.g. infective discitis).

The sagittal MRI of this patient (Figure 63.1) reveals two problems. First, the patient has a congenitally narrow spinal canal. Any disc prolapse is more likely to cause a cauda equina compressive syndrome. Second, the patient has an L4/5 disc prolapse (Figure 63.2) which explains his clinical presentation. This compresses the thecal sac to the extent that little CSF is visible at this level. This compression leads to compromise of the nerve roots which form the cauda equina. Figure 63.3 is at the level of L3/4 disc in the same patient and shows the normal appearance of the thecal sac and spinal canal.

REVISION POINTS

Lumbar disc disease

Incidence

Benign lumbar disc disease is common in clinical practice.

Management

- Patients who present with uncomplicated 'sciatica' or radiculopathic leg pain may generally be managed conservatively for 4–6 weeks. Strong oral analgesics may be required.
- In the absence of 'red flag' conditions or severe neurological deficits, back and leg pain arising from lumbar disc disease generally follows a benign course.
- Investigations (CT or MRI) are then considered if symptoms are severe and persistent.
- More than 80% of patients improve with or without surgery.
- The main aim of surgery (discectomy) is to relieve radiculopathic leg pain. Non-specific back pain is not generally an indication for surgery. Spinal fusion for back pain alone is controversial. Surgical results are inconsistent.

- These patients must be differentiated from those with
  - severe neurological compromise
  - pathologies other than benign disc disease.
- These latter patients require urgent neurosurgical assessment.

Cauda equina syndrome

This is a rare problem – and a surgical emergency. It is characterized by:

- Sphincter disturbances.
- Sexual dysfunction.
- 'Saddle anaesthesia': perianal, buttocks, perineum, genitals, thighs.
- Significant motor weakness usually involving more than one nerve root.
- Bilateral sciatica.
- Bilateral absence of ankle jerks.

Delay in diagnosis and treatment may jeopardize any neurological recovery.

ISSUES TO CONSIDER

- How are the pelvis and the lower limb innervated?
- What other conditions might predispose to the development of a cauda equina syndrome?

FURTHER INFORMATION

www.cauda-equina.org A patient-based website with links and patient perspectives.

www.vh.org/adult/provider/familymedicine/FPH andbook/Chapter16/01-16.html
The Virtual Hospital Site on low back pain.

Acute respiratory failure in a 68-year-old man

Having just finished congratulating yourself for managing your last case so well, you are called to see a 68-year-old man brought into the emergency department by ambulance with severe dyspnoea. He is accompanied by his wife, who states that he has had increasing shortness of breath overnight with some symptoms of an upper respiratory tract infection for the last 1–2 days. Over this time he has also had increasing wheeze and a dry cough with 'tightness' of his chest. He has become somewhat agitated this morning.

He is in obvious respiratory distress, unable to utter more than one or two words at a time.

This man obviously needs urgent assessment and treatment. You only have time to elicit the essential parts of the history while you rapidly examine the patient and start the appropriate management.

Q1 What are the major differential diagnoses to consider?

The patient's breathing is so laboured that he is unable to answer any of your questions.

Q2 What are the main points you would like to know from his wife or the ambulance officer?

The man's wife tells you that he has 'pretty bad' emphysema. He has no known history of cardiovascular disease.

His medications are:
- salbutamol inhaler: 2 puffs prn (1–3 times on a typical day)
- salmeterol: 2 puffs metered dose inhaler bd
- beclometasone: 750 µg metered dose inhaler bd
- ipratropium bromide: 2 puffs metered dose inhaler bd.

He has smoked heavily most of his life, but has reduced his current cigarette consumption to about five a day. He does not drink and has no known allergies.

The ambulance officer states that the man has had an oxygen saturation of about 80% throughout the journey, and that he has been wheezing loudly. He has been given 5 mg nebulized salbutamol in the ambulance.

As you examine the patient, you observe that on 6 l/min of oxygen by face mask, his oxygen saturation is 78%. He seems irritable, obviously dyspnoeic, and grasping the sleeve of your designer shirt, he utters 'help...'.

You persist with the examination. His respiratory rate is 30 breaths per minute with a prolonged expiratory phase. The pulse rate is 110 bpm and regular. His temperature is 36.5°C and the blood pressure 110/75 mm Hg. He is well hydrated and the peripheral perfusion is adequate. His peripheral pulses are all present and of good volume. In the semi-recumbent position his jugular venous pressure (JVP) is 3–4 cm. Both heart sounds appear normal and there are no murmurs. His trachea is in the midline. He is barrel-chested and there are reduced breath sounds throughout. There is a diffuse expiratory wheeze and the percussion note is normal. There are no crepitations. His abdomen is soft and non-tender. The calves are normal and there is no pedal or sacral oedema.

Q3 What investigations should be performed straight away?

An electrocardiogram is performed which shows a sinus tachycardia, and the arterial blood gases (ABGs) show:

Investigation 64.1 Arterial blood gas analysis	
paO$_2$	48 mm Hg
paCO$_2$	65 mm Hg
pH	7.23
Bicarbonate	27 mmol/l

Q4 What does his arterial blood gas show? What should you do immediately with his oxygen therapy?

You adjust his oxygen therapy carefully. He is too dyspnoeic for a peak expiratory flow rate (PEFR) measure. You order an urgent mobile chest X-ray and go on to administer emergency medications to treat this man's condition.

Q5 Describe in detail what you would use to treat this man.

A chest X-ray is performed and is shown in Figure 64.1.

Q6 What does the X-ray show? Does this affect your diagnosis?

The patient starts to improve, but he is still struggling. You call the intensive care team, who admit him to their unit. He receives close monitoring of his gas exchange. He is placed on CPAP (continuous positive airway pressure by mask) to support his ventilation. A radial arterial line is inserted to monitor serial blood gases.

The patient responds to aggressive bronchodilation with continuous nebulized salbutamol and intermittent ipratropium. Oxygen therapy is carefully monitored and adjusted over this period. He is commenced on a course of oral prednisolone 50 mg daily. His blood gases stabilize with improvement in his respiratory condition, achieving his baseline level of function with pO$_2$ 65 mm Hg on room air, pCO$_2$ 42 mm Hg, pH 7.38, bicarbonate 24 mmol/l.

Fig 64.1

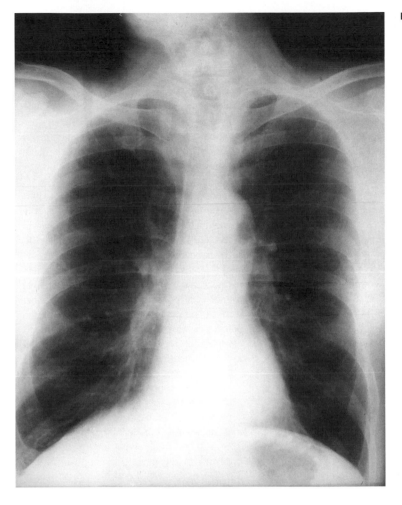

Q7 What follow-up plans will you arrange for this man prior to discharge?

He is discharged after 7 days to complete a 14-day course of prednisolone (dose to be tapered according to clinical progress), a programme to discontinue smoking and arrangements for follow-up appointments with formal pulmonary function testing.

ANSWERS

A1 In the absence of an obvious external cause (e.g. chest trauma), the vast majority of cases of acute shortness of breath in adults will be due to one of four conditions:

- Exacerbation of chronic obstructive pulmonary disease (COPD) or asthma (and their complications, e.g. pneumothorax).
- Pneumonia/lower respiratory tract infection.

ANSWERS – cont'd

- Pulmonary embolus.
- Pulmonary oedema (it is important to look for the underlying causes, e.g. myocardial ischaemia or cardiac arrhythmia).

Even if the cardiorespiratory system is seemingly intact, it is important to consider anaemia and acidosis as causes of shortness of breath but in these instances the onset will be insidious rather than sudden.

A2 You will need to have:
- A brief account of what has happened since the onset of his illness, including his condition on arrival of the ambulance officers and any treatment they gave him so far, to gauge how much and how rapidly he has deteriorated in transit.
- A 'problem list' of his active and inactive medical conditions.
- A list of his current medications.
- Information about any allergies.

A3 The most important immediate investigations are:
- Arterial blood gas analysis.
- Mobile chest X-ray.
- ECG.

All are quick to perform, and can be done while the patient is being examined and treated. Complete blood picture, electrolytes and cardiac enzymes will also be needed.

A4 The ABGs show severe hypoxia. He has an acute respiratory acidosis, with a compensatory increase in bicarbonate. The presence of a low arterial blood pH indicates the pCO_2 is acutely raised, as opposed to the picture in chronic hypoventilation, in which compensatory mechanisms have had sufficient time to bring the pH almost back to normal.

A major error in this patient would be to reduce the rate of oxygen flow. Patients do not lose their hypoxic drive unless they have lost their hypoxia. His pO_2 is 48, i.e. he is definitely still hypoxic, and this is the cause of his agitation and confusion.

- Titrate the O_2 up, aiming for a pO_2 of around 60 mm Hg, but not exceeding 60–65 mm Hg, while watching his pCO_2.
- An arterial line should be inserted as frequent arterial blood gas analysis is required.
- By correlating his haemoglobin–oxygen saturation probe readings with a simultaneous arterial blood gas reading, you can thereafter use the SaO_2 as a guide to what his pO_2 might be. A pO_2 of 60 mm Hg usually corresponds to SaO_2 of about 90%, but in this patient remember acidosis shifts the haemoglobin–oxygen dissociation curve to the 'right', meaning that for any given pO_2, the haemoglobin saturation is lower.
- pCO_2 needs to be followed clinically (drowsiness, vasodilatation, bounding pulses, asterixis) and with periodic blood gases. Remember that good oxygen saturation readings on the pulse oximeter do not mean that the patient's ventilation is adequate – alveolar ventilation is monitored by the pCO_2.
- Venturi masks can be useful in controlling the inspired concentration of oxygen (fraction of inspired oxygen – FiO) in these patients more reliably than ordinary medium capacity O_2 masks (MCOM). Venturi masks deliver gas at a predetermined percentage of oxygen directly to the patient. In contrast, MCOMs deliver oxygen which is mixed with air according to how deeply the patient breathes, and hence the FiO_2 varies with the patient's respiration.

A5 Given the above findings, this man is most likely having an acute exacerbation of his COPD.
- Beta-2 adrenergic agonists are indicated. The conventional way to use them is to nebulize 5 mg (1 ml) of salbutamol, along with 1 ml normal saline (to make up an appropriate volume for nebulization), repeated continuously up to 3 doses in a row (takes about 15 minutes each). The maximal response is usually reached after 3 continuous doses.
- Ipratropium bromide is also useful, suggested to be particularly so for COPD, at a nebulized dose of 250–500 µg every 4–6 hours.

ANSWERS – cont'd

- It is important to remember when using inhaled agents that if the patient's ventilatory status is poor, the dose of nebulized medication actually reaching the airways (rather than being nebulized into the environment for the medical and nursing staff to breathe) may be markedly reduced. In order to overcome this, delivery of undiluted nebulized salbutamol (so that half of what is reaching the airways is not saline), continuous nebulized salbutamol, and occasionally parenteral salbutamol infusion can be used.

- All parenterally administered sympathomimetics and methylxanthines (such as aminophylline) are less effective and more hazardous than the inhaled bronchodilators discussed above, and are nowadays rarely used.

- A short course of systemic corticosteroids has been shown to benefit acute exacerbations of COPD. The current recommendation is to administer a tapered course over roughly 2 weeks, according to the patient's progress. Longer courses have been shown to be of no further benefit. Inhaled corticosteroids currently have no place in the treatment of acute exacerbations of COPD.

- Antibiotics have been shown to produce a small but significant benefit in acute exacerbations of COPD, particularly in patients with severe exacerbation and symptoms of lower respiratory tract infection. However, they are not always indicated. Interpretation of the radiological findings has been shown to be superior to clinical history and examination alone in treatment decision making, and a chest X-ray is mandatory.

- Continuous or Bilevel Positive Airway Pressure (CPAP and BiPAP) are both modalities of 'non-invasive' ventilatory support using a ventilator machine with a mask to apply pressure during inspiration and expiration (non-invasive means not requiring intubation). When used correctly, both these techniques have been shown to reduce the need for intubation, which is associated with a higher incidence of ventilator-related complications and poorer patient outcome. CPAP and BiPAP still require the patient to make a significant respiratory effort, and patients unable to do this require invasive ventilation (intubation).

- Mucolytics and chest physiotherapy have been shown to be ineffective in acute exacerbation of COPD.

A6 The chest X-ray shows flattening of the diaphragms consistent with 'gas trapping', which reflects the inability of gas to escape from the lungs due to airways obstruction. The lung fields are clear, with no evidence of alveolar consolidation or oedema.

This man is having an exacerbation of his COPD, which is commonly triggered by viral airways infection.

He is starting to succumb to respiratory fatigue, and hence hypoventilate. The work of breathing is becoming too much for him. This is reflected by his climbing $paCO_2$, as the carbon dioxide in his alveoli is not being 'washed out' due to inadequate ventilation.

- Remember that cough and wheeze can be due to pulmonary oedema ('cardiac asthma').

Those with low tidal volumes may not have prominent crepitations or wheeze, due to the low volumes of gas reaching the alveoli and low air flows. Thus, the absence of crepitations doesn't exclude cardiogenic pulmonary congestion, and a lack of wheeze doesn't exclude airways disease.

- Remember that hypoxic pulmonary vasoconstriction can cause a raised JVP.

Chest tightness is a symptom commonly described by patients with bronchoconstriction as well as patients with cardiac angina.

For these reasons, acute pulmonary oedema (which may have been precipitated by cardiac ischaemia or infarction) was an important differential diagnosis in this man's presentation, and thus the emergent importance of a CXR and ECG.

A7 This man has had a life-threatening episode of acute respiratory failure. You need to write a letter to his GP explaining what has occurred, and how you wish to taper his oral steroid dose.

Once he has fully recovered, he needs formal pulmonary function tests including:

- Another set of blood gases on room air to ascertain if he has chronic respiratory failure (type 1 or type 2).
- Spirometry before and after administration of B2 agonists in order to ascertain the reversible component of his obstructive airways disease.
- Diffusing capacity of carbon monoxide (DLCO) is a measure of the functional integrity of the alveolar-capillary membrane.

He should then be placed on treatments to optimize his lung function, such as inhaled corticosteroids and B2 agonists if a significant reversible component is shown, and regular follow-up arranged. Most importantly, he must stop smoking.

REVISION POINTS

Acute respiratory failure

- Hypoxia is the enemy.
- It is never correct to reduce oxygen delivery when severe hypoxia is present.
- Not all people with a diagnosis of COPD are CO_2 retainers with 'hypoxic drive'.

Respiratory fatigue, with consequent alveolar hypoventilation, is a common cause for rising pCO_2 in a patient with an acute severe exacerbation of COPD. The correct treatment is delivery of adequate amounts of oxygen, aggressive bronchodilator therapy and ventilatory support as needed.

Adequacy of oxygenation and adequacy of ventilation are *not* the same. They need to be monitored separately (via pO_2 and pCO_2 respectively). Monitoring the adequacy of ventilation and watching for fatigue, both clinically and via pCO_2 measurements, is just as important as assessing the adequacy of oxygenation in acute exacerbations of COPD.

The significance, and even the existence, of losing hypoxic drive to ventilate as a consequence of excessive oxygen therapy in COPD exacerbations is yet to be conclusively demonstrated. The Haldane effect and V/Q mismatch may be the cause of hypercapniea in such cases.

The minimum amount of oxygen should be used to achieve adequate tissue oxygenation. The usual target in these patients with acute on chronic respiratory failure is a pO_2 of 60 +/- 5 mm Hg.

With very few exceptions, impending respiratory arrest in any clinical scenario indicates the delivery of 100% oxygen, even if haemoglobin–oxygen saturation is 100%.

Respiratory fatigue

A large proportion of patients with an acute exacerbation of COPD and a high $paCO_2$ are in respiratory failure due to fatigue as well as severe airways obstruction. As the patient begins to lose the fight against severe airways obstruction, the pCO rises, and pO_2 starts to fall. These patients, such as the one in this case, succumb through respiratory fatigue, not through loss of hypoxic drive.

Achieving adequate tissue oxygenation is an absolute priority in any patient with respiratory failure. The fear of over-correcting hypoxia and removing 'hypoxic drive' often brings about the mistake of inadequate oxygen delivery to patients with an acute exacerbation of COPD.

Hypercapniea occurs due to alveolar hypoventilation. Remember, CO_2 diffuses rapidly across the lung capillary and into the alveoli, and requires fresh inspired air to 'wash out' the CO_2 from the alveolar space. As a patient fatigues and breathing becomes more shallow, a larger proportion of the minute volume is spent moving 'anatomical dead space' without actually reaching and ventilating the alveoli. Hence rapid but shallow breathing still results in hypercapniea.

Recent evidence has examined the mechanisms for the increase in pCO_2 on administration of oxygen therapy in acute exacerbation of COPD. It may occur primarily as a result of haemoglobin losing its affinity for CO_2 once it becomes

continues overleaf

REVISION POINTS – cont'd

oxygenated, thus releasing CO_2 from haemoglobin into plasma (Haldane effect), as well as ventilation–perfusion mismatch due to hypoxic vasoconstriction in the lung. Oxygenated blood also leads to more bicarbonate dissociating into CO_2 and hydrogen ions.

Remember, supplemental oxygen is a 'drug' and it should be used with care – titrate your dose, using clinical and biochemical markers to guide treatment.

ISSUES TO CONSIDER

- What are the normal physiological mechanisms behind respiratory drive?
- What forms of ventilatory assistance are useful in this situation, and how are they used? What are the indications for ventilatory assistance?
- How can you measure the 'work of breathing'?

FURTHER INFORMATION

www.ahrq.gov/clinic/copdsum.htm Management of acute exacerbations of chronic obstructive pulmonary disease. Agency for Healthcare Research and Quality: Evidence report/technology assessment no. 19. AHRQ publication no. 00-E020, September 2000.

Stoller J. Acute exacerbations of chronic obstructive pulmonary disease. New England Journal of Medicine 2002;v364:988–94.

Snow V, Lascher S, Mottu-Pilson C. The evidence base for the management of acute exacerbations of chronic obstructive pulmonary disease. Clinical practice guideline, part 1. Chest 2001;119:1185–9.

Snow V, Lascher S, Mottu-Pilson C. Evidence base for the management of acute exacerbations of chronic obstructive pulmonary disease. Annals of Internal Medicine 2001;134:595–9.

Gomersall C et al. Oxygen therapy for hypercapnic patients with chronic obstructive pulmonary disease and acute respiratory failure: a randomised, controlled pilot study. Critical Care Medicine 2002;30(1):113–16.

A young woman with lower abdominal pain

A 21-year-old woman attends your surgery because she has had some lower abdominal discomfort for the last 12 hours. This discomfort commenced suddenly, but has been constant since that time. Her last menstrual period occurred about 2 weeks ago, at the expected time, and lasted 3 days. She has been sexually active with a new partner for the last 6 weeks and has not been using any contraception.

Q1 What further information would you like from the history and what diagnoses need to be considered?

The aim of the history is to attempt to define the cause of the pain. In this instance further history has proven unhelpful, as it did not assist the clinician in defining the cause.

Q2 What findings on clinical examination would assist you to make a correct diagnosis?

On examination she looks well and does not have a fever. The only abnormal finding is some tenderness in the suprapubic region.

Q3 What investigations should you perform to define the likely cause of the pain?

You arrange some tests, the results of which are shown below:

Investigation 65.1 Summary of results	
Haemoglobin:	140 g/l
White cell count	8.2 x10⁹/l
Blood film:	normal
MSSU:	microscopy normal
Urine culture:	no growth
Cervical swabs:	no evidence of Gram-negative diplococci or chlamydia
Urinary pregnancy test:	negative

A pelvic ultrasound is reported as follows: 'A transabdominal and transvaginal study was performed. The uterus is retroverted but of normal size. The endometrial thickness is 10 mm, consistent with day 14 of the cycle. There are no fibroids. Both ovaries are clearly visible. The right ovary is of normal size and contains a cystic structure 2.3 cm in diameter. The left ovary is slightly enlarged and contains a cystic structure 4.5 cm in diameter which itself has some solid areas within it. Within the cystic area there are some irregular echoes. There is no neovascularization in the region of either cystic structure, and the blood flow to each ovary appears normal. There is no free fluid in the Pouch of Douglas.'

Q4 Interpret these results. What information do they give you? What further investigations may help you formulate your diagnosis?

Q5 How are you going to manage the patient?

The patient's symptoms settled on conservative management and she was then referred to a gynaecologist for an opinion on the management of the ovarian cyst which had the appearance of an uncomplicated dermoid cyst.

ANSWERS

A1 When taking a history from a woman with lower abdominal pain it is important to consider the likely diagnoses and evaluate the possibility of each of the following important conditions:

Pregnancy. The patient may have an ectopic pregnancy or some other pregnancy complication. You need to ask whether contraception has been used, whether the last menstrual period was of normal length and volume and whether she has any symptoms suggestive of pregnancy (nausea, breast tenderness, etc.). Pregnancy always needs to be excluded in women of childbearing age.

Physiological pelvic pain (mittelschmertz). She may have a history of similar symptoms, which might suggest a physiological explanation for the pain. Does she have midcycle pain regularly? If so, the pain could well be due to this now, when the pain is worst at the time of maximum follicular distension prior to follicular rupture.

Ovarian pathology including rupture, torsion or haemorrhage. The type of ovarian cyst would also need consideration – follicular, luteal, endometriotic, dermoid or cystic tumours. History would not enable these to be defined, unless it was known that a cyst had been identified previously. A history of a sudden onset of severe pain would be consistent with a cyst complication.

Pelvic infection, e.g. gonorrhoea or chlamydia. History does not allow this diagnosis to be made or excluded, except that a sudden onset of symptoms would be against this diagnosis.

Urinary tract problems, e.g. infection or a calculus. A history of urinary frequency, dysuria and possibly haematuria should be evident if a urinary tract problem was the cause.

Gastrointestinal tract disease, e.g. acute appendicitis. A history of periumbilical pain preceding a change in position of the pain to the region of the right iliac fossa would be suggestive of this diagnosis.

A2 Clinical examination may be of assistance in making the correct diagnosis, but often clinical examination is of limited value, particularly if the pain is not severe.

ANSWERS – cont'd

Important positive findings would be:

- High fever would be consistent with pelvic infection, although this can also be seen in association with ovarian torsion where the ovary has become necrotic.
- Elevated pulse and low blood pressure would be expected if an ectopic pregnancy had resulted in significant blood loss. If the loss has been minimal, the pulse and blood pressure would be normal.
- Cervical excitation and adnexal tenderness would be consistent with an ectopic pregnancy or pelvic infection.
- Unilateral adnexal tenderness would be consistent with a complication of an ovarian cyst, or an unruptured ectopic pregnancy.
- A low-grade fever, tenderness and guarding, maximal in the right iliac fossa, would suggest acute appendicitis.

An uncomplicated ovarian cyst of less than 5 cm in diameter may not be able to be felt in the appropriate adnexum, unless the patient is very thin and well relaxed.

Abnormal cervical discharge is often not present even when bacteriologic studies have confirmed the presence of gonococcal or chlamydial organisms.

A3 The investigations required are:

- FBE, including WCC – an elevated WCC would suggest infection or necrosis.
- Pregnancy test to exclude a pregnancy complication, or a co-existent pregnancy. (Pregnancy is not always associated with amenorrhoea.)
- Cervical swabs for bacteriologic assessment to exclude gonorrhoea and chlamydia.
- MSU microscopy and culture to exclude a urinary cause for the symptoms.
- Pelvic ultrasound examination, preferably performed vaginally, to assess the ovaries and to allow further evaluation if the pregnancy test is positive. If a cystic structure is found, evidence of neovascularization should be sought, as this would be more common if the cyst was malignant, and the blood supply to and from the ovary should be assessed. In the presence

of torsion, blood flow to and from the ovary is often compromised.

A4 The ultrasound has shown the presence of a probable preovulatory follicle in the right ovary. This may be the cause of the pain, and if so, the pain should settle within the next 24 hours.

The ultrasound has also shown the presence of a probable dermoid cyst in the left ovary. Persistence of the pain could be due to torsion of that ovary, although this clearly has not yet compromised the blood flow to the ovary.

Although the negative cultures for the gonococcus and chlamydia make pelvic infection less likely, they do not exclude it completely. The negative MSU virtually excludes a urinary tract cause for the pain.

The negative pregnancy test excludes a pregnancy-related cause for the pain.

A relevant further investigation would be the performance of a laparoscopy to further evaluate the left ovarian cyst, and to probably deal with it at the same time.

A5 Several treatment options can be considered.

The treatment options are to be conservative, and observe what happens to the pain, or be more radical and perform a laparoscopy to fully assess the left ovary and deal appropriately with what is found.

A conservative policy would assume that the pain is more likely to be that of mittelschmertz, although if midcycle pain has not been a problem in the past, this diagnosis would seem unlikely. It would also assume that the dermoid cyst has not become complicated and is therefore not the cause of the pain. Although the cyst will probably need to be dealt with surgically, probably via the laparoscope, at some time in the future, urgent treatment is not necessary.

A more radical policy would be to perform the laparoscopy at this time and to deal with what is found through the laparoscope or following the performance of a laparotomy have made the diagnosis laparoscopically. A left ovarian cystectomy with conservation of the remaining ovarian substance would probably be possible, and if the pain

ANSWERS – cont'd

was due to torsion, the treatment would be the same as the ovary is clearly still viable because of the demonstration of a normal blood supply.

Because of the timing of the pain, the fact it is not severe, and the fact that ovarian torsion is unlikely to be the cause when normal ovarian blood supply and flow has been demonstrated, a conservative policy in the first instance would be most appropriate. Ultimately a decision will need to be made concerning the surgical management of the probable dermoid cyst of the left ovary.

REVISION POINTS

Dermoid cysts

- often an incidental finding
- can produce pain when torsion occurs
- pathology almost always benign

- best managed by ovarian cystectomy, although unilateral oophorectomy may be required if the cyst is >10 cm in diameter.

ISSUES TO CONSIDER

- What are the various imaging investigations that can be used to make a diagnosis in patients with acute lower abdominal pain? What are the advantages and disadvantages of these investigations?
- Consider the important causes of acute lower abdominal pain and if an imaging investigation is to be used, identify the most appropriate one applicable to each of these.

FURTHER INFORMATION

www.pta.net.au/sgeg/ovcyst.htm From the Sydney Gynaecological Endoscopy Group based at hospitals in New South Wales. Laparoscopic images of ovarian cysts.

www.emedicine.com/med/topic1699.htm Pathophysiology, symptoms, causes, diagnosis, procedures, treatment and follow-up of ovarian cysts.

A young woman with abnormal vaginal bleeding

A 32-year-old woman attends your surgery because she has had some irregular vaginal bleeding for the last 8 days. Her last normal menstrual period occurred at the expected time 3 weeks ago. She is not on the oral contra- ceptive pill and has been trying to conceive for the last 3 years. Neither she nor her husband have had any tests done to see why she has not conceived.

Q1 What further information would you like from the history and why?

Further questioning does not yield any helpful information. The patient last had a PAP smear 18 months earlier and it was normal.

Q2 What findings on clinical examination would assist you to make a correct diagnosis?

Your physical examination of the patient is unremarkable. In particular, abdominal and pelvic examination is normal. The vagina and cervix appear healthy.

Q3 What investigations should you perform to define the likely cause of the bleeding?

You arrange some tests, the results of which are shown below:

Investigation 66.1 Summary of results	
Haemoglobin:	142 g/L
White cell count:	$8.5 \times 10^9/l$
Platelets:	$160 \times 10^9/L$
Urinary pregnancy test:	positive
Serum beta hCG:	1200 U/l
Cervical PAP smear:	no abnormal cells detected. Endocervical cells identified.
Cervical swab:	no evidence of chlamydial infection.

Q4 Interpret these results. What information do they give you? What further investigations may help you formulate your diagnosis?

You note the positive pregnancy test and proceed to a vaginal ultrasound examination (Figures 66.1 and 66.2).

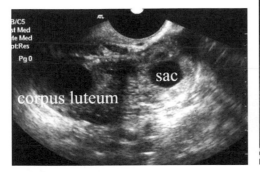

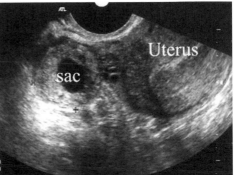

Fig 66.1   **Fig 66.2**

Q5 What does the ultrasound show and what are you going to do now?

ANSWERS

A1 When taking a history from a woman with abnormal vaginal bleeding consider the following:

- Is she pregnant and does she have an ectopic pregnancy or some other pregnancy complication? In someone who has had difficulty conceiving, when a pregnancy is achieved the chance of it being in an ectopic position is increased. You need to ask whether her last menstrual period was of normal volume and duration as it is not uncommon for a 'period' to occur in someone who has conceived although the amount of bleeding at the time of the 'period' is usually less than normally occurs. If she is pregnant the current 8 days of bleeding could be an indication of the pregnancy being in the Fallopian tube, and not the uterus (an ectopic pregnancy), or that one of the various forms of abortion are occurring (threatened, incomplete, complete or missed abortion).

- If she is not pregnant, the most likely causes are a problem at the level of the cervix, or a disturbance of her oestrogen and/or progesterone levels resulting in irregular shedding of her endometrium (DUB = dysfunctional uterine bleeding).

- Is the bleeding from her cervix? For example, a cervical polyp or carcinoma? Check when her last PAP smear was done, whether PAP smears have ever been abnormal, whether there have been previous episodes of abnormal bleeding and whether she has ever had bleeding after sexual activity. Recurrent bleeding, and especially postcoital bleeding, often has a cervical origin.

- Does she have DUB? This would be suggested by the previous menstrual cycles being irregular, or where the definite symptoms associated with ovulatory menstrual cycles (midcycle mucus change, premenstrual bloating of the

A N S W E R S – cont'd

abdomen, premenstrual dysmenorrhoea) are absent.

- Abnormal bleeding in a woman with uterine fibroids is generally heavy bleeding at the time of the period. Bleeding between the periods is only likely if one of the fibroids is in the submucosal position and is being extruded.
- If the bleeding was only in the premenstrual phase, the possibility of it being due to endometriosis or chlamydial infection would need to be considered.

A2 • The clinical examination is often of limited value in making the correct diagnosis in patients with abnormal vaginal bleeding. Even if this patient was pregnant the uterus is not going to be enlarged. If a cervical cancer was present or a uterine fibroid was being extruded, this should be able to be seen unless it is entirely within the cervical canal. If the bleeding is due to DUB, no abnormality will be able to be detected on clinical examination.

- In the absence of pain, even if the bleeding was associated with an ectopic pregnancy, it is likely that the pelvic examination findings will be normal. Where pain is present it is more likely that there will be bleeding into the pelvic peritoneal cavity, under which circumstances it is likely that there will be adnexal tenderness, cervical excitation and a 'boggy' feeling in the Pouch of Douglas.

A3 The investigations required are:
- Complete blood picture.
- Pregnancy test (pregnancy complication?).
- Cervical swabs (exclude chlamydia, although this is unlikely).
- PAP smear (exclude cervical cancer).

A4 She is pregnant.

A vaginal ultrasound examination is required to site the pregnancy and to determine if it is progressing normally. It is normal for an intrauterine pregnancy sac to be visible once the beta-hCG level exceeds 1000 IU/l. If it cannot be seen in the uterus, it is highly likely the diagnosis is an ectopic pregnancy. Sometimes the actual sac containing the fetus can be seen outside the uterus, or a mass of clot and the pregnancy can be seen in one adnexum.

If the vaginal ultrasound shows the sac is in the uterus, the type of 'abortion' then needs to be defined by the ultrasound examination. Types include:
- Threatened abortion: normal sac size, normal fetal size, fetal heart tones present.
- Threatened abortion with increased risk of fetal loss: all the above plus a large amount of intrauterine blood clot, or fetal heart rate less than 100 bpm.
- Inevitable abortion: a very small sac, a normal-sized sac with a very small fetus or a sac with no evidence of a fetus (blighted ovum).
- Incomplete abortion: only placental tissue within the uterus.
- Complete abortion: uterus is empty with no evidence of any remaining fetal or placental tissue.
- Missed abortion: the gestation sac contains the fetus, but the fetus is dead, i.e. no fetal heart tones are present.

A5 The ultrasound shows an empty uterus with a small adnexal mass consistent with a tubal ectopic pregnancy.

There are a number of therapeutic options. In this case the most appropriate option is administration of intramuscular methotrexate (1 mg/kg) along with folinic acid rescue to destroy the ectopic pregnancy. This is associated with a better chance of tubal patency than when any of the surgical options are employed. It is appropriate therapy especially as the beta hCG level is less than 2000 IU/l, the pregnancy sac size is small or not identified, and no fetal heart tones are detected in the ectopic pregnancy itself. Tubal rupture with resulting intraperitoneal bleeding can occur after methotrexate therapy, but is unusual.

Other options include:
- Salpingostomy performed as an open operative procedure or performed laparoscopically.
- Partial salpingectomy performed as an open procedure or laparoscopically (usually the ovary is not removed at the time of removal of the Fallopian tube).

REVISION POINTS

Ectopic pregnancy

Incidence
1:200 pregnancies.

Risk factors
- pelvic inflammatory disease
- previous IUD use
- previous infertility
- pregnancy achieved using IVF or GIFT.

Clinical features
- lower abdominal pain (75%)
- abnormal vaginal bleeding (75%)
- usually amenorrhoea (75%).

Management
- confirm diagnosis:
  - pregnancy test
  - pelvic ultrasound
  - sometimes laparoscopy
- stabilize patient with low hCG levels: methotrexate
- haemodynamically unstable patient or hCG levels >5000 IU/l: surgical intervention.

ISSUES TO CONSIDER

- What types of imaging can be used safely in pregnancy?
- What advice would you give to this woman with regard to her further chances of successful pregnancy?

FURTHER INFORMATION

www.advancedfertility.com/ectopfot.htm
Laparoscopic images of ectopic pregnancy.

www.emedicine.com/EMERG/topic478.htm An article from the emedicine series on ectopic pregnancy.

Index

Numbers in **bold** refer to figures and tables